T0331025

A Guide to Providing LGBTQ+ Inclusive Reproductive Health Care

This evidence-based guide brings together a wide range of information and practical tools for midwives, obstetricians, nurses, health visitors, and birthworkers, empowering them to provide safe and compassionate care throughout the reproductive journeys of lesbian, gay, bisexual, transgender, and queer (LGBTQ+) people. This book may also be helpful to LGBTQ+ people in their own reproductive journeys.

Throughout history, in cultures around the world, LGBTQ+ people have become pregnant, sought abortion care, miscarried, experienced infertility, given birth, and made decisions about infant feeding. Their reproductive journeys are increasingly visible, reflecting the changing social and legal recognition of sexual and gender minority people as parents. LGBTQ+ people require support during these significant life events which is appropriate, expert, and meets their needs. However, healthcare professionals and birthworkers may not always be confident in working with these clients and may lack understanding of LGBTQ+ clients' experiences. There is also often insufficient attention paid to differences in the LGBTQ+ non-gestational parents' experiences. Taking an interdisciplinary approach, this book brings together up-to-date research findings from a range of fields including medicine, psychology, sociology, law, and public health, to provide a knowledge base and tools to support clients at different stages of pregnancy and parenthood. The book follows the reproductive journey, moving from pre-conception and fertility research, through pregnancy and birth, to postnatal physical and mental healthcare. It also addresses termination care and perinatal loss.

The chapters contain vignettes to personalise the issues discussed, highlights key practice recommendations, and suggestions for further reading. This is an essential guide for student midwives and medical students, as well as health visitors, midwives, and obstetricians in practice.

Mari Greenfield (she/they) is a genderqueer dyke who is both a gestational, non-gestational, and foster parent. Mari came into academia after a decade of working as a doula and La Leche Leader, supporting other parents on their breast and chestfeeding journeys.

Kate Luxion (they/them) is a non-binary/genderqueer, bisexual gestational parent who has built both a career in the fine arts and doing research and advocacy around LGBTQ+ reproduction and parenthood. As a Lamaze Certified Childbirth Educator, and trainee lactation consultant, it is important to Kate to ensure that health information is accurate and accessible to both parents and clinicians.

El Molloy (she/her) is a cisgender, pansexual mother and academic whose research focuses on challenging research questions and inequities in access to healthcare. El switched from quantitative to qualitative research after becoming a parent, and as an NCT Breastfeeding Counsellor and researcher she is passionate about informed decision-making for all parents.

Alice-Amanda Hinton (she/they) is a bisexual/queer, non-binary midwife who brings with them 13 years of experience. She is also responsible for Trust-wide guidelines for trans and non-binary staff and patients at King's College Hospital, as well as co-chairing King's and Queers for the Trust LGBT network.

A Guide to Providing LGBTQ+ Inclusive Reproductive Health Care

Pride in Birth

EDITED BY
MARI GREENFIELD,
KATE LUXION,
EL MOLLOY, AND
ALICE-AMANDA HINTON

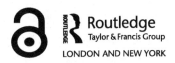
Routledge
Taylor & Francis Group

LONDON AND NEW YORK

Designed cover image: Illustrated by G Sabini-Roberts

First published 2025
by Routledge
4 Park Square, Milton Park, Abingdon, Oxon OX14 4RN

and by Routledge
605 Third Avenue, New York, NY 10158

Routledge is an imprint of the Taylor & Francis Group, an informa business

British Library Cataloguing-in-Publication Data
A catalogue record for this book is available from the British Library

ISBN: 978-1-032-30504-2 (hbk)
ISBN: 978-1-032-30503-5 (pbk)
ISBN: 978-1-003-30544-6 (ebk)

DOI: 10.4324/9781003305446

Typeset in Vectora
by SPi Technologies India Pvt Ltd (Straive)

Contents

Figures

Tables

About the editors

A Guide to Providing LGBTQ+ Inclusive Reproductive Health Care: Pride in Birth brings together a breadth of knowledge from experienced researchers and practitioners. For the editorial team, this includes experiences within both their personal and professional lives.

Mari Greenfield (she/they) is a genderqueer dyke who is both a gestational, non-gestational, and foster parent. Mari came into academia after a decade of working as a doula and La Leche Leader, supporting other parents on their breast and chestfeeding journeys.

Kate Luxion (they/them) is a non-binary/genderqueer, bisexual gestational parent who has built both a career in the fine arts and doing research and advocacy around LGBTQ+ reproduction and parenthood. As a Lamaze Certified Childbirth Educator, and trainee lactation consultant, it is important to Kate to ensure that health information is accurate and accessible to both parents and clinicians.

El Molloy (she/her) is a cisgender, pansexual mother and academic whose research focuses on challenging research questions and inequities in access to healthcare. El switched from quantitative to qualitative research after becoming a parent, and as an NCT Breastfeeding Counsellor and researcher she is passionate about informed decision-making for all parents.

Alice-Amanda Hinton (she/they) is a bisexual/queer, non-binary midwife who brings with them 13 years of experience. She is also responsible for Trust-wide guidelines for trans and non-binary staff and patients at King's College Hospital, as well as co-chairing King's and Queers for the Trust LGBT network.

Separately, we all recognised that there was a gap within education and resources for people working with LGBTQ+ people during the perinatal period. This book is our joint response to this gap.

Contributors

Sophie Zadeh

Dr Sophie Zadeh (she/her) is Associate Professor of Social Psychology at the Thomas Coram Research Unit, University College London, UK. Her research focuses on non-normative families from a social psychological perspective. Sophie has researched single mother, single father, and trans* parent families, and has contributed to studies of lesbian and gay parents and their children. Sophie is currently leading an ESRC-funded project on the perspectives and experiences of donor conceived people, with a focus on young adults. Her first monograph, on single mothers and single fathers "by choice," is under contract with Cambridge University Press.

Susie Bower-Brown

Dr Susie Bower-Brown (she/her) is a Research Associate at the Centre for Family Research, University of Cambridge, UK. Susie's research takes a qualitative, social psychological approach to understanding LGBTQ+ experiences and identities. In 2021, Susie completed her PhD at the Centre for Family Research focusing on the experiences of trans and/or non-binary adolescents and parents. Susie is now conducting research on the experiences of parents in other family forms, including cis same-gender female couples who have used reciprocal IVF.

Ash Bainbridge

Ash Bainbridge (they/he) is a queer student midwife who is passionate about person-centred care and informed choice. They advocate for LGBTQ+ inclusivity in midwifery education and practice, across the childbearing continuum, and for all pregnancy outcomes. Ash is Gender Inclusion Advisor for the safer pregnancy charity MAMA Academy, member of Elsevier's student midwifery advisory board, and Equality Advisory Group representative for Worcestershire Maternity Voices Partnership. Collaborative working with students, midwives, and birth activists is a priority for Ash. As such, they have co-founded the Birth Worker Reading Circle and have served as Co-Editor for *The Student Midwife Journal*. Ash was shortlisted in 2022 for the Mary Seacole Award for Outstanding Contribution to Diversity and

Inclusion at the Student Nursing Times Awards, and was selected for the full The Word Association Mentorship Programme in 2022.

A.J. Lowik

Dr A.J. Lowik (they/them) is the Gender Equity Advisor with the Centre for Gender and Sexual Health Equity in Vancouver, British Columbia. They are a trans scholar and trans health researcher, having earned their PhD from the Institute for Gender, Race, Sexuality and Social Justice at the University of British Columbia in 2021. Dr Lowik's work primarily focuses on trans and non-binary people's reproductive lives, health, decision-making, and experiences accessing reproductive health care. Dr Lowik is a Board Member with the Abortion Rights Coalition of Canada and an Advisory Member on the MindMap BC, Community-Based Research Centre's TestNow, and Trans Healthcare in British Columbia projects and a renowned expert in trans and gender-inclusion. Dr Lowik has worked with researchers, health care and social service organisations, lawyers and policymakers interested in trans- and gender-inclusive research and praxis, policy and practice, and legal reform. They are agender, nonbinary, and queer; they are an unapologetic transfeminist and queer liberationist, who loves cats, puzzles, and fighting the cisheteropatriarchy.

Kayleah Logan

Kay (she/her/they/them) is a former midwife with a postgraduate qualification in reproductive biology. Kay has worked in a range of settings including community, home birthing, on a range of hospital wards, and taught hypnobirthing and parent education. Kay noticed a distinct lack of spaces for LGBTQ+ families throughout her practice and has observed first-hand the impact community networks can have for families and also the role that knowledge has for families in making informed decisions about their perinatal care and the impact of that on satisfaction through pregnancy and birth.

These aspects combined and inspired them to co-found The Queer Parenting Partnership with Kim Roberts, to create a space for LGBTQ+ people to gather knowledge that is culturally appropriate, away from cisheteronormativity, to make informed decisions and network with other families that are similar to them.

Slade Riverfield

Slade (they/them) has worked in the childcare industry for 20+ years and was a finalist in the UK Nanny of The Year Awards 2019, and was nominated for the same award in 2020 and 2021. Slade began their doula training in June 2018. They were motivated to become a doula after supporting a loved one through severe postnatal depression. Before they had finished their first day of training, they already knew they wanted to work specifically with queer families and The Queer Doula was born. Co-creating The Queer Parenting Partnership was the next logical step for them, as queer parents and parents from marginalised groups are consistently left out, let down, or squeezed in as an afterthought and they realised that to effect change, it had to start with themself.

Sofia Klittmark

Sofia Klittmark (she/her) is a midwife (RNM) associated with the Department of Behavioural Sciences and Learning, Linköping University, Sweden. Sofia specialises in LGBTQ+ pregnancy and birth, and supporting LGBTQ+ parents. Her Master's thesis in midwifery was an interview study with LGBTQ+ parents, examining their experiences of reproductive healthcare. Klittmark has worked for three years in a parental support programme within RFSL, the Swedish Federation for Lesbian, Gay, Bisexual, Transgender, Queer and Intersex Rights. Within the project she has developed and facilitated parental support groups online for prospective LGBTQ+ parents from all over Sweden. She has developed information materials and tip sheets on LGBTQ+ issues for midwives, alongside inclusive information and online support materials for LGBTQ+ prospective and new parents, including breast/chestfeeding and how to support induced lactation and co-nursing.

Hanna Grundström

Hanna Grundström (she/her) is a registered midwife who works as an Associate Professor and lecturer at Vrinnevi Hospital in Norrköping and Linköping University, Sweden, with clinical expertise in postpartum care. Her doctoral research investigated the disclosure of invisible experiences, outcomes, and quality of endometriosis healthcare. She has also carried out research about birth experiences, postpartum support, and traumatic births. As a researcher she has worked with quantitative and qualitative research methods. She is involved in several national and international projects about postpartum support and mental health.

Katri Nieminen

Katri Nieminen (she/her) is a senior consultant in obstetrics and gynaecology, with expertise in research on fear of childbirth, traumatic birth, and postpartum experiences, based at Vrinnevi Hospital, Norrköping, and Linköping University, Sweden. Her thesis "Clinical aspects of childbirth-related anxiety" (2016) included studies on internet therapy for fear of childbirth and traumatic birth, and also a health economic analysis about how fear of childbirth influences routine health care. She is experienced in working with health-related questionnaires and quantitative analysis. Over the last year, she has worked as part of a research group with Malmquist and Grundström. The research group has used qualitative and quantitative methods to investigate questions about childbirth anxiety in the LGBTQ+ context.

Josephine Lindén Åsell

Josephine Lindén Åsell (she/her) is a psychology student, currently completing her Master's thesis at Linköping University, Sweden. Her thesis examines birth trauma in LGBTQ+ people. Lindén Åsell has conducted and analysed semi-structured interviews with birth and non-birth LGBTQ+ parents, who experienced the birth of their child as a traumatic event.

Anna Malmquist

Anna Malmquist (she/her) is Associate Professor in Psychology at Linköping University. Her major research area is LGBTQ+ families. Her doctoral thesis (2015) concerned lesbian mothers in Sweden. Malmquist co-edited the first Swedish textbook on LGBTQ+ psychology (2017). Recently she published a book on gay fatherhood in Sweden (2022). In recent years she has worked with Nieminen and Grundström in the field of fear of childbirth and traumatic birth. Together with Nieminen she has conducted a study on fear of childbirth among LGBTQ+ people, showing how minority stress adds a layer of stress for this group of parents. At present, she is running a research project on reproductive health among LGBTQ+ people in Sweden, together with Nieminen, Grundström, and Klittmark.

Alex Howat

Dr Alex Howat (she/her) is a Senior Clinical Psychologist in Children and Young People's Inpatient Mental Health Services in Leeds. She completed a Doctorate in Clinical Psychology between 2018 and 2021, writing her doctoral thesis and subsequently publishing a paper on the experiences of perinatal depression and anxiety of non-birthing mothers in female same-sex parented families. As an ally for the LGBTQIA+ community, she is invested in supporting and promoting issues relevant to this community, particularly through conducting and disseminating research. Dr Howat's research interests include the changes in identity that occur within transitions, particularly the transition to parenthood, as well as the influence of sociocultural and political factors on the experiences of mental health.

Nina A Juntereal

Nina A Juntereal (she/her), BSN, RN is a PhD candidate in Nursing and Hillman Scholar of Nursing Innovation at the University of Pennsylvania. Nina obtained her bachelor of science in nursing with a minor in Nutrition from Penn. Her research interests focus on lactation-related outcomes among diverse childbearing families and critically-ill infants. Nina collaborates with the Children's Hospital of Philadelphia and University of Western Australia to advance the science of lactation for infants prenatally diagnosed with congenital anomalies. Her dissertation research explores the role of antenatal milk expression, the expression of colostrum during the late third trimester of pregnancy for parent-infant dyads. Nina is the Social Media and

Communications Chair of the Governing Committee of the Trainee Interest Group of the International Society for Research on Human Milk and Lactation. Nina also co-teaches a virtual exchange on global heating and healthy climate at the School of Nursing.

Diane L Spatz

Diane L Spatz (she/her), PhD, RN-BC, FAAN is a Professor of Perinatal Nursing and the Helen M. Shearer Professor of Nutrition at the University of Pennsylvania School of Nursing sharing a joint appointment at Children's Hospital of Philadelphia (CHOP) where she is a nurse scientist focused in lactation in the Center for Pediatric Nursing Research and Evidence Based Practice. She is founder of the CHOP Mothers' Milk Bank. In the university portion of her job, she teaches an entire semester course on breastfeeding and human lactation to undergraduate nursing students and developed the Breastfeeding Resource Nurse programme.

Dr Spatz has been PI or co-investigator on over 50 research grants. She has authored/co-authored over 210 peer-reviewed publications, numerous book chapters, and position statements and clinical practice guidelines for five professional organisations as well as a technical brief for the USAID on human milk and breastfeeding in developing countries. In 2004, Dr Spatz developed her 10-step model for human milk and breastfeeding in vulnerable infants. This model has received the prestigious "Edge Runner" designation from the American Academy of Nursing based on the model's outcomes. Dr Spatz is the recipient of numerous awards including the 2016 Lifetime Achievement Award from the National Association of Neonatal Nurses.

Zoe Darwin

Zoe Darwin (she/her) is an Associate Professor in Health Research at the University of Huddersfield. Her main area of research concerns psychosocial aspects of reproduction, including perinatal mental health and wellbeing in all parents and people pursuing parenthood. Zoe's research adopts an applied focus, foregrounding implications for policy and practice, including primary care, maternity settings, health visiting (child health), specialist perinatal mental health services, and the voluntary and community sector. Recent publications include the NHS England improvement good practice guide on involving and supporting partners and other family members in specialist perinatal mental health services; editorials on gestational and non-gestational parents and the invisibility of LGBTQ+ people in perinatal research; a review on assessing mental health in fathers, other co-parents, and partners; and a review on traumatic birth and perinatal mental health in trans and non-binary people.

Lucy Warwick-Guasp

Lucy (she/her) is a trainer and consultant with over 20 years of experience in education and facilitation. In addition to Key Stage 5 leadership and teaching, Lucy spent several years as a Senior Education Officer for Stonewall, developing and delivering two national programmes of work supporting schools and Local Authorities in tackling homophobia and transphobia. Lucy combines her extensive expertise with her lived experience of postnatal depression, and subsequent treatment at Bethlem Mother and Baby Unit, South London and being a same-sex parent. Lucy's current training programmes have been developed over the last few years, working alongside the NHS and non-profit-making organisations specialising in maternal, parental, and perinatal mental health across the UK. These programmes allow participants to explore specific experiences of LGBTQ+ people and discuss how their services can be more inclusive of LGBTQ+ parent families. Alongside delivering training sessions to hundreds of practitioners, Lucy has spoken at several Perinatal Mental Health Conferences and events. These have included the Royal College of Psychiatrists, iHV Institute of Health Visiting, Make Birth Better, The Psychological Society of Ireland (PSI), and Australasian Birth Trauma Association. Her aim is to empower professionals and organisations to feel confident in supporting LGBTQ+ families who are experiencing perinatal mental health issues.

Sarah Arnold

Sarah Arnold (she/her) is a nurse, midwife, and health visitor with almost two decades of experience. She has a passion for inclusivity and person-centred care alongside infant feeding. She has been part of the West Midlands Clinical Senate who review clinical practice, has been an active member of the research and development team at her workplace, and has been the named health visitor for a domestic violence refuge. Here she led on numerous projects including speech and language development with children who are under school age. Sarah has worked with families across the LGBTQ+ community in all of her roles.

Sarah is a mum to four daughters and has personal experience of being part of the LGBTQ+ community and has extensive experience of both using and working in maternity and postnatal services. She is aware of the limitations of both.

She is now working in education after lecturing at a local university for post-graduation health visitor students.

Glossary

TERM	DEFINITION
Additive language	The approach of adding to language to ensure that everyone is included, not replacing terms—for example "fathers AND lesbian non-gestational mothers" or "pregnant women AND other pregnant people"
Allosexual	Someone who experiences sexual attraction towards others. The inverse of asexual
Ally	Someone who is not a member of the LGBTQ+ community, but who actively supports the LGBTQ+ community and members of that community
Aromantic	Someone who experiences low to no romantic attraction. Some aromantic people are asexual, others are allosexual
Asexual, Ace	1. Someone who is asexual and experiences low or no sexual attraction. They may experience romantic attraction and have any orientation or gender 2. Asexuality is also used as an umbrella term, including people who are aromantic and demisexual 3. Grey ace is a form of asexuality, used by people who experience sexual attraction only occasionally or in some circumstances, forming a spectrum of sexual attraction between allosexual and asexual Asexuality comes under the LGBTQ+ umbrella, but not all asexual people may identify as being LGBTQ+
Binder	A strongly elasticated item of clothing designed to flatten and masculinise the chest or breast area. Many transmasculine people wear these all the time

Birth parent	A birth parent is the person who carried, gave birth, and intends to parent a child. Sometimes the term is used within lesbian families to refer to the mother who gave birth. Sometimes it is used by non-binary people and trans men who gave birth to their own children as a gender-neutral way of defining their role. However, it is also commonly used within adoptive families to refer to the adopted child's biological parents. This means it is preferable for professionals to use alternative terms such as gestational parent when referring to LGBTQ+ families to avoid confusion
Biphobia	Fear of, dislike of, prejudice towards, or discrimination against someone who is bisexual
Bisexual	Someone who is sexually and/or romantically attracted to more than one gender
Cis man	A man who was assigned male at birth (from the Latin "same")
Cis woman	A woman who was assigned as female at birth (from the Latin "same")
Cishet	An abbreviation of cisgender and heterosexual, i.e. experiencing romantic and sexual attraction to people of the opposite sex
Cisheterosexism	The privileging of cisgender heterosexual people and relationships above people or relationships that involve other genders or sexual orientations
Cisnormativity	The assumption that everyone is cisgender, and treatment of cisgender people as normal, natural, and more valuable than other gender modalities (thanks to A.J. Lowik for this definition)
Co-mother	A term used to denote either or both parents in a lesbian relationship, or to denote the non-gestational mother
Co-parent or co-parenting	The term co-parent can have different meanings. It can be used to describe any parent (for example a father, co-mother, or any other co-parent). It can be used to describe the relationship between parents in parenting their child. It can also be used to describe arrangements

	where two or more people choose to conceive and raise a child together without necessarily being in a romantic or sexual relationship with each other; for example, where a lesbian couple and a man pursue parenthood together
Coming out	A phrase used to describe the process of telling other people that you are LGBTQ+. LGBTQ+ people usually need to come out multiple times in their lives due to both cisheteronormativity and the process of navigating new spaces, identities, and relationships
Conversion therapy/ conversion practices	This is also sometimes called "reparative therapy" outside the UK. Conversion practices refer to a range of interventions that aim to change a person's sexual orientation or gender identity from any form of non-heterosexual or non-cisgender identity to heterosexual and/or cisgender identities. Practices may include psychological techniques, religious practices, physical and sexual assault. Such practices have been widely discredited by medical and psychological organisations as ineffective, unethical, and actively harmful. These practices are banned in many countries, although in the UK—despite Government promises to introduce legislation to ban conversion therapy in 2021—conversion practices remain legal
Deadname/ deadnaming	A deadname is a birth name that a person no longer uses and which causes them distress. The term originated amongst the transgender community, but has in recent years also been adopted by people who have changed their first or family name following childhood abuse. Recently, some trans people who do not find the term "deadname" accurate have used the term "sweater name"—the idea being that the name was a gift given to you with love, but that no longer fits and is uncomfortable. Deadnaming happens when someone else uses a birth name that a trans person no longer uses. It may be done on purpose, with the intent of denying the person's identity and/or to cause offence as an act of transphobic violence. Deadnaming may also happen

because of institutional transphobia, such as a requirement to use a birth name. Deadnaming may also happen accidentally, if a person is unaware that a trans person has changed their name.

We are unaware of the verb deadnaming being used currently in relation to cis people who have a deadname.

Demisexual	Someone who experiences sexual attraction towards others only in specific circumstances. Common circumstances include only experiencing sexual attraction once an emotional attachment has formed. Demisexual people may be of any sexual orientation
Donor	In this book, the term donor is used to refer to a sperm or egg donor. Donors may be known to the gestational parent, or may be sourced through a fertility clinic with varying levels of anonymity
Donor gametes	Gametes (i.e. egg and sperm) that are used within conceiving. Donor gametes can come from one or more people and would be the gamete(s) that do not originate with either of the parents
Gay	A man or man-aligned person who is sexually or romantically attracted to other men or men-aligned people; in some usage this need not exclude being attracted to people of other genders
Gender	Sex and gender are distinct concepts. Gender is a social construct, and therefore the meaning varies in different societies and at historical times. The construct of gender encompasses the roles, behaviours, activities, expectations, and societal norms associated with each gender in a particular society.

Whilst many societies recognise two genders—man and woman—and associate gender with sex assigned at birth, many societies have recognised more than two genders. Examples include:

- Lakota, Ojibwe, and Navajo, amongst other indigenous American cultures, recognise the existence of Two-Spirit people
- South Asian cultures, such as India, Pakistan, and Bangladesh, where Hirja is a third gender

	— South Pacific cultures, where some Polynesian cultures, such as Samoan fa'afafine and fa'afatama, recognise people assigned male at birth who take on gender roles and responsibilities commonly adopted by women as a third gender — Sulawesi, Indonesia, where the Bugis people recognise five genders — Thailand, where Kathoey (sometimes called Ladyboys) are recognised as a third gender — Modern Western societies, where there is increasing recognition for non-binary people. Non-binary gender identities are multiple and heterogeneous—non-binary is an umbrella term, not a third gender
Gender affirming care	Therapeutic and/or medical care that is focused on ensuring that the individual is able to discuss, discover, and act on types of care that affirm their gender. Types of care that might be utilised include talk therapies, hormonal therapies, and/or surgical care. Gender affirming care is accessed by both cisgender and transgender individuals. For example, the medical administration of hormones is widespread as a method of contraception, to assist in symptoms associated with the perimenopause and menopause, to cisgender individuals whose hormones fall outside of the range considered normal, and to some transgender individuals
Gender diverse/ gender expansive/ gender non-conforming	These are umbrella terms that describes those who do not conform to social expectations of gender identities and/or gender expressions. The term gender non-conforming is less commonly used now. These terms are controversial within the LGBTQ+ community, with some people finding them liberating whilst others feel they are based in cisnormativity and sexism
Gender dysphoria	When a person experiences discomfort or distress because there is a mismatch between their gender and their assigned gender at birth. Not all trans people experience gender dysphoria

Gender euphoria	Where a person experiences joy and happiness when their gender is affirmed and experienced in a positive way. Cis and trans people can experience gender euphoria
Gender expression	How a person presents themselves in terms of the clothing, make up, accessories, etc. they wear, how they speak, mannerisms, etc. This can fluctuate over time. Gender expression does not always match gender identity
Gender reassignment	A range of social, hormonal, surgical, and therapeutic treatments and interventions which support an individual's transition from the gender they were assigned at birth to their gender. It is another way of describing a person's gender transition. "Gender confirmation" often replaces this term. Gender reassignment is also the wording used in the Equality Act 2010 to define the protected characteristic that protects trans people from discrimination
Gender Recognition Certificate	A Gender Recognition Certificate (GRC) is a legal document that helps to acknowledge the change in a person's legal gender, while also helping to facilitate the updating of other legal documents such as a birth or adoption certificate, marriage documentation, pension documentation, among other documents. These updates can include ensuring that the proper gender and/or sex markers are used to align with who the individual is
Gender transition	The process of changing gender presentation or sex characteristics to be consistent with gender identity. Transition can be social (using a new name and pronouns) and changing gender presentation (i.e. clothes, hairstyle). Transition can also be medical, and may include taking hormonal medication and/or various surgeries. This process may take many years and for some people may be lifelong
Genderqueer	Used by some people as an alternative term for non-binary. Genderqueer people may have a range of gender identities and expressions

Gestational parent (also referred to as carrying parent or birthing parent)	A person who is or was pregnant with the baby or babies that they intend to birth and parent. Sometimes this is a preferred term for pregnant trans men or non-binary people. It may also be used within lesbian couples to denote which mother-to-be is pregnant
Heterosexual/ straight	A man or woman who has an emotional, romantic, and/ or sexual attraction towards people of the other binary gender. Sometimes abbreviated to het or hetero
Heteronormative/ heteronormativity	The assumption that binary gender identity and heterosexual orientation are the norm, and the subsequent treatment of heterosexuality as normal, natural, and more valuable than other sexualities
Homophobia	Fear of, dislike of, prejudice towards, or discrimination against someone who is gay or lesbian
Intended parent	In the context of surrogacy, the "intended parent(s)" are the individual or couple who enter into an agreement with a surrogate with the explicit intention of having a child who the intended parent(s) will assume legal and social parenthood of, and who the surrogate will not raise. They or their partner are likely to have provided genetic material necessary for conception, although this is not universally the case
Intersectionality	A term introduced by Crenshaw in 1989 to discuss ways in which different aspects of social identity or characteristics (e.g. race, ethnicity, gender, sexuality, class) combine and overlap (or intersect) to create different experiences of discrimination and inequalities
Intersex	People with variation in sex characteristics (e.g. chromosomes, hormones, primary or secondary sexual characteristics) which do not fit the typical definitions of male and female; people who are intersex may or may not identify with being part of the wider LGBTQ+ community. Also sometimes referred to as differences in sexual development (DSD), or historically, and offensively, as disorders in sexual development

Intersex surgeries/ genital mutilation	Intersex people are recognised in very few countries—in most countries an intersex baby is recorded as either male or female at birth. In countries which do allow for a third option, such as the UK where "not defined" is permitted, knowledge that this category exists may not be widespread, and therefore the category may be underused.
	In many countries, where genitals are visibly different, surgery is performed on intersex babies and young children to alter the appearance of their genitalia so that it conforms with their birth registration documents. This practice is sometimes referred to as "intersex genital mutilation" or "non-consensual intersex medical interventions." Many intersex adults are critical of the existence of such practices. Surgical procedures frequently impact sensory function in the genital area, affecting intersex people's ability to experience sexual pleasure, and causing pain or discomfort during sexual activities, as well as causing physical and emotional trauma
Lesbian	A woman or woman-aligned person who is sexually or romantically attracted to other women or women-aligned people; in some usage this need not exclude being attracted to people of other genders
LGBTQ+	Lesbian, Gay, Bisexual, Transgender, Non-binary*, Queer, Intersex, and/or Asexual; sometimes referred to as sexual and gender minorities. (*Not all non-binary individuals identify as transgender, so are included within the T and the "+" elements of the acronym, with more explicit inclusion in the definition to allow for this clarification.)
Man	Someone whose gender is man
Man-aligned	A person who does not identify their gender as man, but who experiences many aspects of life in the same way as a man, is frequently perceived by others as being a

man, and who therefore feels solidarity with issues affecting men resulting in either a political alignment with that gender, or an internal sense of connection to that gender

Minority stress model (MSM)	A formalisation of minority stress theory[1, 2], which illustrates the role of stigma and discrimination in enabling health disparities within minoritised communities. The initial model was focused on lesbian, gay, and bisexual individuals (i.e. sexual minorities), but has since been expanded to include gender minorities as well

Misgendering

Accidentally or deliberately identifying someone as the wrong gender. This can happen in a variety of ways:

- Through use of the wrong pronoun
- Through lacking adequate options on official forms or documentation (i.e. no gender-neutral options)
- Use of old and incorrect documentation
- Deadnaming
- Signage which enforces the wrong gender identity (for example gendered toilet signs, "women's" health department, etc.)

Monogamy

When two people agree to be each other's only sexual or romantic partners

Non-binary

An umbrella term for people whose gender is something other than man or woman. Many different non-binary identities exist

Non-gestational parent (also referred to as non-carrying parent or non-birthing parent)

Often used in LGBTQ+ families to refer to a parent who was not themselves pregnant, but who was involved in planning to have the baby(s). Whilst most commonly used within two-women families where there are children who were conceived within the relationship, the term is also used by other LGBTQ+ families.

The non-gestational parent may not have a genetic relationship to their children, or may be the biological parent to their child in some cases, including (but not limited to):

— Egg-sharing between a two-women couple
— Trans women who have conceived with a partner who has a uterus
— Non-binary people who find the term non-gestational parent more accurate than father

Outed, Outing

When a lesbian, gay, bi, or trans person's sexual orientation or gender identity is disclosed to someone else without their consent

Pansexual

Someone for whom sexual or romantic attraction is not connected to the person's sex or gender identity

Parent

Someone who has a combination of legal responsibility for a child alongside biological connection or social responsibility for them. Some parents have all three forms of connection

Polyamory/ethical non-monogamy/ENM

When a person has more than one sexual or romantic partner, with the knowledge and consent of all involved

Pronouns

Pronouns are words like I/we, she/her, he/him, or they/them. Many pronouns in English are gendered. Because of this, the correct use of pronouns tends to be particularly important to trans and non-binary people, and to same-sex couples when discussing their partner(s). Some people may choose a gender-neutral pronoun such as they/them or pronouns which are less familiar, such as zie/zir or xe/xem. These are sometimes called neopronouns

Queer

An umbrella term for anyone who is not cishet. Individuals may vary with the extent to which they use this term (and indeed any of the terms listed here) with queer having been used pejoratively

Same-gender relationship	Describing a romantic and/or sexual relationship between people who share the same gender identity; they may or may not have the same biological sex
Same-sex couple	Describing a romantic and/or sexual relationship between people of the same biological sex
Sex	In humans, biological sex is usually considered to be made up of five characteristics:

1. Genetics (chromosomes)
2. Hormones
3. Expression of hormones
4. Internal genitalia
5. External genitalia

Humans typically have 23 pairs of chromosomes, one of which determines a person's genetic sex. Typically, females have XX chromosomes and males have XY chromosomes, however there is a wide range of other combinations found in humans meaning, for example, that a cisgender woman can have XY chromosomes.

A range of hormones play a role in determining a person's sex—most notably oestrogen, progesterone, and testosterone. All humans produce these hormones in varying quantities with several of the sex-based distinctions based on the expected balance of hormone production and metabolism. These expectations translate to males assumed to have higher testosterone than most females, and most females assumed to have higher oestrogen and progesterone than most males. However, the ranges that are considered "normal" for males and females vary slightly by country, and the "normal" male and female ranges of some of these hormones overlap.

Internal genitalia are the anatomical features which relate directly to reproduction, including ovaries, testes, uterus, fallopian tubes, etc., while the external genitalia include vulva, clitoris, labia, testes, scrotum, and penis. These are sometimes referred to as primary sex characteristics, with an examination of the external genitalia being the metric used for assigning sex at birth. Secondary sexual characteristics are the physical features which develop in response to hormones, and include vocal pitch, facial hair, muscle and fat distribution, breasts, hip width, and menstruation. How these characteristics develop vary by individual based on their unique levels of genetic, hormonal, and environmental experiences.

Intersex people can be those whose chromosomes, hormones, or sexual characteristics fall outside of those typically associated with males and females. There is not a universal agreement about the specific combination of genetic, hormonal, and physical characteristics required to define a person's sex as female, male, or intersex. In addition, most estimates of the number of intersex people rely on intersex variations noted at birth, but not all anatomical variations are apparent at birth, hormonal variations are usually noticed during puberty, and most people assume rather than know their chromosomal make-up. This means that estimates of the number of people who are intersex vary quite widely, from 1.7% of the population[3] to 0.018%[4]

Sexual orientation

A person's emotional, romantic, and/or sexual attraction to another person. Examples are opposite gender (straight/heterosexual), same gender (lesbian, gay), more than one gender (bi or pansexual).

Sexual orientation can change over time, and people may choose to define their identity using a variety of terms. Always use the terms that people choose

Sperm donor

A person who provides sperm to someone who wishes to conceive a child, either directly or through a third party, commonly including fertility clinics. Sperm donors may be unknown to the recipient, or known to them at the time of conception. Unknown donors' identities may later be available to the child. They may have contact with any resulting child but do not raise them and

	should not be referred to as parents or by parental titles by professionals
Surrogate	A surrogate carries a baby on behalf of the intended parent(s). The surrogate may be genetically related to the baby or may be carrying a baby created with a donated egg. Many surrogates and intended parents prefer that the surrogate is not genetically related to the baby, believing this will make it easier for the surrogate to separate from the baby after the birth, however using donated eggs carries additional health risks for the surrogate.
	In some counties surrogates are paid for carrying a child whilst in other countries this is illegal. In some countries, working with a surrogate is a popular way for gay men to have children, whilst in other countries it is illegal. Legal and ethical considerations surrounding surrogacy can differ widely among different countries and circumstances
Third-party reproduction (also referred to as donor-assisted reproduction)	Where reproduction involves a third party, for example a donor that provides donor gametes or a surrogate that provides gestation, carrying the pregnancy
TNB	TNB is an acronym for "trans non-binary" It is used in two ways: 1. As an umbrella term to refer to people who are either binary transgender or non-binary. In this context it refers to all people who are not cisgender 2. To refer to people who identify simultaneously as transgender and non-binary
Trans/transgender	Someone whose gender is not the same as that which they were assigned at birth; this includes binary trans people (trans men and trans women) as well as non-binary people. Trans is an adjective—do not misuse it as a verb (i.e. "transgendered" is incorrect usage)
Trans man	A man who was assigned as female at birth; he may have reproductive anatomy to become pregnant, give birth, and to lactate

Trans woman	A woman who was assigned as male at birth; she may retain her own fertile gametes, or may have stored gametes with a fertility clinic
Transfeminine	A term that encompasses both trans women and non-binary people who have moved or are moving towards a feminine gender or gender presentation (as defined by the individual)
Transmasculine	A term that encompasses both trans men and non-binary people who have moved or are moving towards a masculine gender or gender presentation (as defined by the individual)
Transnormativity	A specific ideological accountability structure to which transgender people's presentations and experiences of gender are held accountable (thank you to A.J. Lowik for this definition)
Transphobia	The fear of, dislike of, or prejudice against someone who identifies as trans. Includes the denial or refusal to accept a person's gender, and the denial that non-binary identities exist
Woman	Someone whose gender is woman
Woman-aligned	A person who does not identify their gender as woman, but who experiences many aspects of life in the same way as a woman, is frequently perceived by others as being a woman, and who therefore feels solidarity with issues affecting women, resulting in either a political alignment with that gender, or an internal sense of connection to that gender

REFERENCES

1. Brooks VR. *Minority Stress and Lesbian Women*. Lexington Books; 1981.
2. Meyer IH. Prejudice, Social Stress, and Mental Health in Lesbian, Gay, and Bisexual Populations: Conceptual Issues and Research Evidence. *Psychol Bull*. 2003;129(5):674–697. doi:10.1037/0033-2909.129.5.674
3. Fausto-Sterling A. The Five Sexes. *The Sciences*. 1993;33:20–24.
4. Sax L. How Common is Intersex? A Response to Anne Fausto-Sterling. *The Journal of Sex Research*. 2002;39:174–178.

Introduction

Mari Greenfield, Kate Luxion, El Molloy, and Alice-Amanda Hinton

The four of us work with new and expectant parents in different roles—as a midwife (AAH), doulas (MG), breastfeeding counsellors (MG, KL, EM), and antenatal teachers (KL). We are also all part of the LGBTQ+ community. In our work, we have found a significant lack of knowledge and understanding about how to work with LGBTQ+ people—people like us. Frequently we have found that although perinatal services and individual colleagues have wanted to provide good and equitable care for LGBTQ+ people, they have not known how to do so. A few great resources exist, but they are mostly very specialist. We wanted to be able to refer anyone working in any capacity, with LGBTQ+ people who were becoming parents to a single resource which encompasses the whole perinatal period, from before conception to post-birth, but there was a gap where that resource should be.

This book is our answer to that gap. We have brought together leading researchers and practitioners from around the world, each an expert in their field, to create a book that covers as many aspects of the perinatal journey as possible. We hope the book will be useful to a wide range of healthcare professionals and birth workers, from obstetricians, midwives and health visitors to psychologists, doulas and those who offer community services to parents postnatally, ie, parent and baby groups.

The book is designed to take you through the reproductive journey, beginning with contraceptive choices, and considering safe and appropriate access to abortion care for unwanted pregnancies; then through conception and additional support for parents who need specialist support; into birth, infant feeding, mental health, and early parenthood. We hope that reading the book as a whole will give you a sense of LGBTQ+ parents' journeys. Equally, each chapter is designed to be standalone, so if you just want to read the chapter that relates to your work, please feel free to do so.

DOI: 10.4324/9781003305446-1

Within the book, authors have shared stories they have experienced, witnessed, and been told about. Some readers, particularly those who are themselves LGBTQ+, may find some of the stories difficult to read. Also, we will at times be discussing the ways in which LGBTQ+ people have sex, where this is different to the cisheterosexist assumptions about sex that healthcare professionals may hold. We make no apology for this, as understanding the lived experiences of LGBTQ+ people is fundamental to providing them with appropriate sexual and reproductive healthcare.

Before beginning to discuss LGBTQ+ people's current experiences, we would like to use the introduction to set the context, beginning with a brief history of LGBTQ+ parenthood.

HISTORY OF LGBTQ+ PEOPLE AND PARENTHOOD

Throughout history, humans have experienced diversity in terms of biological sex, conceptions of gender, how they have enacted their gender, and configurations of intimate relationships. No single societal idea about "gender" or "sexual orientation" can be considered as true. While recent limited narratives have told the story of home and family, centring the nuclear family, this is not representative of the diverse genders and sexual orientations seen within families historically.

Contemporary changes in societal norms has enabled visibility of the varied range of families that are commonplace in Western, educated, industrialised, rich, democratic (WEIRD) countries, including single parent families, step families, polyamorous families, same-sex families, and heterosexual families with stay-at-home fathers. Formerly, WEIRD countries have espoused a strictly binary idea of sex, gender, and gender expression—a model which has spread throughout much of the world through colonialism. In this model, sex is determined solely by visible genitalia at birth, establishing medical and legal personhood under a male/female binary based on this observation alone. Males are all boys, who will grow into men, and must embody masculine characteristics. Their domain is the public sphere, they are responsible for providing for their family, of which they are the head. Females are all girls, who will grow into women, and must embody feminine characteristics. Their domain is the private sphere, where they provide care for family members, under the command of their male partner, father, or other male relative. As such, postcolonial approaches reject imposed narratives of cisheterosexual monogamous nuclear families as the ideal within the global majority. Yet the institutions that exist to support people on their journey to parenthood were created under the cisheteronormative societal norms described above.

MODERN PERINATAL SERVICES

Current health service provision is rooted in models and ways of being which assume all people are cis gender and heterosexual (cisheterocentric). Inevitably this means that perinatal services are structured in ways that prioritise cisheterosexist assumptions about service users and delivery of care. This is evident from the earliest encounters which parents have with perinatal services. These encounters may happen as part of preconception care, where expectations around parenting with medical support for a family frame service offering; or during "booking in" form completion with midwifery services in which data collection assumes gender of pregnant parents. Language which is used within perinatal care and service provision is highly gendered, assumes parent genders and relationship structures, and frequently within both perinatal services research into perinatal experiences there is well-documented resistance to change language or terminology to be more inclusive of non-cis heteronormative parenting because of an unfounded fear that biological women's rights will be diminished and reduced. This itself stands in opposition to all research around any other type of service offering and teaching and research pedagogy where it is understood that making services accessible to everyone does not single out specific groups or individuals, and increases accessibility and equity across the board.

For LGBTQ+ parents, mono-normativity within Western societies adds increased complications. LGBTQ+ parents in a monogamous sexual relationship may still need to record that there are more than two people involved in the creation and raising of their child. Medical information about a sperm or egg donor and/or a surrogate may need to be recorded alongside medical and social information about biological or gestational parents, and social information about a non-biological and/or non-gestational parent. In more complex fertility journeys, a gestational parent or surrogate may be pregnant with a donor egg or embryo, meaning that there could be four people involved in the creation or raising of a child, even though the child is being born into a relationship between two monogamous people. Research has shown that perceived validity of non-biological or non-gestational parents by healthcare professionals involved in delivery of care is a valid fear for many couples. This may exacerbate avoidance or and/or disengagement with health services because of the anticipation of, or due to experiences of stigmatising or discriminatory care.

Non-monogamy in various different forms appears to be more common amongst LGBTQ+ people, perhaps because in recent history their relationships were not codified and sanctioned by the State in many countries.[1] Non-monogamous

LGBTQ+ people who are becoming parents may struggle even more to have the relationships which are important to their baby recognised within perinatal services.

THE EFFECTS OF INEQUALITY

Such difficulties in accessing and navigating services related to perinatal care, continue into the postnatal period and influence how LGBTQ+ parents are perceived within the current legal frameworks. In recent years there have been significant numbers of legal cases within the UK as LGBTQ+ people have tried to establish appropriate parenting rights and legal titles within their family relationships, within a legal system that is designed to reinforce and uphold the structure of "family" as consisting of one biologically female mother and one biologically male father. From cases of contested parental responsibility for non-gestational mothers,[2] to donors seeking an involved parental role,[3] to the use of a surrogates,[4] to trans men who are gestational parents challenging the legal assumption that gestational parents are mothers,[5] and trans women who are biological parents refusing to be labelled as fathers,[6] LGBTQ+ parents are at the forefront of redefining families. In some cases the law around these decisions has been clear for a number of years, yet is still misused and misinterpreted, leading to distress and prolonged unnecessary legal battles, for example where non-gestational parents are denied their legal right to parenthood.[7]

These issues are further complicated for LGBTQ+ people who choose to enter parenthood without a romantic or sexual partner, and/or who may or may not choose to co-parent with a non-romantic partner. In particular, fertility treatment may be difficult to access for these people. In the UK, fertility treatment must be paid for by those who are not having sexual intercourse with an opposite sex partner, whilst for heterosexual couples this treatment can be free (dependent on location and circumstance). Although recent changes to infertility definitions in the USA now encompass the need for donor gametes for a parent, until very recently definitions of infertility in the USA have assumed heterosexuality and defined infertility and the need for donor gametes as an issue exclusive to a biological male-female couple.[8] Fortunately, the newest USA definitions describe infertility as:

> 'A disease, condition, or status characterised by any of the following:
>
> - The inability to achieve a successful pregnancy based on a patient's medical, sexual, and reproductive history, age, physical findings, diagnostic testing, or any combination of those factors.
> - The need for medical intervention, including, but not limited to, the use of donor gametes or donor embryos in order to achieve a successful pregnancy either as an individual or with a partner.

– In patients having regular, unprotected intercourse and without any known etiology for either partner suggestive of impaired reproductive ability, evaluation should be initiated at 12 months when the female partner is under 35 years of age and at six months when the female partner is 35 years of age or older.'[9]

And go on to state that: "Nothing in this definition shall be used to deny or delay treatment to any individual, regardless of relationship status or sexual orientation."[9] Previous definitions have assumed heterosexuality and defined infertility and the need for donor gametes as an issue exclusive to these groups. In contrast, in Poland, single LGBTQ+ people who wish to conceive may face legal barriers to accessing any fertility treatment.[10]

Inequality of opportunity in parenthood extends to adoptive families too. Adoption for same-sex couples in Poland, Hungary, and seven other EU countries is illegal, and predominantly based on rhetoric around the potential damaging exposure of children to LGBTQ+ relationships which are touted by religious and political parties in opposition to all empirical research, which shows that children of LGBTQ+ parents do as well, if not better, emotionally, and academically, in comparison with children raised by heterosexual parents.[11, 12] The stigma and discrimination faced by LGBTQ+ parents, and children of LGBTQ+ parents including any risk to their physical or psychological safety, is itself a factor of structural state-endorsed homophobia. This means that in some cases, in countries where LGBTQ+ parenting is to all intents and purposes, illegal, some parents may choose to co-parent with a person who is not their romantic or sexual partner and may face difficulties in other ways.

Throughout the chapters within this book, we will explore the known narratives of stigma and discrimination that are faced within perinatal care. The cause/basis of these experiences can be a lack of resources, underprepared health services, a need for more health education, among other preventable events and shortages. A key aim of this book is to help untangle existing causes of harm for LGBTQ+ parents within perinatal services highlighting what can be prevented and what should be provided. Using the minority stress model[13, 14] as a framework can help readers to better understand the links between LGBTQ+ people's experiences and the state of perinatal care as cisheteronormative. The minority stress model helps to bridge the connection between the experiential, the emotional, the psychological, and the physical—the complex snapshot of what it means to navigate a healthcare system that is structurally unfit for supporting LGBTQ+ individuals reproductive health and perinatal needs.

The model is discussed more fully in Chapter 13, alongside the important concept of allostatic load[15] (ie, balance within the body as positioned in the social world) as a way of understanding the theory in practice. But it is important to move through the chapters of this text with some understanding of the model as it provides a framework to map the additional stress that is faced by minoritised groups. The minority stress model highlights the connection between the amount of stress that individuals face and the quality of health that they are able to experience. LGBTQ+ people usually face a higher level of daily stress because they are LGBTQ+. This additional "minority stress" might come from knowing they could at any time be fired from their job or refused medical care based solely on their gender and/or sexual orientation. In perinatal care, this additional stress could come from reductions in care quality or receiving less support simply due to the cisheteronormative structure and assumptions present. The idea that the body is binary (ie, sex as essentialist and immutable) and reproduction is inherently heterosexual are such two examples. The harms caused by these ideas can be psychological and/or physical. For example, invasive and harmful surgeries being performed on intersex babies and children to fit binary male/female categories, or the denial of transgender people's existence and reproductive health care needs, such as people being presumed as heterosexual women because they are pregnant. In short, what results is poorer health outcomes, due to the way that the minority stress (ie, additional stressors caused by social and medical systems) cascades through the body, even if a person does not experience inequitable care as it is presently defined.

The minority stress model, through helping to explain these preventable harms, also helps to examine instances of resilience and shows the importance of structural changes necessary to implement and support protective factors through supporting, welcoming, and understanding the diverse families and individuals using perinatal services.

FINAL WORDS

It is our hope that this book helps lay the foundation of providing inclusive perinatal services and for enacting perinatal care that is culturally humble. Culturally humble care means recognising that supporting and learning about LGBTQ+ people is an ongoing process. There is no one-size fits all approach that you can adopt, rather, to achieve equitable and inclusive perinatal care it is necessary to take a patient-centred approach. Chapter authors have woven together the literature and the experiences of the people that they have supported to provide a comprehensive exploration of care needs from conception to the postpartum period. Whether you are directly applying the chapters to clinical practice or using them as information for medical education (clinical and research), it is vital that the framing of perinatal and reproductive health acknowledges the entirety of the population accessing support and services. Keeping these things in mind, we hope you enjoy this book, and use it to create change. We would love for our book to serve as a catalyst for change and expand the understanding of LGBTQ+ perinatal health care needs.

REFERENCES

1. Balzarini RN, Dharma C, Kohut T, et al. Demographic Comparison of American Individuals in Polyamorous and Monogamous Relationships. *The Journal of Sex Research*. 2019;56: 681–694.
2. Cobb J. EWHC 1418, https://vlex.co.uk/vid/re-f-assisted-reproduction-792555017 (2013).
3. Thorpe, Black, Chadwick. EWCA Civ 285, https://vlex.co.uk/vid/v-b-and-c-793414449 (2012).
4. Russell. EWFC 36, https://vlex.co.uk/vid/h-b-1st-2nd-792687645 (2015).
5. McFarlane A. EWHC 1823, https://www.judiciary.uk/wp-content/uploads/2019/09/TT-and-YY-APPROVED-Substantive-Judgment-McF-25.9.19.pdf (2019).
6. Darwin Z, Greenfield M. Gestational and Non-Gestational Parents: Challenging Assumptions. *Journal of Reproductive and Infant Psychology*. 2022;40:1–2.
7. MacDonald. EWHC 1982, https://www.bailii.org/ew/cases/EWHC/Admin/2022/1982.html (2022).
8. Practice Committee of the American Society for Reproductive Medicine. Definitions of Infertility and Recurrent Pregnancy Loss: A Committee Opinion. *Fertility and Sterility*. 2020; 113:533–535.
9. Practice Committee of the American Society for Reproductive Medicine. Definitions of Infertility and Recurrent Pregnancy Loss: A Committee Opinion. *Fertility and Sterility*. 2023; 120:1.
10. Mizielińska J, Stasińska A. Negotiations between Possibilities and Reality: Reproductive Choices of Families of Choice in Poland. *European Journal of Women's Studies*. 2023;30: 148–163.
11. Manning WD, Fettro MN, Lamidi E. Child Well-Being in Same-Sex Parent Families: Review of Research Prepared for American Sociological Association Amicus Brief. *Popul Res Policy Rev*. 2014;33:485–502.
12. Mazrekaj D, De Witte K, Cabus S. School Outcomes of Children Raised by Same-Sex Parents: Evidence from Administrative Panel Data. *Am Sociol Rev*. 2020;85:830–856.
13. Meyer IH. Prejudice, Social Stress, and Mental Health in Lesbian, Gay, and Bisexual Populations: Conceptual Issues and Research Evidence. *Psychological Bulletin*. 2003;129: 674–697.
14. Brooks VR. *Minority Stress and Lesbian Women*. Lexington, MA: Heath, 1981.
15. Sterling P, Eyers J. Allostasis: A New Paradigm to Explain Arousal Pathology. In: *Handbook of Life Stress, Cognition and Health*. John Wiley & Sons, 1988, pp. 629–649.

Chapter 1

Contraception and sexual health

Alice-Amanda Hinton

CHALLENGES LGBTQ+ PEOPLE FACE IN ACCESSING CONTRACEPTIVE AND SEXUAL HEALTH SERVICES

There are many reasons why attending any health care setting can be difficult for LGBTQ+ people. When LGBTQ+ people enter any health care setting they are often aware that their needs are less well understood and evidenced, and that as a consequence the health care they might be offered is less likely to be matched to their needs. This may result in hypervigilance, which can make relationships with health care professionals (HCPs) more difficult.[1, 2] One in seven LGBT people have avoided treatment for fear of discrimination,[1] and 13% experiencing some form of unequal treatment as a result of their identity. Mental health can have an impact, with half (52%) of LGBTQ+ people reporting that they have experienced depression in the last year.[3] A survey of lesbian and bisexual+ (LB+) women found that only 2% would go to their GP for advice about sex with women.[4]

Public health campaigns and information rarely include images of or references to queer lives, which can lead to LGBTQ+ people feeling a sense of not belonging in a health care environment. Indeed, the ways in which some information is presented may not only fail to be inclusive, but signal that services are only for cisgender or heterosexual people, as Figure 1.1 below shows.

Accessing any form of health screening for trans and non-binary people can be particularly challenging. In countries which allow self-identification in health records, trans and non-binary people may face difficulties in accessing appropriate screening tests,[5] or be called for inappropriate screening tests. In my clinical practice I have met trans masculine people who have been unaware whether or not they still have a cervix requiring screening following gender affirming hysterectomy. Poor communication from HCPs which leaves patients unaware of

DOI: 10.4324/9781003305446-2

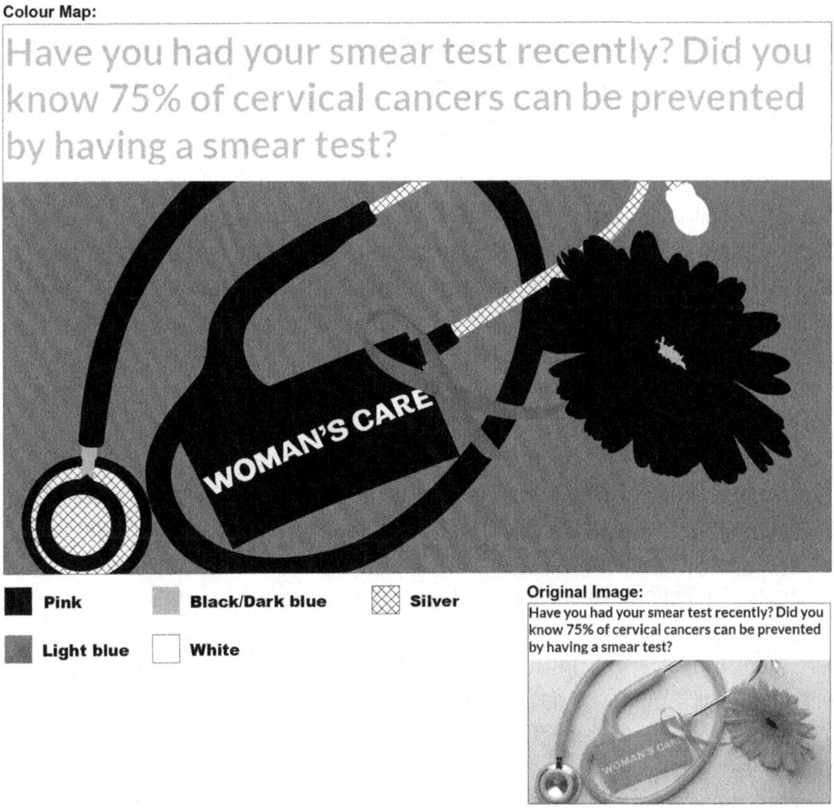

Colour Map:

Have you had your smear test recently? Did you know 75% of cervical cancers can be prevented by having a smear test?

■ Pink   ■ Black/Dark blue   ▨ Silver   ■ Light blue   □ White

Original Image:

Have you had your smear test recently? Did you know 75% of cervical cancers can be prevented by having a smear test?

Figure 1.1 An advert for cervical screening, with colour map, consisting of a pink stethoscope labelled "woman's care" and a pink gerbera flower.

which health screenings would be appropriate puts their health at risk. Later detection of issues such as abdominal aortic aneurysm, cervical and breast cancers result in poorer outcomes because of the more advanced stages at time of presentation.

Accessing contraceptive and sexual health services, where their genitals and information about their sexual and/or romantic relationships are relevant to the discussion, may pose even greater challenges to trans and non-binary people than accessing other forms of health care. Official documentation in sexual health services often fails to make space for non-normative lives—gender is often assumed to be binary, sexual orientation is assumed to fall into a limited range of definitions and to be fixed, and relationships are assumed to be monogamous.

The health care concerns of LGBTQ+ people may also not match the priorities of mainstream sexual health services resulting in marginalisation even where direct discrimination is not experienced. For example, lesbian, bisexual or pansexual cis women might be anxious about transmitting human papilloma virus (HPV)—the high-risk strains of which are the highest cause of cervical cancer—to other partners who have vaginas. There is very little information available about those risks and health care providers may be unfamiliar with answering those concerns. There is some evidence that LGBTQ+ populations overlap with populations who engage in bondage, dominance, and sadomasochist (BDSM) activities.[6] LGBTQ+ people may therefore wish to discuss with HCPs transmission risks of sexually transmitted infections (STIs) during BDSM activities, or using when using specific kinds of sex toys, but again, as little research exists, HCPs are unlikely to be able to offer informed advice.[4] Where information for LGBTQ+ people is provided, categorisations tend to be blunt and to equate sex with gender, such as "'men who have sex with men'," "'men who have sex with women'," and "'women who have sex with men'." Sexual health information is rarely provided for women who have sex with women, perhaps the lower chance of transmission of some sexually transmitted infections means they are perceived as a group who have fewer sexual health needs. Where HCPs are aware that a cis man is bisexual or pansexual, they may just provide copies of information for "'men who have sex with men'" and "'men who have sex with women'," which does not provide adequate information for men who have sex with more than one gender. For transgender and non-binary people, or for those with transgender or non-binary partners, these binary groupings may be inappropriate and even harmful.

Experiencing sexual violence is a known risk factor for unwanted pregnancies, sexually transmitted infections, and poorer quality sexual health.[7] Gender and sexual minorities are more likely to experience sexual violence than cisheterosexual people, with bisexual women and trans people shouldering an especially heavy burden.[8] Forty-two percent of LB+ women report having experienced sexual violence.[9] This figure may be even higher when multiple minority identities intersect, for example amongst disabled and/or racially and ethnically minoritised LGBTQ+ people.

As a result of both personal and collective community experiences of marginalisation, ignorance and discrimination, LGBTQ+ people may delay or avoid health care screening and treatment.[3, 5, 9] The greater the gap between the perceived "fit" of the individual into the acceptable cisheterosexist archetypes, the lower the uptake of screening and treatment is likely to be, with negative health sequelae.

MISINFORMATION ABOUT SEXUAL HEALTH

When LGBTQ+ people do access sexual health services they are frequently given incorrect information. Research shows that up to 37% of cis women who exclusively have sex with other people who have vaginas have been told that they do not need cervical screening tests.[10] This is medically incorrect, and is highly dangerous misinformation to communicate as delays to the detection of HPV presence or changes to cervical cells can result in cervical cancer being detected at a more advanced stage when treatment may be more invasive or less effective. As a result, LGBTQ+ people may be forced to gain more expertise in their own health care needs, drawing on community knowledge rather than HCP information as a coping strategy for the dearth of evidence-based information.[9]

Other misinformation may be based on HCPs making incorrect assumptions about sexual practices. The kind of sex which LGBTQ+ people are having is often poorly understood, and HCPs may know little about common sexual practices, such as muffing[11] and vaginal fisting.[12] Because these sexual practices are viewed as non-normative, there is little or no research evidence about the sexual health issues associated with them, making it difficult for HCPs to give accurate information. Frequently recommended safer sex practices which are appropriate for LGBTQ+ sexual practices, such as hygiene for dildoes and sex toys, wearing gloves, and using dental dams for oral sex are poorly researched. Some of these safer sex methods also have a low acceptability rate amongst LGBTQ+ people, with 93% of LB+ women sometimes or never using barrier methods and contraception where necessary, and only 7% always doing so.[9] Similarly, an assumption that all trans men are dysphoric about their vaginas, and so will not use their vaginas for sex, appears to be widespread, despite the fact that it is not accurate for all trans men.[13] Further, HCPs may view LGBTQ+ sex as transgressive or even immoral. Relationship structures and sexual partnerships may not fit the conventional nuclear family model, and this may be pathologised and regarded as increasing risk factors, despite the mitigation of often greater literacy in sexual health.

Further misinformation can be related to the cisheterosexist assumptions underlying health care systems. Where sexual health screening tests are sex-dependent, transgender people may not receive invitations to screenings, for example, in the UK, trans women are not routinely called for prostate checks and trans men are not routinely called for mammograms or cervical smear tests—if, as discussed earlier, poor communication has meant they are unaware they proactively need to book such screening tests this can result in poorer outcomes (eg, barriers to and experiences of trans men in smears).[14, 15]

Bisexual people can face a discrete set of difficulties when accessing sexual health services. Their sexual orientation may be inferred as heterosexual or lesbian/gay, based on the relationship they disclose to the HCP, resulting in bi-invisibility. Bisexual people may also be viewed as vectors of disease from gay men to the supposedly "safer" heterosexual population, or lesbian women.[8] This means that sexual health services aimed at LGBTQ+ people may appear less welcoming to bisexual people, and may be seen as only catering to gay cisgender men. Research shows that whilst 36% of gay and lesbian people did not disclose their sexual orientation to their HCP, that number rises to 67% for bisexual people.[16]

Stigma about LGBTQ+ people's sexual health also has a negative impact on cis women who have sex with men particularly in relation to HIV and pre-exposure prophylaxis (commonly referred to as PrEP). The association of gay men's sex with the risk of HIV transmission and therefore the need to discuss PrEP results in appropriate information not being provided to cis women. For example, West African women have a higher incidence of HIV. There is a common understanding of management of existing HIV infection and of preventing vertical transmission (from mother to baby) within perinatal services. However, there is little knowledge about PrEP amongst perinatal specialists and it is not routinely discussed or recommended at postnatal appointments when appropriate contraception is discussed and recommended.[17] Reasons behind this lack of knowledge may be rooted in an association of PrEP with promiscuity—something which is more acceptable within specialist gay men's sexual health services than within perinatal services.

MISINFORMATION ABOUT CONTRACEPTION

Unless appropriate education is provided about LGBTQ+ people's contraceptive needs, HCPs may be reliant on societal stereotypes to inform their predictions of the contraceptive services LGBTQ+ people may need. One such assumption is that LGBTQ+ people will not start a family, or that if they do so they will not want or be able to have biological children. In some countries, this assumption may be reinforced by laws which limit LGBTQ+ people's access to reproductive services,[18] and even laws which insist on sterilisation of transgender people as a prerequisite for gender affirming treatments.[19] Being unable to obtain appropriate contraceptive advice or contraception can lead to increased chances of unwanted pregnancies, and therefore to a greater need for pregnancy termination and abortion services. Evidence shows that this disproportionately affects some groups of LGBTQ+ people, with rates of abortion being higher in young women who later identify as lesbian or bisexual and amongst trans masculine people than amongst cisheterosexual women.[20]

The available evidence contradicts this assumption, showing that a large percentage of LGBTQ+ adults would like to become parents.[21–31] Whilst fewer LGBTQ+ people may intend to act on this desire and become parents, this is usually linked to barriers to achieving parenthood.[18, 32]

Most people accessing contraceptive services will be engaging in sex with at least one person of a different sex. HCPs may infer that this kind of sex denotes the person's sexual orientation. This leads to difficulties for people of all non-heterosexual identities, and in particular results in the invisibility of bisexual and pansexual identities. Misidentifying someone's sexual orientation may lead to gaps in the advice, information or treatment provided.

Little research has been carried out into the effects of Gender Affirming Hormone Therapy (GAHT) on fertility. Without a strong evidence base, HCPs may not be able to provide transgender people with accurate information on the need for contraception—a problem which is exacerbated by the division of medical disciplines in many health care systems between gender-affirming care and other services. Fertility and contraceptive advice may therefore be given to transgender people by gender-care specialists who have limited knowledge of fertility and contraception.[33, 34] Trans women are frequently advised that taking oestrogen will result in infertility,[35] and trans men have reported being given dangerously inaccurate information, including that testosterone is 100% effective as a contraceptive, and that taking testosterone will result in permanent infertility or lowered fertility.[36] This information is not supported by any available evidence.[37] Recent research suggests that testosterone therapy may in fact preserve fertility for longer for some trans men, as when testosterone use does result in anovulation, ovarian reserves may remain at a higher level than would have been expected in relation to chronological age.[38, 39] It is therefore possible that some trans men may remain fertile past the normal age of menopause for cis women, into a period where trans men may assume their age means that conception is not a risk, and therefore that contraception is unnecessary. We have found no evidence that trans men are counselled about this possibility.

In a current research project, a trans woman reported that she had been prescribed oestrogen and had used it for several months before her gender-care HCPs asked about parenting intentions. When she said that she planned to become a parent in the near future, she was advised that taking oestrogen would permanently impair her fertility. The only option she was given was to cease oestrogen use for 6 months, and to then deposit her sperm in a fertility storage facility, at which point her sperm was fertility tested. She described the 6 months of ceasing oestrogen therapy as the most difficult of her life. Six months later when she moved countries, she found that exporting her sperm was bureaucratically complicated and very expensive. A few years later, when she and her wife wished to conceive, they decided to try to conceive through sexual intercourse at home, without ceasing oestrogen therapy. This was successful.[40]

Discussions of contraceptive use form a routine part of postpartum care in many countries.[41] Postnatal conversations around contraception and family planning within the perinatal setting routinely assume a monogamous cisgender heterosexual relationship. Even when the patients' notes clearly indicate that the patient is in a monogamous cisgender lesbian relationship, HCPs may be so accustomed to providing advice based on assumptions of heterosexual sexual activity that they give inappropriate advice. In recent research, one lesbian reported that:

> The doctor said 'We need to talk about contraception. What sort of contraception are you going to be using after you've given birth? And Kate said 'Yeah, no, she's good, but she's not that good'. He went 'Oh my goodness'. And he just left.[40]

MISTREATMENT AS PART OF SEXUAL HEALTH AND CONTRACEPTION SERVICES

Misinformation and incorrect assumptions on the part of HCPs can result in LGBTQ+ people experiencing suboptimal treatment. This can happen despite the HCP wishing to provide the best care, as is shown in the case study below:

CASE STUDY 1

A lesbian patient presents for the removal of a persistent and painful ovarian cyst, accompanied by her partner. During the surgery to remove the cyst, the gynaecologist also removes the ovary to prevent further cysts occurring, and in case it might be cancerous. When the patient is later informed that her ovary was removed, she is very distressed, as ovarian removal was not discussed beforehand, and she would not have consented to this. The gynaecologist explains that he removed it rather than biopsied it because the patient had disclosed she was a lesbian, so he assumed that she would not want to have children. The patient actually very much wished to become pregnant. She later faced significant fertility challenges, and was not able to have the family she wanted.

We must also acknowledge that homophobia and transphobia sometimes mean that HCPs choose to provide suboptimal care to or mistreat LGBTQ+ people. One example of how this might appear is shown in the real-life case study below:

CASE STUDY 2

A trans man presents at gynaecological services with severe endometriosis and pain. It is clear that a hysterectomy because of the endometriosis is the only clinically appropriate option, and the patient's history reveals no contraindications. The senior gynaecologist later describes the case in the coffee room, and states he has not recommended a hysterectomy because he was not going to give

'free gender affirming care to a trannie'

This is overheard by junior doctors who are horrified because the clinical indicators are clear, and no other course of treatment is clinically appropriate. They feel unempowered to challenge the more senior member of staff or to intervene in any way.

When LGBTQ+ people access any reproductive health services, they will come with not only their own experiences of mistreatment, but with knowledge about the mistreatment that other LGBTQ+ people have experienced from health care services.

RESULTS—BROKEN TRUST

Experiences of misinformation and mistreatment amongst the LGBTQ+ community lead LGBTQ+ people to mistrust HCPs generally. For transgender and non-binary people this may be even more acute, as accessing gender-affirming care in most countries requires generalist HCPs to make referrals to specialist services, and there is good evidence of gatekeeping and delays in referrals.[2] Not only does this have implications for mistrust when LGBTQ+ people access contraceptive and sexual health services, but it also then has implications for pregnancy care. Lacking trust in HCPs who provide perinatal care can amplify fears, leading to tokophobia.[42] As we will see later in this book, this in turn can increase the risks of stillbirth, birth trauma rates, perinatal mental health, and can determine whether care is sought if postnatal mental health problems develop.

RESULTS—SEXUAL HEALTH IS LATER REPRODUCTIVE HEALTH

An individual's lifelong sexual health is linked with their future reproductive, pregnancy and birth choices.[43] Contracting some sexually transmitted infections (STIs) can impact future fertility, as can delaying or not obtaining treatment for them.[43, 44] For lesbian and bisexual women, trans men, and non-binary people who have a vagina, pelvic inflammatory disease (PID) can have a significant effect on future fertility. A very high proportion of PID is associated by untreated chlamydia and gonorrhoea

> of women who received a diagnosis of acute PID, approximately 50% have a positive test for either of those organisms[45]

As well being linked to PID, chlamydia can cause damage to the fallopian tubes without any symptoms

> Untreated, about 10–15% of women with chlamydia will develop PID. Chlamydia can also cause fallopian tube infection without any symptoms. PID and 'silent' infection in the upper genital tract may cause permanent damage to the fallopian tubes, uterus, and surrounding tissues, which can lead to infertility.

Bacterial vaginosis occurs more commonly in cisgender lesbian and bisexual women than in cisgender heterosexual women (no research has included trans men or non-binary people who have vaginas).[46] Research shows the comparative rates to be 25.7% amongst lesbians and 14.4% in heterosexual women.[47] To date, no research has established why this is, or which safer sex practices would be both effective and acceptable to advise lesbian and bisexual women to consider. Having bacterial vaginosis can predispose people to contracting other STIs. If someone with bacterial vaginosis (which can be asymptomatic) becomes pregnant, they are at a much greater risk of experiencing a late miscarriage or preterm birth than someone who does not, with the reported odds ratio being 1.4:7.0.[48] Some sexual health screening takes place at pregnancy booking, but in the UK, contrary to a widespread assumption, a comprehensive sexual health screening does not take place. For example, screening for syphilis, Hep B, and HIV are usually offered, but screening for chlamydia, gonorrhoea, and herpes are not. Midwives tend not to be vocal about recommending regular sexual health screening for all sexually active patients.

If LGBTQ+ people are not able to access routine sexual health screenings, they are less likely to be aware that they have chlamydia, potentially compromising their own or their partners' future fertility. They are also less likely to be aware they have asymptomatic bacterial vaginosis, potentially compromising the health of any future children.

Conversely, some groups of LGBTQ+ people may be more likely than their cisheterosexual counterparts to access sexual health services. Some cis gay and bisexual men see sexual health screening as a routine part of life (for example when collecting data for the Gay Men's Sexual Health Survey, a repeating survey of gay and bisexual men's sexual health in London, a gay man found it extraordinary that someone might not be aware of their HIV status, and wouldn't test regularly).

The term reproductive health is often taken to refer exclusively to cis women, but sperm quality also affects reproductive choices. What is often termed "male factor" infertility accounts for half of all infertility problems in heterosexual couples.[49] One of the few areas of evidence concerning LGBTQ+ health which has been well studied are the rates of alcohol,[3] recreational drug use,[50] and smoking,[51] all of which LGBTQ+ people do more, and all of which can have a significant impact on sperm viability. For trans feminine people and gay and bisexual men who want to have a family, information about the impact on sperm quality is unlikely to have been part of advice around health improvements, as it is commonly assumed that they will not have children.

CHALLENGES HCPS FACE IN PROVIDING LGBTQ+ PEOPLE WITH CONTRACEPTIVE AND SEXUAL HEALTH SERVICES

LGBTQ+ people do not face difficulties with access, misinformation and mistreatment because HCPs wish to exclude them. Rather, HCPs face challenges in providing contraceptive and sexual health care to LGBTQ+ people. These challenges fall into three main categories; education, information, and health care systems.

Education

HCPs are used to thinking about contraceptive and sexual health advice based on risk assessments which group sexual behaviours into broad categories, using a flowchart or algorithm model for both assessment and treatment. In this model a HCP who will usually not have met the individual before will take a patient's history and mentally stratify the person into a risk group. This is a useful skill where health services are under-resourced and have a heavy workload. If the HCP does not have sufficient education about sexual and gender minorities to accurately assess risk for those groups, they may fall back on common societal stereotypes. Research shows that many HCP students feel underprepared for working with LGBTQ+ patients, and that their lecturers feel underprepared to teach HCP students about this.[52–54]

LGBTQ+ HCPs exist, and in the absence of a robust educational programme about LGBTQ+ people's health needs, this person may be assumed by other HCPs to be a good source of information to ensure services are appropriate. Several problems arise from this assumption. First, if the workplace is not conducive to constructive criticism, or if the workplace is not an environment where LGBTQ+ HCPs can be fully open about their LGBTQ+ identity, they will not be able to challenge assumptions, model behaviours, or be willing to share their lived experiences. This can lead to assumptions being made that services are accessible, because the LGBTQ+ person has not said they are inaccessible.

Second, simply being an LGBTQ+ person does not give a HCP expertise in the needs and experiences of all LGBTQ+ people who use the service. Not only may the issues faced by lesbians accessing sexual health services be quite different to those faced by a gay man, intersecting inequalities also affect experiences, so a Black lesbian may have significantly different experiences of obtaining contraceptive information than a white lesbian.

Third, over reliance on LGBTQ+ staff to champion LGBTQ+ equality, without recognition of the labour this entails can lead to the LGBTQ+ HCP experiencing burnout. Simultaneously, if the knowledge and experience in caring for LGBTQ+ people is held by the one LGBTQ+ HCP and they then leave, the collective knowledge and experience of the team may reduce suddenly.

Information

HCPs face a difficult balance in giving evidence-based statistical and generalised information whilst also giving personalised care. If the evidence base for the provision of statistical and generalised information doesn't exist, then the care that the HCP can provide is compromised. There are significant gaps in the evidence base for LGBTQ+ sexual and reproductive health. For example, information about transmission rates of sexually transmitted infections between women, broken down by the type of sexual activity they engage in, is simply not available. Robust data about the contraceptive efficacy of different variations of testosterone and oestrogen for transgender people is also not available. Where gaps in information exist, HCPs may over-rely on the small amount of information they do have, leading to the provision of inappropriate health care, as seen in the case study below:

CASE STUDY 3

A cis bisexual man and his cis bisexual woman partner attended a sexual health clinic I worked at. Assumptions were made that, because they were presenting as a couple, they must be heterosexual. All of the initial conversations they wanted to have with HCPs were about reproductive health and pregnancy. However, as soon as they disclosed that they were both bisexual, the conversation turned to how high risk they were as a couple. These conversations were not based on behaviours they discussed, nor on their actual sexual history, but on their identities. When HCPs base risk discussions on identity, stereotypes are very present and misinformation is more likely. These people's identities were assumed to give information about their sexual behaviour, rather than the HCPS asking about their actual behaviours. The couples' priorities were about starting a family, and that was the conversation they wanted to have.

Gaps in information may also occur on an individual level, as LGBTQ+ people may choose to selectively disclose their history. This can be because of previous poor experiences (this couple were perhaps less likely to disclose their identities in future), internalised homo/transphobia, a desire to help HCPs by making themselves fit into the expected boxes, or a desire to not be a source of gossip. As a result, HCPs may be treating LGBTQ+ people whilst believing they are treating cisheterosexual people. In turn this leads to some HCPs believing they have no LGBTQ+ clients.

Health care systems

Gaps in education and information are not the only factors at play. The systems that HCPs work within shape the possibilities they consider. If data collection systems only allow "man/woman" and conflates sex with gender to make cisnormative assumptions, then an HCP who spends all day putting information into this system will think in the same binary and cisnormative way. I am an LGBTQ+ person and a vocal advocate for changing cis and heteronormative practices, but I have still had to work hard in my clinical practice as a midwife to not refer to all those I care for as women.

In wider society, stereotypes about LGBTQ+ sexual behaviour abound. Gay and bisexual men are often stereotyped as promiscuous, whilst sex between two cis women may be fetishised, as well as being perceived as being less significant than penis-in-vagina sex, more like "a kiss and a cuddle" rather than a full, healthy sex life. This can lead to a perception that lesbian women have no sexual health or contraceptive needs. Bisexual women may be assumed to be heterosexual if they have a visible cis opposite sex partner, with their identity hidden and invalidated, leading to their sexual health needs relating to sex they have with women being invisibilised and ignored.

WAY FORWARD

The World Health Organisation states that

> "Reproductive and sexual healthcare as a human right"
>
> (page 12, 1.1)[55]

Furthermore, they say that sexual health and reproductive health are closely linked. In recognition of this, amongst their sustainable development goals, the United Nations have set

> "a specific target to ensure universal access to sexual and reproductive health-care services by 2030"
>
> (target 3.7)[56]

To make this a reality for LGBTQ+ people, we need to change the ways in which contraceptive and sexual health services are delivered to LGBTQ+ people, whether we are aware that they are LGBTQ+ or not.

First, we need to change the information available to HCPs about different kinds of sexual practices amongst LGBTQ+ people, including polyamorous relationships and kink practices. Not only do HCPs need good quality information about what LGBTQ+ people do, they need evidence-based information about the sexual health implications of those practices, which means that research specifically examining transmission risks for LGBTQ+ people is required.

The process of updating the evidence-base about LGBTQ+ sexual health is going to take time, but there are things that can help improve services for LGBTQ+ people in the interim, on a policy level, an organisational level, and an individual practice level.

Policy

A number of specific services and campaigns to address the sexual health needs of LGBTQ+ people already exist. Examples include:

— "Are you ready for your screen test" LGBT Foundation cervical campaign and toolkit to dispel the myths around lesbian and bisexual women and cervical screening https://lgbt.foundation/screening
— CliniQ—a trans led holistic sexual health, mental health and wellbeing service for all trans people, partners, and friends https://cliniq.org.uk/
— 56T at Dean Street—an expert sexual health clinic in London who focus on the needs of the LGBTQI+ community https://www.dean.st/
— Clinic T—a trans and non-binary friendly sexual health and contraception service in Brighton https://brightonsexualhealth.com/service/clinic-t/
— Butterfly—the axess sexual health clinic for trans and non-binary folk https://www.axess.clinic/services/butterfly-clinic/
— Birmingham LGBT—a user-led organisation aimed at improving the health and wellbeing of LGBTQ+ people that includes sexual health services https://blgbt.org/services/sexual-health-services/
— Pitstop clinics—drop-in STI testing and advice for LGBTQ+ people in Woolwich https://metrocharity.org.uk/sexual-health/pitstop-clinics
— LGBT Foundation's "Get tested with us" service—offering free sexual health tests for LGBTQIA+ people and men who have sex with men living in Greater Manchester, aged 18+ https://lgbt.foundation/testing
— "Best for my chest" campaign run by Live Through This—a cancer support and advocacy charity for the LGBTIQ+ community https://livethroughthis.co.uk/bestformychest/
— "Remove the doubt campaign"—an NHS campaign in collaboration with OUTpatients, aimed at giving lesbians, bisexual women, and trans and non-binary people with a cervix the knowledge and confidence to attend cervical screenings https://livethroughthis.co.uk/removethedoubt/

Key learning points from these services include the importance of including LGBTQ+ people in the development of any education, guidance, or policies in a recognised and therefore paid role. National and local guidelines which are easy to use and well publicised, as well as cooperation between different health care settings to ensure policies guidelines and learning are harmonised across the different health care settings. Recording of demographic information about sexual orientation and gender should be consistent and standardised in order to improve future stratified risk-based information available to patients and clinicians.

Specific training for HCPs about how to care for LGBTQ+ people needs to be integral in education and ongoing mandatory training. Additionally, roles which include expertise in LGBTQ+ health issues should be developed within health services. Initially, to meet the current needs of LGBTQ+ people these roles may need to be fulfilled through the commissioning of external "by and for" services due to the dearth of expertise within many health care settings, but with the long-term aim of mainstreaming this expert knowledge to in-house health care services.

The learning from these services can be adapted, and used to create new national or local policies which can drive the improvements in accessibility of services for LGBTQ+ people. It is essential that policy work is accompanied by appropriate training for HCPs already in services, and by organisational changes.

Organisational

Auditing the current accessibility of a service should be undertaken, and should include LGBTQ+ people as part of that evaluation process. Options for this might include carrying out Equality Impact Assessments,[57] conducting "mystery shopper" style research from LGBTQ+ people, or using one of the many toolkits for working through accessibility.[58] When service improvements are identified through one of these processes, they should be implemented. Implementation should be accompanied by a robust training programme. Such training should include good practice examples for HCPs.

Collecting data about sexual orientation and gender is fundamental to knowing who your service users are, and also who is not using your services. Advice should be taken about ways to collect data which do not cause harm to service users, for example by clumsy language (see case study 4).

Continuity of carer has been shown to be beneficial to LGBTQ+ people when accessing contraceptive and sexual health services, as it removes the requirement for them to repeatedly "come out," thus reducing anxiety about encountering homophobia and transphobia. Continuity of carer should be provided to LGBTQ+ people wherever possible.

It is also important to ensure that LGBTQ+ HCPs in contraceptive and sexual health services feel safe at work, and are able to be open about their LGBTQ+ identities. Creating conditions in which LGBTQ+ HCPs are visible will help to (though not ensure) that LGBTQ+ service users are expected within the service and able to be open about their identities.

CASE STUDY 4

A trans man wants to book an appointment online with his local sexual health clinic. The registration form asks for his sex, offering only female and male as options. A box next to this question explains that he must put his sex assigned at birth as that is the medically important information. He knows that ticking a box that states he is female will cause harm to his mental health.

Other alternatives might include asking for gender (man/woman/non-binary/other), and then asking if the person's gender is the same as they were assigned at birth. This would collect better information, and would not compromise transgender people's mental health.

Individual practice

There are many things that individual HCPs can do to improve the services that they provide, regardless of organisational and policy changes. This begins with challenging our own assumptions about gender and sexual orientation, becoming aware that we are offering care to people who we do not know are LGBTQ+.

HCPs are already largely aware of the importance of introducing themselves and of checking the pronunciation of unfamiliar names. Checking pronouns can be incorporated into these practices, and immediately indicates an awareness in the service user that the HCP has some knowledge of LGBTQ+ issues. Ideally, we should then aim to have nuanced and non-judgemental conversations with all service users about the kinds of sex that person is having, and then base our further conversation on that. This requires the HCP to engage in actively listening to patients, mirroring the language they use to describe themselves, their partners and their sexual activities. It can be helpful to seek out good practice examples of both the content of discussions about these subjects, and ways of asking clients for appropriate information, before you need them. When treating transgender people in contraceptive or sexual health services, it is important that you do not automatically treat them as their sex assigned at birth, but also that you also do not medically treat them as a cis person of their acquired gender. Moving away from a binary categorisation can be challenging when organisational systems reinforce this, but is essential if you aim to deliver appropriate care.

Tailoring care to fit the person in front of you rather than using a one-size fits all or crude categorisations is a skill that most HCPs in contraceptive and sexual health services already have, and it is the skill that is fundamental to delivering good quality care to LGBTQ+ people. Improving the care offered to LGBTQ+ patients will improve the care that is offered to cisheterosexual people too, as it relies on caring for the person in front of you rather than an imagined archetype.

Second, when the evidence base for sexual health and contraceptive advice is lacking for LGBTQ+ people, it is important we acknowledge this, and acknowledge that this is unacceptable. Telling service users that we do not have the information they are seeking can be uncomfortable, but if our practice is to remain evidence-based, then it is important that we do so.

Finally, there are practical adaptations that can be made to our practices that may make the delivery of sexual health services more accessible to LGBTQ+ people. These can include offering a smaller speculum, offering the option of the person inserting the speculum themselves, and the option of rectal ultrasound scanning where transvaginal ultrasound is unacceptable. New research looking at options such as analysis of urinary samples for HPV presence and self-sampling (where the patient is follows instructions to swab their own vaginas) may also indicate other adaptations.[59] Even if the person does not accept one of these adaptations, the effort and consideration from the HCP serves as a demonstration of a genuinely more inclusive service, which in itself has a positive effect on the health care experience.

REFERENCES

1. Mann S. A Health-Care Model of Emotional Labour: An Evaluation of the Literature and Development of a Model. *Journal of Health Organization and Management*. 2005;19(4): 304–317.
2. Hunter B, Deery R. *Emotions in Midwifery and Reproduction*. Palgrave Macmillan; 2009.
3. Gooch B, Bachmann CL. *LGBT in Britain: Health Report*. Stonewall; 2017:21. Accessed September 13, 2023. https://www.stonewall.org.uk/system/files/lgbt_in_britain_health.pdf
4. LGBT Foundation. *Beyond Babies and Breast Cancer: Expanding Our Understanding of Women's Health Needs*. LGBT Foundation; 2013:52. Accessed September 13, 2023. https://s3-eu-west-1.amazonaws.com/lgbt-website-media/Files/4d02f34a-74f5-47da-b11a-b78f57b6ee2c/Beyond%2520Babies%2520and%2520Breast%2520Cancer.pdf
5. Berner AM, Connolly DJ, Pinnell I, et al. Attitudes of Transgender Men and Non-Binary People to Cervical Screening: A Cross-Sectional Mixed-Methods Study in the UK. *Br J Gen Pract*. 2021;71(709):e614–e625. doi:10.3399/BJGP.2020.0905
6. Wright S. Second National Survey of Violence & Discrimination against Sexual Minorities. *National Coalition for Sexual Freedom*. Published online 2008. Accessed September 13, 2023. https://evolvingyourman.com/wp-content/uploads/2020/09/2008_bdsm_survey_analysis_final.pdf
7. Jina R, Thomas LS. Health Consequences of Sexual Violence against Women. *Best Practice & Research Clinical Obstetrics & Gynaecology*. 2013;27(1):15–26. doi:10.1016/j.bpobgyn.2012.08.012

8. Flanders CE, Anderson RE, Tarasoff LA, Robinson M. Bisexual Stigma, Sexual Violence, and Sexual Health Among Bisexual and Other Plurisexual Women: A Cross-Sectional Survey Study. *The Journal of Sex Research*. 2019;56(9):1115–1127. doi:10.1080/00224499.2018. 1563042

9. LGBT Foundation. *It's a Question of Sex*. LGBT Foundation; 2020:36. Accessed September 13, 2023. https://dxfy8lrzbpywr.cloudfront.net/Files/ffccfbf7-6dfa-4115-933d-d666d9a13fee/It%27s%2520A%2520Question%2520of%2520Sex%2520Community%2520Report.pdf

10. Light B, Ormandy R. *Lesbian, Gay & Bisexual Women in the North West: A Multi-Method Study of Cervical Screening Attitudes, Experiences and Uptake*. University of Salford; 2011.

11. Bellwether M, ed. *Fucking Trans Women: A Zine about the Sex Lives of Trans Women*. CreateSpace Independent Publishing Platform; 2013.

12. Addington D. *A Hand in the Bush: The Fine Art of Vaginal Fisting*. Greenery Press; 1997.

13. Sevelius J. "There's No Pamphlet for the Kind of Sex I Have": HIV-Related Risk Factors and Protective Behaviors Among Transgender Men Who Have Sex With Nontransgender Men. *Journal of the Association of Nurses in AIDS Care*. 2009;20(5):398–410. doi:10.1016/j.jana.2009.06.001

14. Sbragia JD, Vottero B. Experiences of Transgender Men in Seeking Gynecological and Reproductive Health Care: A Qualitative Systematic Review. *JBI Evidence Synthesis*. 2020; 18(9):1870–1931. doi:10.11124/JBISRIR-D-19-00347

15. Connolly D, Hughes X, Berner A. Barriers and Facilitators to Cervical Cancer Screening Among Transgender Men and Non-Binary People with a Cervix: A Systematic Narrative Review. *Preventive Medicine*. 2020;135:106071. doi:10.1016/j.ypmed.2020.106071

16. UK Government. *National LGBT Survey: Research Report*. Government Equalities Office; 2018.

17. NHS England. Your 6-Week Postnatal Check. Published online April 4, 2023. Accessed September 14, 2023. https://www.nhs.uk/conditions/baby/support-and-services/your-6-week-postnatal-check/

18. Mizielińska J, Stasińska A. Negotiations between Possibilities and Reality: Reproductive Choices of Families of Choice in Poland. *European Journal of Women's Studies*. 2023; 30(2):148–163. doi:10.1177/1350506819887765

19. Lowik A.J. Reproducing Eugenics, Reproducing while Trans: The State Sterilization of Trans People. *Journal of GLBT Family Studies*. 2018;14(5):425–445. doi:10.1080/1550428X.2017. 1393361

20. Hodson K, Meads C, Bewley S. Lesbian and Bisexual Women's Likelihood of Becoming Pregnant: A Systematic Review and Meta-Analysis. *BJOG*. 2017;124(3):393–402. doi:10.1111/1471-0528.14449

21. Baiocco R, Laghi F. Sexual Orientation and the Desires and Intentions to Become Parents. *Journal of Family Studies*. 2013;19(1):90–98. doi:10.5172/jfs.2013.19.1.90

22. Costa PA, Bidell M. Modern Families: Parenting Desire, Intention, and Experience Among Portuguese Lesbian, Gay, and Bisexual Individuals. *Journal of Family Issues*. 2017;38(4): 500–521. doi:10.1177/0192513X16683985

23. Gato J, Leal D, Tasker F. Parenting Desires, Parenting Intentions, and Anticipation of Stigma Upon Parenthood Among Lesbian, Bisexual, and Heterosexual Women in Portugal. *Journal of Lesbian Studies*. 2019;23(4):451–463. doi:10.1080/10894160.2019.1621733

24. Kranz D, Busch H, Niepel C. Desires and Intentions for Fatherhood: A Comparison of Childless Gay and Heterosexual Men in Germany. *Journal of Family Psychology*. 2018;32(8): 995–1004. doi:10.1037/fam0000439

25. Leal D, Gato J, Tasker F. Prospective Parenting: Sexual Identity and Intercultural Trajectories. *Culture, Health & Sexuality*. 2019;21(7):757–773. doi:10.1080/13691058.2018.1515987

26. Riskind RG, Patterson CJ. Parenting Intentions and Desires Among Childless Lesbian, Gay, and Heterosexual Individuals. *Journal of Family Psychology*. 2010;24(1):78–81. doi:10.1037/a0017941

27. Shenkman G. The Gap between Fatherhood and Couplehood Desires Among Israeli Gay Men and Estimations of their Likelihood. *Journal of Family Psychology*. 2012;26(5):828–832. doi:10.1037/a0029471

28. Shenkman G. Anticipation of Stigma upon Parenthood Impacts Parenting Aspirations in the LGB Community in Israel. *Sex Res Soc Policy*. 2021;18(3):753–764. doi:10.1007/s13178-020-00498-y

29. Shenkman G, Bos H, Kogan S. Attachment Avoidance and Parenthood Desires in Gay Men and Lesbians and their Heterosexual Counterparts. *Journal of Reproductive and Infant Psychology*. 2019;37(4):344–357. doi:10.1080/02646838.2019.1578872

30. Simon KA, Tornello SL, Farr RH, Bos HMW. Envisioning Future Parenthood Among Bisexual, Lesbian, and Heterosexual Women. *Psychology of Sexual Orientation and Gender Diversity*. 2018;5(2):253–259. doi:10.1037/sgd0000267

31. Tate DP, Patterson CJ. Desire for Parenthood in Context of Other Life Aspirations Among Lesbian, Gay, and Heterosexual Young Adults. *Front Psychol*. 2019;10:2679. doi:10.3389/fpsyg.2019.02679

32. Wang J, Zheng L. Parenting Desire Among Childless Lesbian and Gay Individuals in China: The Influence of Traditional Family Values, Minority Stress, and Parenting Motivation. *Journal of Family Issues*. 2022;43(9):2438–2455. doi:10.1177/0192513X211030921

33. Fix L, Durden M, Obedin-Maliver J, et al. Stakeholder Perceptions and Experiences Regarding Access to Contraception and Abortion for Transgender, Non-Binary, and Gender-Expansive Individuals Assigned Female at Birth in the U.S. *Arch Sex Behav*. 2020;49(7):2683–2702. doi:10.1007/s10508-020-01707-w

34. Todd NJ. At Risk of Pregnancy? Contraception for Transgender, Nonbinary, Gender-Diverse, and Two Spirit Patients. *BC Medical Journal*. 2022;62(4):69–74. Accessed September 14, 2023. https://bcmj.org/articles/risk-pregnancy-contraception-transgender-nonbinary-gender-diverse-and-two-spirit-patients

35. Human Fertilisation and Embryology Authority. Information for Trans and Non-Binary People Seeking Fertility Treatment. Published online 2021. Accessed May 10, 2023. https://www.hfea.gov.uk/treatments/fertility-preservation/information-for-trans-and-non-binary-people-seeking-fertility-treatment/

36. Gomez AM, Đỗ L, Ratliff GA, Crego PI, Hastings J. Contraceptive Beliefs, Needs, and Care Experiences Among Transgender and Nonbinary Young Adults. *Journal of Adolescent Health*. 2020;67(4):597–602. doi:10.1016/j.jadohealth.2020.03.003

37. Mancini I, Alvisi S, Gava G, Seracchioli R, Meriggiola MC. Contraception across Transgender. *Int J Impot Res*. 2021;33(7):710–719. doi:10.1038/s41443-021-00412-z

38. Marschalek J, Pietrowski D, Dekan S, Marschalek ML, Brandstetter M, Ott J. Markers of Vitality in Ovaries of Transmen after Long-Term Androgen Treatment: A Prospective Cohort Study. *Mol Med*. 2020;26(1):83. doi:10.1186/s10020-020-00214-x

39. Yaish I, Tordjman K, Amir H, et al. Functional Ovarian Reserve in Transgender men receiving Testosterone Therapy: Evidence for Preserved Anti-Müllerian Hormone and Antral Follicle Count under Prolonged Treatment. *Human Reproduction*. 2021;36(10):2753–2760. doi:10.1093/humrep/deab169

40. Greenfield M. *LGBTQ+ Mums Research*. Best Beginnings; 2023. doi: 10.5281/zenodo.8326480

41. *WHO Recommendations on Maternal and Newborn Care for a Positive Postnatal Experience*. World Health Organization; 2022.

42. Størksen HT, Garthus-Niegel S, Vangen S, Eberhard-Gran M. The Impact of Previous Birth Experiences on Maternal Fear of Childbirth. *Acta Obstet Gynecol Scand*. 2013;92(3):318–324. doi:10.1111/aogs.12072

43. Youatt EJ, Harris LH, Harper GW, Janz NK, Bauermeister JA. Sexual Health Care Services Among Young Adult Sexual Minority Women. *Sex Res Soc Policy*. 2017;14(3):345–357. doi:10.1007/s13178-017-0277-x

44. Tsevat DG, Wiesenfeld HC, Parks C, Peipert JF. Sexually Transmitted Diseases and Infertility. *American Journal of Obstetrics and Gynecology*. 2017;216(1):1–9. doi:10.1016/j.ajog.2016.08.008

45. Centers for Disease Control and Prevention. *Pelvic Inflammatory Disease (PID)*; 2022. Accessed September 14, 2023. https://www.cdc.gov/std/treatment-guidelines/pid.htm

46. Takemoto MLS, Menezes MDO, Polido CBA, et al. Prevalence of Sexually Transmitted Infections and Bacterial Vaginosis Among Lesbian Women: Systematic Review and Recommendations to Improve Care. *Cad Saúde Pública*. 2019;35(3):e00118118. doi:10.1590/0102-311x00118118

47. Evans AL, Scally AJ, Wellard SJ, Wilson JD. Prevalence of Bacterial Vaginosis in Lesbians and Heterosexual Women in a Community Setting. *Sexually Transmitted Infections*. 2007;83(6):470–475. doi:10.1136/sti.2006.022277

48. Hay P. Bacterial Vaginosis. *Medicine*. 2014;42(7):359–363. doi:10.1016/j.mpmed.2014.04.011

49. Oud MS, Smits RM, Smith HE, et al. A De Novo Paradigm for Male Infertility. *Nat Commun*. 2022;13(1):154. doi:10.1038/s41467-021-27132-8

50. UK Data Service. *Crime Survey for England and Wales 2013–2014: Teaching Dataset*. Accessed September 14, 2023. http://doc.ukdataservice.ac.uk/doc/7911/mrdoc/pdf/7911_csew_2013-14_teaching_dataset_user_guide.pdf

51. Office for National Statistics. *The Odds of Smoking by Sexual Orientation in England, 2016*. Office for National Statistics; 2018. Accessed September 14, 2023. https://www.ons.gov.uk/peoplepopulationandcommunity/healthandsocialcare/healthinequalities/adhocs/009373theoddsofsmokingbysexualorientationinengland2016

52. Bradbury-Jones C, Molloy E, Clark M, Ward N. Gender, Sexual Diversity and Professional Practice Learning: Findings from a Systematic Search and Review. *Studies in Higher Education*. 2020;45(8):1618–1636. doi:10.1080/03075079.2018.1564264

53. Arias T, Greaves B, McArdle J, Rayment H, Walker S. Cultivating Awareness of Sexual and Gender Diversity in a Midwifery Curriculum. *Midwifery*. 2021;101:103050. doi:10.1016/j.midw.2021.103050

54. Brown M, McCann E, McCormick F. *Making the Invisible Visible: The Inclusion of LGBTQ+ Health Needs and Concerns within Nursing and Midwifery Pre-Registration Programmes*. Queen's University Belfast and Trinity College Dublin; 2021. Accessed September 19, 2023. https://www.qub.ac.uk/schools/SchoolofNursingandMidwifery/FileStore/Filetoupload,1222743,en.pdf

55. World Health Organization. *Selected Practice Recommendations for Contraceptive Use*. 3rd ed. World Health Organization; 2016. Accessed September 19, 2023. https://apps.who.int/iris/handle/10665/252267

56. World Health Organization, UNDP/UNFPA/UNICEF/WHO/World Bank Special Programme of Research Development and Research Training in Human Reproduction (HRP). *Sexual Health and Its Linkages to Reproductive Health: An Operational Approach*. World Health Organization; 2017. Accessed September 19, 2023. https://apps.who.int/iris/handle/10665/258738

57. Equality and Human Rights Commission. *Equality Impact Assessments*; 2017. Accessed September 19, 2023. https://www.equalityhumanrights.com/en/advice-and-guidance/equality-impact-assessments

58. Darwin Z, Greenfield M. Diversity of Family Formation: LGBTQ+ Parents. In: Borg Xuereb R, Jomeen J, eds. *Perspectives on Midwifery and Parenthood*. Springer International Publishing; 2022:163–179. doi:10.1007/978-3-031-17285-4_13

59. Thorpe E. ACES (Alternative Cervical Screening): Acceptability of a Urine Self-Test for Cervical Screening in the LGBTQ+ Population. Manchester Cancer Research Centre. Published n.d. https://www.mcrc.manchester.ac.uk/aces-alternative-cervical-screening-acceptability-of-a-urine-self-test-for-cervical-screening-in-the-lgbtq-population/

Chapter 2

LGBTQ+ fertility and conception

Susie Bower-Brown and Sophie Zadeh

INTRODUCTION

Although rates of adoption are overall higher in LGBTQ+ populations than non-LGBTQ+ populations,[1] many LGBTQ+ individuals wish to pursue parenthood through gestation. The reasons for this may be numerous, ranging, for example, from the anticipation of structural barriers in access to adoption services,[2, 3] to a preference for biologically related children.[4] Among those pursuing parenthood through birth, some will not need or want to access fertility services. For example, cis bisexual parents in a different-gender relationship, or those in relationships in which one or more partners are TNB, may not require the use of fertility treatment involving donor gametes and/or surrogacy. Other prospective parents, such as single parents and cis men/cis women couples, do require the use of donor gametes or a surrogate. Such journeys to parenthood may still take place entirely outside of the clinical context for a range of reasons, such as wanting more choice or information about the donor than is permitted by legislation[5, 6] and due to the high financial cost of conception within a fertility clinic.

This chapter focuses on LGBTQ+ prospective parents who either require or prefer to access fertility services to conceive, a population that is increasing in the UK year on year.[7, 8] It will highlight the structural and interpersonal barriers that impact LGBTQ+ prospective parents' access to fertility treatment, before focusing on the experiences of LGBTQ+ individuals who have used fertility services, including experiences of decision-making about fertility and conception and experiences of fertility treatment and clinical care. We will provide examples of positive and negative experiences of reproductive care from our research with TNB parents, and outline their recommendations for practice. Our discussion is primarily focussed on experiences with UK fertility services, but where relevant, prospective parents' experiences in other contexts are also highlighted.

DOI: 10.4324/9781003305446-3

FERTILITY, CONCEPTION, AND MINORITY STRESS

In order to contextualise the material we present in this chapter, we begin by briefly outlining the minority stress model, which is described in further detail in Chapter 13. Research has consistently identified worse mental health outcomes within LGBTQ+ populations than non-LGBTQ+ populations.[9] This association is theorised within the minority stress model[10] which explains the relationship between stigma, discrimination, stress, and health outcomes within LGB populations. The model suggests that stigma leads to stress, which in turn leads to negative health outcomes. In support of this model, research has consistently found associations between stigma and mental and physical health.[11] The model distinguishes between different types of stigma, referred to as "distal" and "proximal" stressors, respectively. Distal stressors refer to external prejudice events (including discrimination and violence) and proximal stressors refer to internal stigma processes (including expectations of rejection, concealment, and internalised stigma). The model highlights the importance of coping and social support (at both individual and community levels), as these can moderate the link between stressors and adverse outcomes. The model has since been extended to TNB populations, referring more specifically to "gender minority stress".[12]

As the chapter progresses, the relevance of the model to LGBTQ+ prospective parents' experiences of fertility treatment – which can include numerous challenges, and varying levels of support – will become clear. We turn first to barriers to treatment.

BARRIERS TO TREATMENT

In 2008, the UK's Human Fertilisation and Embryology (HFE) Act was amended to reflect the fact that clinical considerations about a "child's need for a father" in deciding whom to offer fertility treatment were misaligned with empirical evidence, which has consistently shown the number or gender of parents to be less relevant for children's psychological, social and emotional adjustment than are high quality parenting and positive parent-child relationships.[13-15] Changes to the HFE Act in 2008 also enabled both members of cis women couples to be registered on their child's birth certificate; the process for cis men couples who had used surrogacy remained lengthier, requiring a parental order. This was because under UK law, the person who gives birth to a child was – and today remains – recognised as their "mother".[16]

Under the 2008 legislation, access to surrogacy by single LGBTQ+ people remained complex, requiring them to obtain a parental order to become the legal parent of a child born through surrogacy. The HFE Act 2008 (Remedial) Order 2018 brought the experiences of single people using surrogacy in the UK in line with cis men couples who become parents through this means. However, legislation in the UK remains obstructive to TNB parents, particularly among those who have given birth, who are not always able to be listed using the appropriate parental designation on their child's birth certificate, irrespective of whether they have a Gender Recognition Certificate[17] (eg, the case of trans father Freddy McConnell). Current UK legislation also fails to accommodate families in which there are more than two parents, such as polyamorous parenting families and families with co-parenting arrangements. It is also worth remembering that legislation in other jurisdictions may shape the experiences of LGBTQ+ parents in the UK, particularly in cases of cross-border reproductive care. For example, agreements with donors and surrogates that are legally recognised in the UK may not be recognised elsewhere, with potential consequences for the legal status of children born overseas.[18, 19]

Although UK legislation permits access to fertility treatment for LGBTQ+ prospective parents in principle, the legal complexities that may accompany the path to parenthood for LGBTQ+ individuals are vast. Empirical evidence has also shown that interpretations of the law by practitioners are not always accurate, and that discrimination within fertility services may mean that treatment that is permitted by law is not always accessible to LGBTQ+ prospective parents. For example, welfare of the child assessments conducted by clinical staff and allocation of the limited government funds for treatment remain underpinned by normative assumptions about parenting in different family types. [19, 20] In terms of the former, our research has shown that the mandatory counselling for those seeking fertility treatment with donor gametes may result in discrimination against TNB parents and denial of access to services[3] (Table 2.1). In terms of the latter, although LGBTQ+ individuals of all incomes report similar levels of desire for parenthood,[22] access to fertility treatment that is funded by the UK's National Health Service (NHS) by LGBTQ+ prospective parents varies by nation, with 11% of IVF cycles for cis women couples being funded in England, compared to 40% in Scotland and 21% in Wales.[7] This "postcode lottery" of treatment funding has been identified as a barrier for many LGBTQ+ prospective parents.[23]

The Government's 2016 Report on Transgender Equality identified that public service provision for TNB people is characterised by widespread transphobia, and that the NHS is "letting down trans people".[24(pp.3)] In terms of fertility services specifically, TNB prospective parents clearly face several additional barriers to treatment when compared to cis LGBTQ+ parents. For instance, there are currently

Table 2.1 Negative experiences of fertility services reported by trans and/or non-binary (TNB) parents

Negative experiences of fertility services	Example quotation from TNB parents
Distal stressors	
Denial of care	The first clinic we went to rejected us for what we considered to be spurious grounds…We felt it was a little bit eugenic to be honest. (trans woman)[1]
Cisgendered language	Nothing was gender neutral, none of the language. Everything assumed that the mum was having a baby with a man. (non-binary person)
Clinicians' lack of knowledge	The language they used [at the clinic] was a bit clumsy or a bit invasive…sort of straight people trying their best but not quite getting it. (non-binary woman)
Inappropriate paperwork	We had to ask [the fertility clinic] to change some of their forms actually because on their forms the sperm donor form to fill in is has father's signature on it…to this day I don't know if they did. (trans woman)
Unfriendliness towards TNB patients	I did speak to a private fertility clinic to see about sperm storage, but I was incredibly anxious and I rang up and the woman on the phone…said "oh, unless its through the NHS we can't help you" and just really upset me and so I never considered it again. (trans woman)
Exclusion of non-birth parents	You end up feeling useless and just excluded from spaces that you want to be included in. (trans woman)
Proximal stressors	
Avoiding clinics due to discrimination	We tried to have IVF, and the NHS told us "go practice for another month and tell us how you get on". The then ex-husband has no penis so we can try for a month of Sundays and get nowhere…We [decided to] do home insemination and cut out the NHS and the medical side of things. (genderfluid person)
Identity concealment	Because we'd had a bad experience, we then censored ourselves a little bit [in IVF counselling], we treated it as "no, this is a test we have to pass" rather than a counselling that we benefited from. (trans woman)
Fear of discrimination	If I went through the adoption route or surrogacy, I would be subjecting myself to systems that weren't designed for me, and would potentially be quite scary and unpredictable and might just reject me outright. (trans man)

Participants' gender identities are included after each quotation in Tables 2.1, 2.3, and 2.4, as they described them themselves.

no national guidelines on gamete freezing/storage provision for TNB people,[25] meaning that gamete freezing represents an additional financial barrier for many TNB individuals.[26] Relatedly, TNB people are often not given appropriate information about fertility preservation if they pursue a medical transition.[27] Toze describes that hysterectomies have been regularly recommended for trans men on medical grounds, despite limited evidence of their efficacy, thus limiting the possibility for trans men to later pursue pregnancy.[28] In general, research has identified a lack of information amongst both clinicians and the TNB community about reproduction and contraception.[29] TNB people assigned female at birth may rely on testosterone as a contraceptive,[30] resulting in unplanned pregnancies.[31] This evidence overall highlights the importance of providing accurate information about reproduction and contraception.

Such findings are also reflective of a broader lack of knowledge about TNB health amongst health care professionals.[32] An Australian survey found the number of TNB individuals who had been offered fertility counselling before their medical transition and who had frozen their gametes remained very low, despite an overwhelming consensus that this should be available freely.[33] For some TNB individuals, the lack of education about, and financial barriers to, gamete preservation may limit their opportunities for becoming a parent before they even start their journey to parenthood.[26, 34]

The barriers identified thus far (ie, restrictive legislation, lack of education, denial of services, and financial barriers) can be seen as "distal stressors" or "distal barriers" when viewing experiences through the minority stress lens. Several "proximal barriers" for LGBTQ+ parents can also be identified; in other words, anticipated stigma may limit the extent to which LGBTQ+ individuals can imagine, and thus pursue, parenthood. For instance, quantitative studies have found that desire for parenting is negatively associated with distal stressors (ie, experiences of stigma, prejudice, discrimination) among lesbian populations.[i,35,36] These same studies also found that the desire for parenting is associated with internalised stigma, a proximal stressor, highlighting that both factors are relevant. Among TNB populations, some trans men and women see their gender as a barrier to becoming a parent,[37] with cisnormative understandings of parenthood in society having been shown to limit opportunities for TNB individuals to imagine themselves as parents.[38] Moreover, TNB adults perceive fertility clinics to be unwelcoming spaces,[34] and fear of discrimination in fertility clinics may dissuade TNB parents from pursuing parenthood via a clinic.[39] We will further explore these distal and proximal stressors throughout the rest of the chapter as we turn to discuss LGBTQ+ parents' decision-making about, and experiences of, fertility treatment.

DECISION-MAKING AROUND FERTILITY AND CONCEPTION

After having decided to pursue gestational parenthood, LGBTQ+ individuals face many complex decisions about their route to parenthood.[40] These decisions range from whether to conceive within a clinic or not, which treatment route to take, and, if using donor gametes, which type of donor to use, and where to access gametes for conception. Many LGBTQ+ families will have more than one prospective parent with the same reproductive capacity (ie, two potential gestational parents or two potential sperm providers), and choices must be made about which parent will be biologically related to their child. Numerous factors, which we outline below, have been found to influence all of these decisions.

Many LGBTQ+ prospective parents will have to decide between different routes to parenthood and, as previously discussed, the specific pathway to parenthood pursued depends not only on individual choices, but also on biological, social, financial, and legal constraints.[41] Several studies have found that, somewhat paradoxically, complex fertility treatments may be seen as the easiest route to parenthood,[2, 3] in many cases due to fear of discrimination in the adoption system.[42] Research suggests that this fear may be especially pronounced for cis men, due to gender discrimination in adoption services.[43] Research with lesbian, bisexual and queer (LBQ) parents in Australia has shown that the most common reason for conceiving via a fertility clinic is to ensure legal recognition of parenting relationships,[44] demonstrating that clinical conception may be protective for those LBGTQ+ parents who are able to access it.

Technological developments and changes in social policy have resulted in an increasing range of advanced fertility treatments for LGBTQ+ parents. [45] One novel route to parenthood that is growing in popularity and visibility is reciprocal IVF (also called shared biological motherhood).[46] This route to parenthood allows couples with two potential birth parents to "share" biological parenthood: one partner's egg is extracted, and the other partner carries this egg; resultantly, each parent has either a genetic or gestational link to the child. Reciprocal IVF can be used as an example to provide insight into the many factors which impact decision making around parenthood. For instance, some LGBTQ+ parents choose reciprocal IVF due to medical reasons (such as the gestational parent having a low egg count), but most couples choose reciprocal IVF for non-medical reasons.[47] Couples who choose reciprocal IVF for non-medical reasons must balance the increased medical risks involved in having both parents as medical patients, with the perceived benefits of having respective gestational and genetic connections with the child.[48] One recent

UK study, to which one of us (SBB) contributed, explored experiences of cis women within two-mother families, and their reasons for choosing reciprocal IVF over other treatment routes. Mothers reported choosing reciprocal IVF so that they could both be seen as "legitimate" parents, to share the journey of motherhood with their partner, and to build strong bonds within their family. [49] Examples of these reasons, taken from Shaw et al.'s study,[49] can be seen in Table 2.2. Notably, mothers' expectations of reciprocal IVF (eg, that it would prevent jealousy between mothers) were not always borne out in reality, demonstrating the importance of longitudinal research on LGBTQ+ families formed by assisted reproduction.

Table 2.2 Two-mother families' reasons for using reciprocal IVF

Motivations to use reciprocal IVF	Example quotations
Becoming mums together	We both had to do injections, we both had to do scans, it was very much like we were in this together and it felt like we were making a baby. 'Cos obviously you wish every day that you could just go upstairs, have sex and fall pregnant, but it's really not that fun at all. (gestational mother)
Legitimacy: "Who's the real mum?"	We are parents because I gave birth, and it's [partner's] DNA. So, no one in the world can doubt that we are both parents. (gestational mother)
Choices and constraints	When we were having to pay that amount of money, we wanted the most success. (gestational mother) My age meant that I would be more likely to provide more eggs, and her womb was in a better condition than mine. So it kind of dictated which way round we did it. (genetic mother)
Biological connections strengthen family connections	If you had your own genetic baby there could be room to feel jealous or some sort of partition in your family like that and I think having each other's eggs completely negates that because, because he's part of her. (genetic mother)

Note: These findings come from a thematic analysis of interview data from 28 mothers in two-mother families conceived via reciprocal IVF. These findings are published in the following paper, which is available open access. This project[49] was funded by the ESRC: Shaw K, Bower-Brown S, McConnachie A, Jadva V, Ahuja K, Macklon N, Golombok S. "Her Bun in My Oven": Motivations and Experiences of Two-Mother Families who have Used Reciprocal IVF. *Family Relations*. 2023;72(1):195–214. https://doi.org/10.1111/fare.12805.

Although reciprocal IVF offers couples the opportunity for both members of a couple to be involved in the clinical route to parenthood, many LGBTQ+ families must make the choice around who will undertake which aspect of the process. Research has explored the factors related to decision making about gestational parenthood and these include fear of childbirth, differing parental desire for genetic relatedness and parental gender identity/expression.[50] Importantly, parental experiences of gender may impact decision-making around gestational parenthood among cis women, trans men and non-binary people alike.[50–52] Such findings highlight that societal assumptions about gender and pregnancy are not only cisnormative, but also gender normative, in that pregnancy is assumed to be not just for women but specifically for feminine women.[53]

However, TNB potential parents may also have to consider additional factors in decision-making when compared to cis women, and research has highlighted that balancing transition goals (ie, beginning/continuing to take testosterone) and reproductive goals (ie, pursuing pregnancy) can be challenging for TNB birth parents.[34, 51, 52] Notably, a recent case report highlighted that reciprocal IVF may be a particularly effective route to parenthood for some trans men/non-binary people partnered with cis women; a trans man's egg was extracted and his partner (a cis woman) carried the pregnancy.[54] Importantly, this allowed for the trans man to continue to use testosterone throughout the pregnancy, demonstrating that recent technological advancements may allow TNB parents to conceive in ways that align with both their transition goals and reproductive goals.

In couples with two individuals who could potentially carry a pregnancy, research has found that many couples may swap the person who is pregnant if having more than one child.[49, 55] Similar findings are echoed with cis men couples conceiving via surrogacy, with one survey finding that most couples create embryos with both partners' sperm, and choose one partner's embryo for their first child, keeping the other partner's in case of a second child.[56] One study of cis men couples using surrogacy found that most couples chose to transfer two embryos, despite increased medical risks, and this was related to the costs involved and the desire to conceive twins.[57] More research is needed on the factors influencing decision-making around sperm provision in LGBTQ+ parent families.

A key reason for LGBTQ+ parents to use a fertility clinic is due to the need for donor gametes. LBQ women have identified a number of benefits associated with accessing donor gametes through fertility clinics, including that sperm is screened for infections, that it may be more successful than self-insemination or conception via intercourse, and that it ensures the child would be able to identify their donor in the future.[44] In terms of choosing donor sperm, many LGBTQ+ families have been found to pick a sperm donor with the same characteristics as the non-genetically related parent,[58] a process referred to as "donor matching". Additionally, cis LBQ mothers have been found to often choose the same donor if they have multiple children, with the hope of strengthening connections between siblings.[58] Although research on this topic has primarily focussed on cis women's use of donor sperm, studies of cis men who have conceived via surrogacy have found that they tend to minimise the genetic contribution of the egg donor, by depersonalising the donor and separating the donation from the person.[59]

Some LGBTQ+ parents may also become donors themselves on the journey to parenthood. For example, cis women in same-gender couples are much more likely to use egg sharing programmes than heterosexual women;[7] in these schemes, patients can donate their eggs to other patients so as to reduce their cost of treatment. The discrepancy in egg sharing between heterosexual women and LGBTQ+ parents may be related to the lack of NHS funding for LGBTQ+ fertility treatment, but more research is necessary to ascertain whether this is the case.

In 2005, legislation was introduced in the UK which removed donor anonymity; subsequently, all children conceived via fertility clinics in the UK after 1 April 2005 will be able to access the donor's identifying information when they turn 18. Although distinctions between anonymous, known and identifiable donation remain relevant within the context of fertility clinics, it is becoming increasingly common for LGBTQ+ parents to seek a co-parent or sperm donor online[5] and in online settings, distinctions between different types of donor are less clear.[60] One study of women who had searched for a sperm donor online found that they reported several advantages, including detailed donor information, having the opportunity to meet the donor, and reduced financial costs.[61] However, disadvantages included the absence of health screening and "dishonest donors" (ie, men whose motivations were unclear or who were looking for sex). TNB people have also been found to access donor sperm outside of a clinic and undergo insemination at home.[39] For some parents this may be a deliberate choice (eg, so their child can have contact with their donor) whereas for others, this may be due to the prohibitively high costs involved in clinical conception and fears of discrimination from fertility clinics.[3, 39]

EXPERIENCES OF FERTILITY TREATMENT AND CLINICAL CARE

We now turn to the research that has explored LGBTQ+ parents' experiences of accessing fertility treatment. After overcoming many barriers and making multiple, often complex, decisions about treatment, LGBTQ+ parents come into contact with a number of health care providers and professionals. Although experiences are mixed, fertility clinics are generally not designed to cater to LGBTQ+ bodies, identities and families.[62] Providers have been found to rely on cisheteronormative assumptions and lack training and awareness of issues pertaining to LGBTQ+ fertility and family formation.[3, 39, 62–65] Distinctions have been made between experiences at structural and interpersonal levels, with lesbian non-gestational mothers reporting exclusion by service structures but inclusion by health care staff.[66] One study analysed the LGBT content of fertility clinic websites in the US, finding that whilst just over half contained LGBT content, the most mentioned terms were "lesbian", "LGBT", and "gay".[67] Websites infrequently used the terms "trans" and "bisexual", demonstrating a lack of consideration of the specific needs of bisexual and trans parents. We will now outline the research on the experiences of these different groups of LGBTQ+ parents.

Studies of cis women have shown that they lack support when accessing fertility treatment, as well as experiencing inappropriate mandatory processes designed for heterosexual parents, such as fertility counselling.[64] Research in Scotland with LGB women found that their sexual orientation affected their experience of fertility treatment, with participants reporting that they were asked intrusive questions about their sexual history and their future child's lack of a father.[68] Several participants reported receiving higher quality care in private fertility clinics than in the NHS – indeed, among those responding to the UK Government's National LGBT Survey, spontaneous reports of negative experiences of care and informal discrimination in the NHS were common.[69] Such findings highlight that an individual's income may affect the quality of care that they receive. Lesbian mother families have also been found to minimise experiences of stigma from health care providers in fertility clinics,[70] suggesting that discrimination may be more widespread than is immediately evident.

TNB parents' experiences within clinics have generally been found to be negative, and generally these experiences are related to cisnormative assumptions about bodies, ie, that women are pregnant and that men provide sperm.[71] Across several studies, identified experiences include encountering inappropriate paperwork, having to accept suboptimal treatment, and being denied fertility treatment due to transphobia.[3, 39, 65] Importantly, research with TNB pregnant parents has reported that conception outside of a clinical setting is positive and straightforward,[39, 51] demonstrating that TNB conception does not need to be a negative experience. Taken together, these findings evidence the need to improve fertility services for TNB individuals, and to ensure inclusivity and sensitivity in treatment provision overall.[72, 73] Although less commonly identified, positive experiences with clinicians include proper pronoun/name use, familiarity with gender diversity, and warmth towards TNB individuals.[51, 65, 74]

Most research has focused on distal stressors (ie, experiences of discrimination and stigma), but there is some research that has identified LGBTQ+ parents' experiences of proximal stressors within the clinical context. One example is the finding that some cis women conceal their sexual orientation by bringing a male friend along to the fertility clinic.[75] TNB prospective parents also report concerns about confidentiality when pursuing gamete freezing,[76] highlighting the importance of understanding how fear of discrimination impacts LGBTQ+ individuals' access to fertility services. Our research on TNB parents in the UK explored parents' strategies of navigating discrimination, finding that parents used both pioneering and pragmatic strategies, meaning that in some cases parents asserted their identities and aimed to change spaces to be more inclusive, while in others they concealed their identities to avoid discrimination.[3]

More research on parents' experiences of proximal stressors is, however, needed. The experiences of some groups also remain understudied. Research has primarily focussed on the experiences of gestational parents, but research has reported feelings of exclusion among cis and trans non-gestational mothers on the journey to parenthood.[49, 71, 77] Less research has been conducted on LGBTQ+ parents' experiences of surrogacy than their experiences of IVF or donor insemination. Cis gay men who have pursued surrogacy report a lack of knowledge from fertility clinics and hospitals, about both LGBTQ+ parenthood and surrogacy itself.[63] There is also a dearth of research on the fertility and conception experiences of bisexual parents. Given that bisexual mothers have been found to have poorer mental health than lesbian mothers during the perinatal period, and report feelings of invisibility and exclusion,[78] it seems particularly important to further research their experiences.

Most research on LGBTQ+ parents and prospective parents has focussed on white, middle class, cis women in two-mother families. It has thus been suggested that it is important for researchers to look at LGBTQ+ parents' experiences through an intersectional lens.[79] Our research on TNB parents took an intersectional approach,[3] and we found that parents who were facing multiple oppressions (ie, racism, ableism, classism) and who differed furthest from others' expectations of a "good" parent (ie, in terms of parental age and family set-up) had the most negative experiences. Other research with single fathers who became parents through surrogacy has found that they face "multiple marginalities" of being single, male, and gay.[19, 20] Several unique barriers to fertility care for ethnic minority groups have been identified,[81] and in general, IVF birth rates are lower for Black and Asian patients in the UK.[82] Taken together, these findings reinforce the value of understanding LGBTQ+ parents' experiences intersectionally, and point to a need for further research.

EXAMPLES OF POSITIVE AND NEGATIVE EXPERIENCES

In Tables 2.1 and 2.3, we have included some examples of positive and negative perinatal experiences from TNB parents in the UK. These quotations come from our research, which consisted of an interview study, funded by the Wellcome Trust, with 13 TNB parents. The findings have also been published in two academic articles which can be accessed online, cost-free.[3, 71] Overall, participants reported more negative experiences than positive experiences, and reported experiencing both distal and proximal stressors. In terms of positive experiences, participants reported that some clinicians were inclusive, responsive, and knowledgeable. The parents within the study were also asked about their recommendations for improving reproductive care for TNB parents (see Table 2.4). Some of these recommendations are specific to TNB populations, whereas others, such as the importance of inclusive language, staff education, and equitable access to treatment, are relevant to the LGBTQ+ population more generally.

Table 2.3 Positive experiences reported by trans and/or non-binary (TNB) parents

Positive experiences of fertility services	Example quotation from TNB parents
Correct pronoun use	People in hospital were so cool and I didn't even get misgendered once. (trans man)
Attempts at inclusiveness	They were obviously trying to openly be like "oh yeah we support LGBT parents" but I think a lot of cases people will say LGBT but they forget what the T is…but like I said, I felt like they were making an effort and I felt like they weren't being bigoted. (non-binary woman)
Inclusive systems	I wasn't the first trans man to give birth in this hospital trust area, so they had actually already changed the IT systems. (trans man)
Responsiveness	[We said] we only wanted them to ask questions about us being trans if they were directly related…they were very understanding. She said, if I say anything inappropriate "just kick me" (trans woman)
Clinician knowledge of TNB health	The fertility clinic I went to…they were totally unphased by it. They were just like "yeah, we just need your hormone levels to come back at this and then everything's fine". (trans man)

Table 2.4 Trans and/or non-binary (TNB) parents' recommendations for inclusive practice

TNB parents' practice recommendations	Example quotation from TNB parents
Awareness of gender diversity	It would have just been nice if the NHS had recognised that there's more than two gender identities. (genderfluid person)
Evidence informed practice	There could be a maternity service conceived and developed with [the gender clinic]…it could provide a blueprint for sections or protocols at least to use in mainstream maternity clinics. (neither gender person)
Inclusive language	A basic understanding of inclusive language is a thing that would really benefit trans people within the NHS. (non-binary person)
Staff education	I think [fertility clinics] probably need to send their nurses on training courses, I would say. (trans woman)
Gender neutral spaces	Making the spaces inclusive to everyone…you can be supportive of people giving birth without making everything woman focussed. (trans woman)
Improved access to NHS funded treatment	Access to fertility care needs to be trans inclusive. I think the criteria at the moment for getting it on the NHS is quite rigid and doesn't really fit if you're not in a heterosexual couple…and if you're not cis. (trans man)
Improved access to gamete storage	I think sperm storage should be a basic part of care, similarly egg storage if requested for trans men. (trans woman)

CONCLUSION

In this chapter, we have outlined LGBTQ+ individuals' experiences of fertility and conception, including barriers to treatment, factors influencing decision-making, and experiences of accessing fertility care. LGBTQ+ parents clearly undergo complex decision-making processes when considering their route to parenthood, and whilst access to assisted reproduction for LGBTQ+ populations has never been higher, the legal, social, biological, and financial barriers outlined in this chapter mean that many LGBTQ+ individuals are still not able to access appropriate and inclusive reproductive care. Given that LGBTQ+ individuals often report more positive experiences of conception outside of a clinical setting, improving access to, and the quality of, fertility services for LGBTQ+ prospective parents is crucial. Clinicians need ongoing training about LGBTQ+ identities and experiences, so that they can meet the needs of this growing group of parents. This is particularly the case, given that novel clinical treatments may now allow LGBTQ+ parents to pursue parenthood in ways that align with their goals and preferences. Among researchers, it is clear that we need to explore further the experiences and needs of diverse groups of LGBTQ+ parents, many of whose experiences remain so far understudied. As explained by the TNB parents within our research, reproductive care for LGBTQ+ populations must be accessible, inclusive, and evidence-based.

NOTE

   i   When reporting research findings in this chapter, we generally use the language on sexual orientation and/or gender identity of participants, as it is described within the study.

REFERENCES

   1.   Goldberg S, Conron KJ. *How Many Same-Sex Couples in the US are Raising Children?* 2020. https://williamsinstitute.law.ucla.edu/wp-content/uploads/Parenting-Among-Same-Sex-Couples.pdf

   2.   Blake L, Carone N, Raffanello E, Slutsky J, Ehrhardt AA, Golombok S. Gay Fathers' Motivations For and Feelings about Surrogacy as a Path to Parenthood. *Human Reproduction*. 2017;32(4):860–867. https://doi.org/10.1093/humrep/dex026

   3.   Bower-Brown S, Zadeh S. "I Guess the Trans Identity Goes with Other Minority Identities": An Intersectional Exploration of the Experiences of Trans and Non-Binary Parents Living in the UK. *International Journal of Transgender Health*. 2021;22(1–2):101–112. https://doi.org/10.1080/26895269.2020.1835598

   4.   Herbrand C. Co-Parenting Arrangements in Lesbian and Gay Families: When the 'Mum and Dad' Ideal Generates Innovative Family Forms. *Families, Relationships and Societies*. 2018;7(3):449–466. https://doi.org/10.1332/204674317X14888886530269

   5.   Jadva V, Freeman T, Tranfield E, Golombok S. "Friendly Allies in Raising a Child": A Survey of Men and Women Seeking Elective Co-Parenting Arrangements via an Online Connection Website. *Human Reproduction*. 2015;30(8):1896–1906. https://doi.org/10.1093/humrep/dev120

   6.   Nordqvist P. Origins and Originators: Lesbian Couples Negotiating Parental Identities and Sperm Donor Conception. *Culture, Health and Sexuality*. 2012;14(3):297–311. https://doi.org/10.1080/13691058.2011.639392

   7.   HFEA. *Family Formations in Fertility Treatment 2018*. 2020 https://www.hfea.gov.uk/about-us/publications/research-and-data/family-formations-in-fertility-treatment-2018/

   8.   Horsey K. *Surrogacy Trends for UK Nationals*. 2021. https://www.mysurrogacyjourney.com/blog/surrogacy-trends-for-uk-nationals-our-exclusive-findings/

   9.   King M, Semlyen J, Tai SS, Killaspy H, Osborn D, Popelyuk D, Nazareth I. A Systematic Review of Mental Disorder, Suicide, and Deliberate Self Harm in Lesbian, Gay and Bisexual People. 2008. In *BMC Psychiatry* (Vol. 8). BMC Psychiatry. https://doi.org/10.1186/1471-244X-8-70

10. Meyer IH. Prejudice, Social Stress, and Mental Health in Lesbian, Gay, and Bisexual Populations: Conceptual Issues and Research Evidence. *Psychological Bulletin*. 2003;129(5): 674–697. https://doi.org/10.1037/2329-0382.1.S.3

11. Meyer IH, Frost DM. Minority Stress and the Health of Sexual Minorities. *Handbook of Psychology and Sexual Orientation*. 2013. https://doi.org/10.1093/acprof:oso/97801997 65218.003.0018

12. Testa RJ, Habarth J, Peta J, Balsam K, Bockting W. Development of the Gender Minority Stress and Resilience Measure. *Psychology of Sexual Orientation and Gender Diversity*. 2015;2(1):65–77.https://doi.org/10.1037/sgd0000081

13. Bower-Brown S, McConnachie AL. *LGBT Parent Families: What do we Know? And What do we Need to Know? The Constellation Project*. 2020

14. Golombok S. *We are Family: What Really Matters for Parents and Children*. Scribe. 2020

15. McCandless J, Sheldon S. The Human Fertilisation and Embryology Act (2008) and the Tenacity of the Sexual Family Form. *The Modern Law Review*. 2010;73(2):175–207. https://doi.org/10.2307/824017

16. *McConnell and YY v. Registrar General*, Pub. L. No. EWCA Civ 559 IN (2020).

17. Wilder BL. Evolution of the Birth Certificate: A Tale of Gender, ART, and Society. *Journal of the American Academy of Matrimonial Lawyers*. 2021;33(2):543–570.

18. Jadva V, Prosser H, Gamble N. Cross-Border and Domestic Surrogacy in the UK Context: An Exploration of Practical and Legal Decision-Making. *Human Fertility*. 2021;24(2):93–104. https://doi.org/10.1080/14647273.2018.1540801

19. Zadeh S, Jadva V, Golombok S. Documenting Families: Paper-Work in Family Display among Planned Single Father Families. *Sociology*. 2022. 1–17. https://doi.org/10.1177/0038038 5211073238

20. Lee E, Sheldon S, Macvarish J. After the "Need for··· A Father": "The Welfare of the Child" and "Supportive Parenting" in Assisted Conception Clinics in the UK. *Families, Relationships and Societies*. 2017;6(1):71–87. https://doi.org/10.1332/204674315X14303 090462204

21. Zadeh S, Foster J. From 'Virgin Births' to 'Octomom': Representations of Single Motherhood via Sperm Donation in the UK News. *Journal of Community and Applied Social Psychology*. 2016;26:551–566. https://doi.org/10.1002/casp

22. Family Equality. LGBTQ Family Building Survey, 2019. https://www.familyequality.org/resources/lgbtq-family-building-survey/

23. BPAS Fertility. *BPAS Fertility Investigation: NHS-Funded Fertility Care for Female Same-Sex Couples*, 2021.

24. Women and Equalities Committee. *Transgender Equality*. 2016 https://publications.parliament.uk/pa/cm201516/cmselect/cmwomeq/390/390.pdf

25. HFEA. *Information for Trans and Non-Binary People Seeking Fertility Treatment*. (n.d.) https://www.hfea.gov.uk/treatments/fertility-preservation/information-for-trans-and-non-binary-people-seeking-fertility-treatment/

26. Chen D, Kyweluk MA, Sajwani A, Gordon EJ, Johnson EK, Finlayson CA, Woodruff TK. (2019). Factors Affecting Fertility Decision-Making Among Transgender Adolescents and Young Adults. *LGBT Health*. 6(3):107–115. https://doi.org/10.1089/lgbt.2018.0250

27. Pyne J. *Transforming Family: Trans Parents and their Struggles, Strategies, and Strengths*. 2012.

28. Toze M. The Risky Womb and the Unthinkability of the Pregnant Man: Addressing Trans Masculine Hysterectomy. *Feminism & Psychology*. 2018;28(2):194–211. https://doi.org/10.1177/0959353517747007

29. Krempasky C, Harris M, Abern L, Grimstad F. Contraception Across the Transmasculine Spectrum. *American Journal of Obstetrics and Gynecology*. 2020;222(2):134–143. https://doi.org/10.1016/j.ajog.2019.07.043

30. Gomez AM, Đỗ L, Ratliff GA, Crego PI, Hastings J. Contraceptive Beliefs, Needs, and Care Experiences Among Transgender and Nonbinary Young Adults. *Journal of Adolescent Health*. 2020;67(4)597–602. https://doi.org/10.1016/j.jadohealth.2020.03.003

31. Light A., Wang LF, Zeymo A, Gomez-Lobo V. Family Planning and Contraception Use in Transgender Men. *Contraception*. 2018;98(4):266–269. https://doi.org/10.1016/j.contraception.2018.06.006

32. Bachmann CL, Gooch B. *LGBT in Britain: Trans Report*.2018. https://www.stonewall.org.uk/sites/default/files/lgbt-in-britain-trans.pdf

33. Riggs DW, Bartholomaeus C. Fertility Preservation Decision Making Amongst Australian Transgender and Non-Binary Adults. *Reproductive Health*. 2018;15(1):1–10. https://doi.org/10.1186/s12978-018-0627-z

34. Tasker F, Gato J. Gender Identity and Future Thinking About Parenthood: A Qualitative Analysis of Focus Group Data With Transgender and Non-binary People in the United Kingdom. *Frontiers in Psychology*. 2020;11(May):1–15. https://doi.org/10.3389/fpsyg.2020.00865

35. Amodeo AL, Esposito C, Bochicchio V, Valerio P, Vitelli R, Bacchini D, Scandurra C. Parenting Desire and Minority Stress in Lesbians and Gay Men: A Mediation Framework. *International Journal of Environmental Research and Public Health*. 2018;15(10). https://doi.org/10.3390/ijerph15102318

36. Scandurra C, Bacchini D, Esposito C, Bochicchio V, Valerio P, Amodeo AL. The Influence of Minority Stress, Gender, and Legalization of Civil Unions on Parenting Desire and Intention in Lesbian Women and Gay Men: Implications for Social Policy and Clinical Practice. *Journal of GLBT Family Studies*. 2019;15(1):76–100. https://doi.org/10.1080/1550428X.2017.1410460

37. Tornello SL, Bos H. Parenting Intentions among Transgender Individuals. *LGBT Health*. 2017;4(2):115–120. https://doi.org/10.1089/lgbt.2016.0153

38. von Doussa H, Power J, Riggs, D. Imagining Parenthood: The Possibilities and Experiences of Parenthood Among Transgender People. *Culture, Health and Sexuality*. 2015;17(9):1119–1131. https://doi.org/10.1080/13691058.2015.1042919

39. Riggs DW, Pfeffer CA, Pearce R, Hines S, White FR. Men, Trans/Masculine, and Non-Binary People Negotiating Conception: Normative Resistance and Inventive Pragmatism. *International Journal of Transgender Health*. 2020. 1–12. https://doi.org/10.1080/15532739.2020.1808554

40. McInerney A, Creaner M, Nixon E. The Motherhood Experiences of Non-Birth Mothers in Same-Sex Parent Families. *Psychology of Women Quarterly*, 2021;45(3):279–293.https://doi.org/10.1177/03616843211003072

41. Costa PA, Tasker F. "We Wanted a Forever Family": Altruistic, Individualistic, and Motivated Reasoning Motivations for Adoption Among LGBTQ Individuals. *Journal of Family Issues*. 2018;39(18):4156–4178.

42. Goldberg A, Tornello S, Farr R, Smith JAZ, Miranda L. Barriers to Adoption and Foster Care and Openness to Child Characteristics Among Transgender Adults. *Children and Youth Services Review*. 2020;109(October 2019):104699. https://doi.org/10.1016/j.childyouth.2019.104699

43. Smietana M, Thompson C, Twine FW. Making and Breaking Families – Reading Queer Reproductions, Stratified Reproduction and Reproductive Justice Together. *Reproductive Biomedicine and Society Online*. 2018;7:112–130. https://doi.org/10.1016/j.rbms.2018.11.001

44. Power J, Dempsey D, Kelly F, Lau M. Use of Fertility Services in Australian Lesbian, Bisexual and Queer Women's Pathways to Parenthood. *Australian and New Zealand Journal of Obstetrics and Gynaecology*. 2020;60(4):610–615. https://doi.org/10.1111/ajo.13175

45. Inhorn MC, Birenbaum-Carmeli D. Assisted Reproductive Technologies and Culture Change. *Annual Review of Anthropology*. 2008;37:177–196. https://doi.org/10.1146/annurev.anthro.37.081407.085230

46. Golombok S, Shaw K, McConnachie A, Jadva V, Foley S, Macklon N, Ahuja K. Relationships between Mothers and Children in Families Formed by Shared Biological Motherhood. *Human Reproduction*. 2023;1–10.

47. Bodri D, Nair S, Gill A, Lamanna G, Rahmati M, Arian-Schad M, Smith V, Linara E, Wang J, Macklon N, Ahuja KK. Shared Motherhood IVF: High Delivery Rates in a Large Study of Treatments for Lesbian Couples Using Partner-Donated Eggs. *Reproductive BioMedicine Online*. 2018;36(2):130–136. https://doi.org/10.1016/j.rbmo.2017.11.006

48. Pennings G. Having a Child Together in Lesbian Families: Combining Gestation and Genetics. *Journal of Medical Ethics*. 2016;42(4):253–255. https://doi.org/10.1136/medethics-2015-103007

49. Shaw K, Bower-Brown S, McConnachie A, Jadva V, Ahuja K, Macklon N, Golombok S. "Her Bun in My Oven": Motivations and Experiences of Two-Mother Families who have Used Reciprocal IVF. *Family Relations*. 2023;72(1):195–214. https://doi.org/10.1111/fare.12805

50. Malmquist A, Nieminen K. Negotiating Who Gives Birth and the Influence of Fear of Childbirth: Lesbians, Bisexual Women and Transgender People in Parenting Relationships. *Women and Birth*. 2021;34(3):e271–e278. https://doi.org/10.1016/j.wombi.2020.04.005

51. Fischer OJ. Non-Binary Reproduction: Stories of Conception, Pregnancy, and Birth. *International Journal of Transgender Health*. 2021;22(1–2):77–88. https://doi.org/10.1080/26895269.2020.1838392

52. Hoffkling A, Obedin-Maliver J, Sevelius J. From Erasure to Opportunity: A Qualitative Study of the Experiences of Transgender Men Around Pregnancy and Recommendations for Providers. *BMC Pregnancy and Childbirth*. 2017;17(Suppl 2). https://doi.org/10.1186/s12884-017-1491-5

53. Ryan M. The Gender of Pregnancy: Masculine Lesbians Talk about Reproduction. *Journal of Lesbian Studies*. 2013;17(2):119–133. https://doi.org/10.1080/10894160.2012.653766

54. Greenwald P, Dubois B, Lekovich J, Pang JH, Safer J. Successful In Vitro Fertilization in a Cisgender Female Carrier Using Oocytes Retrieved From a Transgender Man Maintained

on Testosterone. *AACE Clinical Case Reports*. 2023;8(1):19–21. https://doi.org/10.1016/j.aace.2021.06.007

55. Malmquist A. Women in Lesbian Relations: Construing Equal or Unequal Parental Roles? *Psychology of Women Quarterly*. 2015;39(2):256–267. https://doi.org/10.1177/03616843 14537225

56. Hemalal S, Yee S, Ross L, Loutfy M, Librach C. Same-Sex Male Couples and Single Men Having Children Using Assisted Reproductive Technology: A Quantitative Analysis. *Reproductive BioMedicine Online*. 2021;42(5):1033–1047. https://doi.org/10.1016/j.rbmo.2020.08.032

57. Lindheim SR, Madeira JL, Ludwin A, Kemner E, Parry JP, Sylvestre G, Pennings G. Societal Pressures and Procreative Preferences for Gay Fathers Successfully Pursuing Parenthood through IVF and Gestational Carriers. *Reproductive Biomedicine and Society Online*. 2019;9:1–10. https://doi.org/10.1016/j.rbms.2019.09.001

58. Nordqvist P. Bringing Kinship into Being: Connectedness, Donor Conception and Lesbian Parenthood. *Sociology*. 2014;48(2):268–283. https://doi.org/10.1177/0038038513477936

59. Riggs DW. Making Matter Matter: Meanings Accorded to Genetic Material Among Australian Gay Men. *Reproductive Biomedicine and Society Online*. 2018;7:150–157. https://doi.org/10.1016/j.rbms.2018.06.002

60. Ravelingien A, Provoost V, Pennings G. Creating a Family through Connection Websites and Events: Ethical and Social Issues. *Reproductive BioMedicine Online*. 2016;33(4):522–528. https://doi.org/10.1016/j.rbmo.2016.07.004

61. Jadva V, Freeman T, Tranfield E, Golombok S. Why Search for a Sperm Donor Online? The Experiences of Women Searching For and Contacting Sperm Donors on the Internet. *Human Fertility*. 2018;21(2):112–119. https://doi.org/10.1080/14647273.2017.1315460

62. Epstein R. Space Invaders: Queer and Trans Bodies in Fertility Clinics. *Sexualities*. 2018;21(7):1039–1058. https://doi.org/10.1177/1363460717720365

63. Fantus S. Experiences of Gestational Surrogacy for Gay Men in Canada. *Culture, Health and Sexuality*. 2021;23(10):1361–1374. https://doi.org/10.1080/13691058.2020.1784464

64. Gregory KB, Mielke JG, Neiterman E. Building Families Through Healthcare: Experiences of Lesbians Using Reproductive Services. *Journal of Patient Experience*. 2022;9:23743735 2210894. https://doi.org/10.1177/23743735221089459

65. James-Abra S, Tarasoff LA, Green D, Epstein R, Anderson S, Marvel S, Steele LS, Ross LE. Trans People's Experiences with Assisted Reproduction Services: A Qualitative Study. *Human Reproduction*. 2015;30(6):1365–1374. https://doi.org/10.1093/humrep/dev087

66. Cherguit J, Burns J, Pettle S, Tasker F. Lesbian Co-Mothers' Experiences of Maternity Healthcare Services. *Journal of Advanced Nursing*. 2013;69(6):1269–1278. https://doi.org/10.1111/j.1365-2648.2012.06115.x

67. Wu HY, Yin O, Monseur B, Selter J, Collins LJ, Lau BD, Christianson MS. Lesbian, Gay, Bisexual, Transgender Content on Reproductive Endocrinology and Infertility Clinic Websites. *Fertility and Sterility*. 2017;108(1):183–191. https://doi.org/10.1016/j.fertnstert.2017.05.011

68. Equality Network. *Lesbian, and Bi+ Women's Experiences of Reproductive Health and Fertility Services in Scotland*. 2021.

69. Government Equalities Office. *National LGBT Survey*. 2018.

70. Malmquist A, Nelson KZ. Efforts to Maintain a "Just Great" Story: Lesbian Parents' Talk about Encounters with Professionals in Fertility Clinics and Maternal and Child Healthcare Services. *Feminism and Psychology*. 2014;24(1):56–73. https://doi.org/10.1177/095935351 3487532

71. Bower-Brown S. Beyond Mum and Dad: Gendered Assumptions about Parenting and the Experiences of Trans and/or Non-Binary Parents in the UK. *LGBTQ+ Family: An Inter-disciplinary Journal*. 2020;1–18. https://doi.org/10.1080/27703371.2022.2083040

72. Moseson H, Zazanis N, Goldberg E, Fix L, Durden M, Stoeffler A, Hastings J, Cudlitz L, Lesser-Lee B, Letcher L, Reyes A, Obedin-Maliver J. The Imperative for Transgender and Gender Nonbinary Inclusion: Beyond Women's Health. *Obstet Gynecol*. May 2020;135(5): 1059–1068. https://doi.org/10.1097/AOG.0000000000003816

73. Obedin-Maliver J, Makedon HJ. Transgender Men and Pregnancy. *Obstet Med*. 2016;9(1): 4–8. doi: 10.1177/1753495X15612658.

74. Light A, Obedin-Maliver J, Sevelius JM, Kerns JL. Transgender Men who Experienced Pregnancy after Female-to-Male Gender Transitioning. *Obstetrics and Gynecology*. 2014; 124(6):1120–1127. https://doi.org/10.1097/AOG.0000000000000540

75. Chapman R, Wardrop J, Zappia T, Watkins R, Shields, L. The Experiences of Australian Lesbian Couples Becoming Parents: Deciding, Searching and Birthing. *Journal of Clinical Nursing*. 2012;21(13–14):1878–1885. https://doi.org/10.1111/j.1365-2702.2011.04007.x

76. Kirubarajan A, Barker LC, Leung S, Ross LE, Zaheer J, Park B, Abramovich A, Yudin MH, Lam JSH. LGBTQ2S+ Childbearing Individuals and Perinatal Mental Health: A Systematic Review. *BJOG: An International Journal of Obstetrics and Gynaecology*.2022. https://doi.org/ 10.1111/1471-0528.17103

77. Abelsohn KA, Epstein R, Ross LE. Celebrating the "Other" Parent: Mental Health and Wellness of Expecting Lesbian, Bisexual, and Queer Non-Birth Parents. *Journal of Gay & Lesbian Mental Health*. 2013;17:387–405. https://doi.org/10.1080/19359705.2013.771808

78. Ross LE, Siegel A, Dobinson C, Epstein R, Steele LS. "I Don't Want to Turn Totally Invisible": Mental Health, Stressors, and Supports among Bisexual Women during the Perinatal Period. *Journal of GLBT Family Studies*. 2012;8(2):137–154. https://doi.org/10.1080/15504 28X.2012.660791

79. Hafford-Letchfield T, Cocker C, Rutter D, Tinarwo M, McCormack K, Manning R. What do We Know about Transgender Parenting?: Findings from a Systematic Review. *Health and Social Care in the Community*. March 2019;1–15. https://doi.org/10.1111/hsc.12759

80. Maya T, Adital BA. Single Gay Fathers via Surrogacy: The Dialectics between Vulnerability and Resilience. *Journal of Family Studies*. 2021;27(2):247–260. https://doi.org/10.1080/ 13229400.2018.1551148

81. Kirubarajan A, Patel P, Leung S, Prethipan T, Sierra S. Barriers to Fertility Care for Racial/ Ethnic Minority Groups: A Qualitative Systematic Review. *F&S Reviews*. 2021;2(2):150–159. https://doi.org/10.1016/j.xfnr.2021.01.001

82. HFEA. *Ethnic Diversity in Fertility Treatment 2018*. 2021. https://www.hfea.gov.uk/about-us/publications/research-and-data/ethnic-diversity-in-fertility-treatment-2018/#Section8

Chapter 3

LGBTQ+ pregnancy loss

Ash Bainbridge

"There is as much diversity in death, as there is in life."
– Jessica Clasby-Monk, *The Legacy of Leo*

INTRODUCTION

Opportunities for LGBTQ+ people to build families via pregnancy have grown over the last two decades[1] and, tragically, some of these pregnancies end in loss. Bereaved parents deserve compassionate, empathetic, and supportive care that respects who they are, their pregnancy journey, and relationships to their child(ren). In the UK at the time of writing, formal midwifery and medical education does not include care for bereaved LGBTQ+ parents and the NHS guide "Having a baby if you're LGBT+" does not mention pregnancy loss at any gestation.[2] A small but growing body of research focuses on pregnancy loss experiences in distinct LGBTQ+ communities with the rates unevenly spread between the community's sub-groups. The most in-depth and nuanced analyses of pregnancy outcomes focus on the experiences of lesbian and bisexual cisgender women in committed relationships.[3–7] Little to none focus on pregnancy outcomes for individuals with an intersex assignment at birth, intersex identity and/or lived experience, asexual sexual orientation, or who belong to polyamorous relationship structures.

To bridge this gap, this chapter will discuss LGBTQ+ experiences of pregnancy loss by exploring how current definitions and methods of data capture are barriers that render LGBTQ+ losses invisible; how the frequency of pregnancy loss is impacted by minority stressors and culturally incompetent health care; and how intrapersonal and interpersonal stigma cultivates silence around pregnancy loss in LGBTQ+ communities. The chapter will then explore positive and negative experiences of bereavement support for both gestational and non-gestational parents, how routes to conception and pregnancy loss are interconnected

DOI: 10.4324/9781003305446-4

experiences for LGBTQ+ families, and how hormone therapy impacts experiences of pregnancy and loss.

In this chapter, an intersectional lens is applied and this application is vital. Pregnancy losses experienced by LGBTQ+ people are affected by intersecting axes of power, privilege, marginalisation, and oppression, both historical and present. LGBTQ+ identity neither eclipses, nor negates other identity characteristics. How these characteristics interlock and overlay influences how someone perceives themselves, their pregnancy loss experience, health care, and health care providers.[8] A holistic, person-centred approach should be adopted where sexual orientation and gender identity are a critical, but not the sole lens through which a pregnancy is viewed.[9] Intersectional research findings on LGBTQ+ pregnancy loss experiences are scant.

Where possible, attempts have been made to locate research evidence from outside the Global North, and, when writing, to distinguish between distinct LGBTQ+ communities. For consistency, a parent who is expecting a child and carrying the pregnancy is referred to as a "gestational parent", and a parent expecting a child and not carrying the pregnancy as a "non-gestational parent". For accuracy, where relevant, gendered and LGBTQ+ specific language is taken from the original source referenced (eg mothers,[10] gender-expansive,[11] gender variant,[12] birth parent,[13] etc.).

DEFINITIONS OF PREGNANCY LOSS

In this chapter, pregnancy loss refers to the unplanned end of a pregnancy at any gestational age: an umbrella term for miscarriage (early, late, and missed; ectopic and molar pregnancies; loss following IUI and IVF), and stillbirth (early, late, and term). Parameters delineating miscarriage and stillbirth are currently inconsistent, as detailed in Table 3.1.

Such disparities in definition – both published and as they have evolved since – complicate comparison drawing in relation to miscarriage and stillbirth. This landscape is even more complex for LGBTQ+ families due to the absence of disaggregated data on loss prevalence and inconsistencies when considering who is and who is not a legible data subject.[23, 24] For example, when requesting personal data on sexual orientation, often forms employ "bisexual" as a catch all, for all sexual orientations that are not heterosexual. In perinatal services where gendered language is default, data fails to capture pregnancy loss experiences specific to trans men, transmasculine persons, non-binary people, and intersex people who do not identify as women. These distinct experiences may be recorded and then inaccurately assigned as women's.

Table 3.1 Parameters delineating miscarriage and stillbirth by county

Place or Agency in alphabetical order	Definition (antenatal and intrapartum death)	
	Miscarriage	Stillbirth
Australia[14]	≤19+6 weeks or <400g birthweight	≥20+0 weeks or ≥400g birthweight
China[15–17]	≤20+0 weeks or ≤23+6 weeks or ≤28+0 weeks	≥20+0 weeks or ≥24+0 weeks or ≥28+0 weeks
Mexico[18]	≤20+6 weeks	≥21+0 weeks
UNICEF[19]	≤27+6 weeks	≥28+0 weeks
United Kingdom[20]	≤23+6 weeks with no signs of life (eg, voluntary muscle movement, umbilical cord pulsation, heartbeat presence at birth regardless of whether the placenta is still attached or umbilical cord has been cut)	≥24+0 weeks with no signs of life
United States[21]	≤19+6 weeks (usually) or <350g birthweight if gestational age unknown	≥20+0 weeks (usually but not always) or ≥350g birthweight if gestational age unknown
World Health Organisation (WHO)[22]	≤21+6 weeks or <500g birthweight or <25cm body length	≥22+0 weeks or ≥500g birthweight or ≥25cm body length
WHO for international comparison purposes[22]	≤27+6 weeks or <100g birthweight or <35cm body length with birthweight prioritised over gestational age	≥28+0 weeks or ≥100g birthweight or ≥35cm body length with birthweight prioritised over gestational age

In the UK, this inaccuracy is acknowledged and knowingly perpetuated in evidence-based recommendations. For instance, the National Institute for Health and Care Excellence's (NICE) clinical guideline on the diagnosis and initial management of ectopic pregnancy and miscarriage reads: "we use the terms 'woman' and 'women', based on the evidence used in its development. The recommendations will also apply to people who do not identify as women but are pregnant or have given birth".[25] Evidence that applies to a percentage of the pregnant population does not automatically apply to the whole population, and health care needs during pregnancy loss differ. Such heteronormative and cisnormative language surrounding pregnancy loss blunts the accuracy and relevance of clinical guidelines and policy, dilutes health care providers' understanding of differing reproductive loss experiences and needs, and hinders access for LGBTQ+ individuals to grieve and cope.[26]

A recent update to the style guide for all NICE publications, however, suggests a shift towards better LGBTQ+ inclusion.[27] This update recommends using additive language when guidance applies to varying populations ("This guideline is for pregnant women and pregnant people") and specific language when discussing specific populations ("use man, woman, or trans person, trans man or trans woman if you are referring to someone whose gender identity differs from the sex they were registered with at birth").[27] Beginning to use language that more accurately reflects the populations to whom recommendations refer means NICE can improve bereavement care for LGBTQ+ families by influencing how policy is written at national and local Trust level, how health care training and curricula develop, and by highlighting research gaps where distinctions between different pregnancy populations and their outcomes have not previously been considered.

In England and Wales, the legal definition of a stillborn child as contained in the Births and Deaths Registration Act 1953 section 41 and amended by the Stillbirth (Definition) Act 1992 section 1(1) is exclusionary: "a child which has issued forth from its mother after the 24th week of pregnancy and which did not at any time breathe or show any other signs of life".[28, 29] Here, only one identity and role for the person who carries and births the baby who has died is acknowledged. Stillborn babies can be – and are – born via surrogacy; by trans men, non-binary and gender non-conforming people; and by people not identifying as mothers. As a result, all these babies who die – if their parents' identities and roles are not accurately recognised – are rendered legally invisible.

RECOMMENDATIONS

- Broaden and standardise pregnancy loss definitions and parameters.
- Where safe to do so, employ accurate representative methods of data collection and analysis to capture and begin to understand LGBTQ+ pregnancy outcomes and loss experiences. Write-in boxes offer one approach if information provided is analysed meaningfully and included in subsequent counts.

In documentation (policy, audit, research, service user leaflets, etc.), use language that accurately reflects the population in question.

FREQUENCY OF PREGNANCY LOSS

Globally, an estimated 23 million miscarriages occur each year, affecting one in ten people who conceive in their lifetime.[30] In many low-income and lower middle-income settings, miscarriages and stillbirths are not counted uniformly, or at all.[31] The most recent available data of national stillbirth rates shows the countries with the lowest stillbirth rates per 1,000 total births were Monaco (1.4), Japan (1.5), South Korea (1.7), San Marino (1.8), and Iceland (1.9).[32] Countries with the highest national stillbirth rates per 1,000 total births were Afghanistan (28.4), South Sudan (28.8), Central African Republic (29.8), Pakistan (30.6), and Guinea-Bissau (32.2).[32] In the UK, an estimated one in four pregnancies end in loss between conception and birth, 250,000 pregnancies end in miscarriage, and 11,000 end in emergency admissions for ectopic pregnancies.[33–36] In 2021, a rise in stillbirth rates was seen in England and Wales: from 3.8 per 1,000 births in 2020 to 4.1 per 1000 births in 2021.[37] This rise is the first year-on-year increase in stillbirths since 2014.[37] LGBTQ+ pregnancies are encompassed in these statistics, but their number is unknown. The national, governments-commissioned audit programme that collects information about late-term fetal losses, stillbirths, and neonatal and maternal deaths MBRRACE-UK does not capture data on gender identity or sexual orientation, and so hinders the identification and development of interventions to prevent outcome disparities for LGBTQ+ families.[38]

In addition to miscarriage and stillbirth, other reproductive losses are not routinely captured in data and research. These include unsuccessful IUI and IVF cycles, infertility, and sterility.[1, 39] For LGBTQ+ families, the anticipation of a pregnancy, even if the pregnancy does not occur, can be felt as a loss.[1, 39] Other losses rendered invisible include offshore surrogacy arrangements ending in loss and outcomes when LGBTQ+ people choose not to engage with perinatal services. While not a type of pregnancy loss itself, the loss of a child via adoption and fostering processes may impact future experiences of pregnancy loss and should be considered when planning (bereavement) care provision.[40]

As discussed in the Introduction and Chapter 13, LGBTQ+ people experience daily stressors as a result of their sexual and/or gender diversity. Despite NHS guidance to the contrary,[41] research findings from a systematic review and meta-analysis support a link between psychological and emotional stress before and during pregnancy, and miscarriage; such stress may increase the risk of miscarriage by ~42%.[42] A US-based study documented that bisexual and lesbian women have an increased risk of miscarriage and stillbirth in comparison to heterosexual women, a disparity linked with exposure to a greater variety and higher number of stressors.[43] Swedish studies found lesbian, bisexual, and/or trans people experienced stress caused by a lack of control during the fertility process and birth.[44, 45] For those whose gender identity and/or sexual orientation is fluid, changes here are associated with elevated levels of stress and depression that may impact pregnancy outcomes.[43, 46]

In the UK, Black and Black Mixed Heritage women are 43% more likely to suffer a miscarriage than white women,[47, 48] and in England and Wales are nearly 50% more likely to suffer a stillbirth.[49] Higher levels of miscarriage and stillbirth are also reported amongst Romany Gypsies and Travellers resident in Britain compared to the general population.[50] A UK population-based cohort study concluded that babies of Asian ethnicities are also at "excess risk of stillbirth", as are babies born to parents of Bangladeshi, Black, and Pakistani ethnicity living in the most deprived areas.[51] This data capture is crucial for identifying those at increased risk due to race and ethnicity, and inequalities in health care and treatment rooted in racism. Yet all gestational parents are assumed to be cisgender women and data on sexual orientation is absent. Subsequently, possibilities for identifying and learning how to tackle outcome inequities and inequalities based on where race, gender, and sexual orientation intersect are blocked.

In the United States, a quantitative survey of pregnancy outcomes for transgender, non-binary, and gender-expansive individuals assigned female or intersex at birth provides data showing that for those who describe their ethnicity as Black, African American, Middle Eastern, and North African, miscarriage rates are equal to or exceed rates of livebirth, as shown in Table 3.2.[11]

Additional community-based and community-led research is needed to determine the incidence, prevalence, and patterns of pregnancy loss for Black LGBTQ+ parents and LGBTQ+ People of Colour: to improve and provide more equitable access to health services, improve the care received inside these services, and improve pregnancy outcomes.[52]

Table 3.2 Pregnancy outcome by ethnicity for transgender people in the US

Description of ethnicity	Pregnancy outcome	Percentage	Number
Black or African American	Miscarriage	63%	5
	Livebirth	31%	1
Middle Eastern or North African	Miscarriage	38%	3
	Livebirth	38%	3
Multiple racial identities	Miscarriage	41%	28
	Livebirth	35%	24

LGBTQ+ parents may hold disabled identities: physical, cognitive, sensory, and/or complex. The ITEMS research project – running between September 2020 and April 2021 in the UK – provided insight into trans and non-binary birth parent experiences of perinatal services, and made recommendations for service improvement.[13] In this survey, 29% of trans and non-binary respondents considered themselves to be a disabled person; these disabilities included impairments, long-term conditions, and mental health conditions.[13] Research conducted in the Global North suggests a gestational parent's disability is associated with an increased risk for perinatal complications, including miscarriage and stillbirth.[53, 54] Here, however, all participants were assumed to be cisgender women, a cisnormative methodology that erased any disabled trans and non-binary pregnancy loss experiences.

For both younger (<20 years) and older (>45 years) LGBTQ+ parents, the age of a gestational parent is potentially a compounding risk factor for miscarriage and stillbirth. Young gay men, young lesbians, and cisgender women who have sex with women are up to three times more likely to be involved in a teenage pregnancy than their heterosexual counterparts.[55] Moreover, lesbian and bisexual adolescents are at greater risk of unwanted pregnancies.[56] Teenage pregnancies have been shown as more likely to end in miscarriage: the risk of pregnancy loss in mothers <20 years is 15.8% compared to a risk of 9.8% for mothers aged 25–29.[10] Positive associations have also been identified between adolescent miscarriage and adolescent suicide attempts.[57] The intersection of LGBTQ+ identity and adolescence could mean LGBTQ+ young people are not only at a higher risk of pregnancy loss, but also of harming themselves in the event of a pregnancy loss.

Young LGBTQ+ people are at a higher risk of substance abuse, sexually transmitted infections, anxiety, depression, of being in the juvenile justice and/or foster care/child welfare system, suicide attempts, and suicide as compared to the general population.[55, 57, 58] All these factors have been identified as potential risks for miscarriage and/or stillbirth.[59–65] This information is critical when planning clinical, social, and public health care provision for LGBTQ+ teenagers across the (pre-) pregnancy continuum: from contraceptive advice, health screenings, and pre-conception care to providing specialist support and suicidality screening to those who experience pregnancy loss.

When transitioning to parenthood, the average age of a homosexual couple is thought to be slightly older than that of a heterosexual couple, and a study has shown this to be the case in Sweden.[66] The risk of miscarriage is greatest for gestational parents >45 years (53.6%).[10] This intersection of LGBTQ+ identity and age is significant in light of a broader trend of advancing parental ages; the average age for birthing a child now stands at 30 or above (with exceptions to this trend seen in Colombia and Mexico).[67–69] More research is needed to ascertain how best to care for this pregnant population, both to improve pregnancy outcomes when risks are currently increased and to provide suitable support in the event of a loss.

Those who experience imprisonment during pregnancy are less able to access to prenatal care and experience higher rates of pregnancy complications compared with those in the community.[70] A study describing the number of admissions of pregnant people to US jails and the outcomes of pregnancies that ended in jail found that only 64% (n=144) resulted in live births: 18% (n=41) ended in miscarriage, 1.8% (n=4) in ectopic pregnancies, 0.9% (n=2) in stillbirths, and 0.5% (n=1) in neonatal death.[71] In the UK, pregnant women are five times more likely to suffer a stillbirth than women in the general population.[72, 73] In June 2020, a stillborn baby was birthed at Her Majesty's Prison Styal. The baby's mother Louise was a lesbian who had unknowingly been raped and did not believe she was pregnant when entering prison.[72] As Louise had not knowingly had sexual intercourse with anyone with sperm, the possibility of pregnancy was dismissed by both Louise and the nurse when she experienced a bloated abdomen, vaginal bleeding, and excruciating pain.[74] Investigation by the Prisons and Probation Ombudsman found the UK prisons' initial and secondary health assessment templates do not facilitate the discovery of pregnancy in someone who is unaware, or in denial, that they are or might be pregnant.[74] When interviewed, the consultant obstetrician said that while complete certainty is not guaranteed, Louise's baby appeared to have been alive when labour commenced and she likely died during premature labour or the labour process.[74] Appropriate triaging based on a full clinical picture, instead of eliminating possibilities based on sexual orientation and reported sexual activity, may have meant Louise birthed a live baby in a hospital and received appropriate medical care.[74]

SUPPORT AND STIGMA DURING PREGNANCY LOSS

Pregnancy loss can be associated with significant stigma. This stigma is related to patriarchal systems of power and deep-rooted expectations of reproduction imposed on cisgender women.[75] Pregnancy loss can be experienced as a personal failure to fulfil these societal expectations. For all gestational parents the resulting stigma may be intrapersonal, where stigmatising perspectives are internalised by an individual and self-imposed, and/or interpersonal, where stigmatising perspectives are imposed on an individual by others.[75] This stigma fuels the silence around miscarriage and stillbirth, rendering pregnancy loss a lonely, isolated experience for all parents.[76]

LGBTQ+ families face additional stigma. Societally, the desire for children can be dismissed and problematized with LGBTQ+ families seen as illegitimate.[77–79] An emphasis on "vertical" biology in the context of family building negatively correlates with "horizontal" community support for LGBTQ+ families.[80, 81] LGBTQ+ gestational parents may not believe they can rely on support from the LGBTQ+ community owing to the gendered nature of childbearing,[82] a lack of familiarity and lived experiences with childbearing,[5] and stigmatisation that they are choosing to do something they should not be doing.[12] A study of male and gender variant gestational parents' experiences highlighted perceptions of judgement when someone deviated from expected community norms; some chose to distance themselves from their trans and gender non-conforming friends.[12] By separating from community and chosen family, these individuals remove a crucial source of support in the event of a loss. This source may be the only one available to them given community reluctance to engage with perinatal services,[13] and with support from birth families/families of origin far from guaranteed.

Studies exploring lesbian experiences of pregnancy loss reveal varied challenges navigating support spaces. One mother faced marginalisation from her lesbian peers after choosing gestational parenthood; she was called a "breeder" (an insulting term reserved for heterosexual parents) and so sought community in a group for lesbian mothers.[6] After her baby died, she no longer felt comfortable in this community and joined a local bereaved parents' support group where she concealed her sexuality.[6] This mother suffered "multilevel stigma"[83] and marginalisation: in a heterosexist society that questions lesbian entitlement to parenthood;[7] amongst her peers for choosing gestational motherhood; in a lesbian parenting community where the other babies had been born alive; and in a bereavement support group where heterosexual relationships were default. Such inability to publicly mourn a pregnancy loss or access necessary support is termed "disenfranchised grief".[6, 84] By obstructing vital support, such layered disenfranchisement after pregnancy loss can lengthen and intensify grief, significantly harm self-esteem, isolate, and increase feelings of depression, all alongside experiencing the emotional loss of a child.[7]

By contrast, some bereaved lesbian couples describe feeling a connection with heterosexual couples who have also experienced pregnancy loss.[5] Other bereaved LGBTQ+ parents, however, believed their loss experiences incomparable with those of their cisgender and/or heterosexual counterparts, and so could not be understood by them.[85] The (perceived) need to educate in non-LGBTQ+ specific spaces prevents emotional and community needs from being met for some LGBTQ+ parents.[85] Others describe finding comments on their pregnancy loss from cisgender and/or heterosexual family members and friends condescending, which led to feelings of isolation, alienation, and silencing.[85] For some lesbian mothers, support after loss came from high-quality clinical care.[6] One mother received unwavering support from multiple sources and believed this care made her experience "more manageable".[6] Empathetic, compassionate, and person-focused care affects how LGBTQ+ bereavements are experienced both in terms of information gathering, emotional understanding, processing, and future family planning.[85]

RECOMMENDATIONS

- Identify who in the local community offers pregnancy loss support where LGBTQ+ parents are welcome. Ask if other LGBTQ+ parents attend, or have attended in the past. Spaces run by non-LGBTQ+ individuals may claim to be safe and inclusive because they want or aspire to be, not because they are. Such spaces should be screened to prevent a bereaved parent from exposure to potential additional harm when seeking support.
- Understand families may choose not to join general loss support groups for fear they would have to explain experiences with perinatal loss and/or justify their relationship when grieving and vulnerable.
- Create a list of LGBTQ+ groups and services (in person and on-line) that support parents suffering miscarriage, stillbirth, and other forms of pregnancy loss.

BRIDGING CONCEPTION AND LOSS

In LGBTQ+ pregnancies, the route to conception and pregnancy loss are inextricably linked. As explored in Chapter 2, conception challenges may be severalfold and differ depending on gender identity, sexual orientation, reproductive health and history, family structure, available social and financial support, and country of residence. If someone does not fall pregnant or their baby dies, this outcome can be unexpected and devastating; the resulting feelings of grief and loss have been labelled as "profound".[86, 87]

Planning and coordination complexities faced by cisgender lesbian and bisexual women when achieving conception compound pregnancy loss experiences, a phenomenon termed "amplification".[3-5, 40, 88, 89] Despite significant emotional, logistical, and often financial investment, as well as planning in the form of decision making, negotiation, and compromise, these women share not feeling in control of how and when pregnancy occurs.[5] Such hopes, deliberation, and uncertainty raise the stakes of a pregnancy and drain resources, which – in the event of loss – results in amplified grief.[4, 5, 23] Descriptors for this grief include "excruciating", "indescribable", and "horrible" as these parents recall feeling "suddenly that the world has ended", "utter devastation", and existing on "autopilot".[4-6]

The cost of conception is referred to as a "hidden loss" for LGBTQ+ parents. The extent of financial investment varies widely between countries, counties, and jurisdictions based on which reproductive technologies and surrogacy options are available – if any – and how much they cost. Some bereaved LGBTQ+ parents describe the discomfort conveyed by others when they spoke about the cost of pregnancy, even though financial concerns were extremely important to these grieving parents.[40] For one mother, concerns about the money invested in a pregnancy that ended in loss and concerns about the money she needed to invest in another pregnancy journey were so severe she feared the stress may cause another loss.[40]

Investments are also involved when conception occurs via surrogacy. Gay men entering parenthood via surrogacy whose pregnancies end in losses may experience a traumatic lack of power and control. With their status as parents and grief unacknowledged, they describe grief as disassociating, feeling at the mercy of others, and in limbo, and summarise the experience as "bloody tremendously hard".[90, 91] A harmful lack of empathy and support from professionals – both in surrogacy agencies and health care settings – was felt by fathers when they were not given the information they needed, informed about the surrogate's health and wellbeing, or allowed to meet or say goodbye to their babies, and when conversations quickly turned to "trying again".[90, 91] The emotional consequences of focusing solely on the physiological aspects of a pregnancy and loss without attending to the emotional safety, health, and wellbeing of non-gestational parents are significant.[90] When surrogacy agencies and health care settings facilitated such distance, depersonalisation, and disenfranchisement, the distress of these fathers increased.[91]

NON-GESTATIONAL PARENTS AND PREGNANCY LOSS

Research of pregnancy and pregnancy loss is "centred within a heteronormative framework"[92] and primarily focuses on gestational parents' outcomes and experiences, leaving non-gestational parents and how they could best be supported behind. The body of literature investigating the pregnancy loss experiences of LGBTQ+ gestational parents is smaller than that of their cisheterosexual counterparts, and the experiences of LGBTQ+ non-gestational parents is smaller still. Research that is available highlights that LGBTQ+ non-gestational parents' experiences of perinatal loss are varied,[93–95] and the lack of consideration or care for a bereaved non-gestational parent is a stressor that compounds distress.[3]

An international mixed methods study of lesbian and bisexual women's experiences of pregnancy loss found that 85% of mothers – including non-gestational mothers – described the impact of loss on their lives as "significant" or "very significant".[4] These mothers describe how health care professionals did not recognise their partners as parents, asked them to leave during examinations, and, following a stillbirth, would not allow them to answer questions concerning autopsy or funeral arrangements.[40]

Experiences shared elsewhere include the harm caused by death certificates not accommodating non-gestational parents' information.[6,40] For one lesbian mother with her own history of pregnancy loss, this legal exclusion was experienced as multi-layered loss: "In losing our daughter and in making the decision that it wouldn't be safe for me to carry again, and because we live in [a state that prohibits listing two same-sex parents on a birth certificate], I lost not only a biological and a physical connection and the possibility of breastfeeding my, our first child … I also lost the ability to have legal [rights to our future children], to have my name on this child's birth certificate".[40] For this parent, the consequence of this erasure was grief that required her to process both the death of her baby in the present, and the loss of a legally recognised relationship with future children as a non-gestational mother.

Outside such systems and inside communities, the significance of pregnancy loss for non-gestational parents may not be recognised by acquaintances and friends. One lesbian mother explains how her friends – both heterosexual and non-heterosexual – were surprised by how, as the non-gestational parent, she didn't recover from her loss more quickly; they more consistently inquired after her partner's health and wellbeing.[40] In the workplace, experiences can be particularly difficult for non-gestational parents due to heteronormative attitudes and policies questioning parental legitimacy. Challenges in accessing leave, misgendering leave entitlements, and failing to accommodate for high attachment to unborn babies in early gestation may all compound distress.[5, 80, 91] The result is loneliness, invisibility, and isolation,[96] all experienced with both actual and feared risks of exposure to conversations about other people's pregnancies in physical workplace settings.[80]

This difference in support and the perception of support that is required by gestational and non-gestational parents can be mirrored within the dynamic of a bereaved couple. Differences have been underscored in how those who belong to couples experience and express grief following pregnancy loss.[6] Gestational mothers describe grieving openly, while non-gestational mothers hide their grief and "act strong" for their partners.[5] Non-gestational mothers recall needing to multitask: to work through their own grief, support their partner through her grief, and learn more about their individual styles of grieving.[6] Professional external support is understood to help partners empathise with each other's experiences, and to do so openly.[6] In the UK, the ability to access such support as a non-gestational parent via the NHS is unclear, and remains unclear in the current "maternal mental health series" policy ambition as outlined in the NHS Long Term Plan.[97, 98]

RECOMMENDATIONS

- Do not assume a non-gestational parent's gender and/or sexuality.
- Include adoption and fostering in antenatal history taking. With informed consent, take pre-conception histories that include the reproductive, adoption, and fostering histories of the gestational parent and non-gestational parent(s).
- With the pregnant person's informed consent, communicate with non-gestational parents compassionately, in a timely manner, and in a way that encourages and facilitates discussion, acknowledging their role in care planning and provision.
- In the event of a miscarriage or stillbirth, if a birth setting provides a Certificate of Life and/or memory box, ensure any references to parents accurately represent the family whose baby has died.
- Provide both gestational and non-gestational parents – regardless of their gender and sexuality, and their baby's gestational age – access to parental and bereavement leave. Allow flexibility in hours, workload, and tasks following pregnancy loss.
- While taking care to avoid asking inappropriate questions or making assumptions, sensitively acknowledging the extent of investment involved in conception may help contribute to holistic, personalised bereavement care by recognising unique adversities, thereby potentially assuaging feelings of loneliness and "othering".

TESTOSTERONE AND PREGNANCY LOSS

One treatment for gender dysphoria – an experience that can be distressing and lead to depression, anxiety, self-neglect, self-harm, and low self-esteem – is hormone therapy. Testosterone therapy in trans men and non-binary people can suppress ovulation and alter ovarian histology.[99, 100] Oestrogen therapy in trans women and non-binary people can impair spermatogenesis and lead to testicular atrophy.[101] More research is needed to understand how frequently these effects occur, and to what extent when they do. Anecdotal evidence suggests medical advice concerning the impact of hormone therapy on fertility and future pregnancies falls generally into one of three boxes: the impact will be full, long-lasting, and potentially irreversible; the impact may not affect future fertility and contraception advice is provided; the impact is not mentioned at all. Such inconsistent advice based on a lack of evidence is a reproductive justice issue: fully informed decisions about reproductive health care and family planning cannot be made. For example, after seeking and receiving medical advice, some trans and non-binary people undertake gamete preservation treatments that are costly, require significant time without hormone therapy, and, for trans men and people registered female at birth, are physically invasive. All these factors can cause considerable distress. Other trans and non-binary people will not undertake these treatments based on different information received.

How gender-affirming hormone therapy influences pregnancy outcomes is unknown, and taking testosterone in pregnancy is not recommended within UK guidelines.[102] Due to this lack of evidence, some trans, non-binary, and gender non-conforming people delay commencing hormone therapy until their fertility goals are achieved; others delay pregnancy.[11, 103] Experiencing pregnancy while pausing, delaying, reversing, and/or hiding aspects of transition can increase gender dysphoria, all in addition to the adverse impact of testosterone or oestrogen cessation on mood.[103, 104] The effects of such intense gender dysphoria on pregnancy outcomes are unknown, although this may be comparable to the aforementioned effects of stress and stressors.

A national quantitative study in the United States explored pregnancy intentions and outcomes among 1,694 transgender, nonbinary, and gender-expansive people assigned female or intersex at birth.[11] Among survey respondents who had ever used testosterone, only 58% discussed the potential interactions between testosterone use and pregnancy with their health care provider. Of the pregnancies where the pregnant person reported using testosterone at the time when they became pregnant, 50% ended in miscarriage. While this study is to date the largest report of pregnancies experienced by gender diverse populations, the relevant sample size is very small (n=46). Other limitations include relying on participants accurately recalling testosterone initiation and cessation dates, and an absence of data on testosterone dosage and regimen compliance. Further research is needed in this area.

When discussing pregnancy and loss, the impact of hormone therapy is important not only for the physiological effects of testosterone therapy experienced by an individual person, but also for how that person's body is perceived by health care providers and written about in health care systems, as shown in the following case study.

CASE STUDY—SAM[105]

Sam, a 32-year-old trans man, entered triage with an 8-hour history of severe, intermittent lower abdominal pain, in hypertensive crisis, and with a positive home pregnancy test. Sam shared with the nurse in triage that he was trans, had previously used testosterone and antihypertensives, had stopped using both medications after losing insurance coverage, and that menstruation had ceased years prior. Sam also explained how he may have peed himself that morning. He was assessed to be an obese man with untreated chronic hypertension. Amongst other tests, a sample for human chorionic gonadotropin (hCG) testing was sent.

Several hours later, an emergency physician evaluated Sam. The serum hCG test result was positive, indicating pregnancy. On examination, Sam's abdomen was obese and gravid. Sam's clinical picture now suggested possible labour, placental abruption, and/or preeclampsia. Advanced pregnancy was confirmed via ultrasound with fetal cardiac activity unclear. A pelvic exam assessed Sam's cervix to be 4–5cm dilated and an umbilical cord was palpated in the vagina. Sam was transferred to theatre where no fetal heartbeat could be detected on ultrasound. He was transferred to a delivery suite where he birthed a stillborn baby.

Even though Sam explicitly stated that he was a trans man and the nurse recognised the possibility of pregnancy when she requested a serum hCG test, Sam's gender presentation meant that he was not evaluated using pregnancy algorithms in the way a cisgender woman presenting with a similar clinical picture would have been. If Sam had been evaluated in this way, the cord prolapse may have been detected in time to prevent fetal death.[105] Care pathways that enable trans men and non-binary people with uteruses to be evaluated for pregnancy, training for health care professionals that teaches how to care for populations based on clinical presentation instead of assumptions, and better understandings of how hormone therapy affects physical appearance, menstruation, and reproductive capacity will save lives.

RECOMMENDATIONS

- During pre-conception and antenatal care, discuss the potential for impaired pregnancy while using testosterone.
- In the event of miscarriage or stillbirth, if necessary, reassure the parent that a link between hormone therapy and pregnancy loss is unclear.
- Recognise limitations of current classification methods and consider each clinical presentation in its entirety.
- Update algorithms and records to recognise human diversity, documenting sex at birth, gender identity, and legal sex as three separate categories.

Provide staff education on the needs of trans people receiving hormone therapy, including writers of policies, algorithms, and systems.

CONCLUSION

This chapter has explored LGBTQ+ experiences of pregnancy loss with a focus on gestational and non-gestational journeys, intersectionality, and, where possible, research findings generated both in and beyond the UK. Current limitations in definitions, data capture methods, documentation, and algorithms have been outlined, as well as the impacts of minority stressors, culturally incompetent health care, and insufficient evidence about the effects of gender affirming hormone therapies. Positive and negative examples of bereavement support, care planning, and provision have been discussed, as well as how a pregnancy's conception affects the experience and processing of its unexpected end. Throughout, the need for a higher volume of more nuanced, community-led, and funded research into pregnancy loss experiences is clear, particularly in the LGBTQ+ community's sub-groups where any such evidence is yet to be generated.

REFERENCES

1. Craven C. *Reproductive Losses: Challenges to LGBTQ Family-Making*. Routledge; 2019.
2. NHS. Having a Baby if You're LGBT+. Published online 2021. Accessed July 25, 2022. https://www.nhs.uk/pregnancy/having-a-baby-if-you-are-lgbt-plus/
3. Craven C, Peel E. Queering Reproductive Loss: Exploring Grief and Memorialization. In: Lind E, Deveau A, eds. *Interrogating Pregnancy Loss: Feminist Writings on Abortion, Miscarriage, and Stillbirth*. Demeter Press; 2017:225–245.
4. Peel E. Pregnancy Loss in Lesbian and Bisexual Women: An Online Survey of Experiences. *Human Reproduction*. 2010;25(3):721–727. doi:10.1093/humrep/dep441
5. Wojnar D. Miscarriage Experiences of Lesbian Couples. *Journal of Midwifery & Women's Health*. 2007;52(5):479–485. doi:10.1016/j.jmwh.2007.03.015
6. Cacciatore J, Raffo Z. An Exploration of Lesbian Maternal Bereavement. *Social Work*. 2011;56(2):169–177. doi:10.1093/sw/56.2.169
7. Wojnar D, Swanson KM. Why Shouldn't Lesbian Mothers who Miscarry Receive Special Consideration? A Viewpoint. *Journal of GLBT Family Studies*. 2006;2(1):1–12. doi:10.1300/J461v02n01_01
8. Parent MC, DeBlaere C, Moradi B. Approaches to Research on Intersectionality: Perspectives on Gender, LGBT, and Racial/Ethnic Identities. *Sex Roles*. 2013;68:639–645. doi:10.1007/s11199-013-0283-2
9. Richards C, Barrett J. Introduction to Gender Diversity. In: *Trans and Non-Binary Gender Healthcare: For Psychiatrists, Psychologists, and Other Health Professionals*. Cambridge University Press; 2021:1–13.
10. Magnus MC, et al. Role of Maternal Age and Pregnancy History in Risk of Miscarriage: Prospective Register Based Study. *British Medical Journal (Online)*. 2019;364. doi:10.1136/bmj.l869
11. Moseson H, et al. Pregnancy Intentions and Outcomes Among Transgender, Nonbinary, and Gender-Expansive People Assigned Female or Intersex at Birth in the United States: Results from a National, Quantitative Study. *International Journal of Transgender Health*. 2021;22(1–2):30–41. doi:10.1080/26895269.2020.1841058
12. Ellis SA, Wojnar DM, Pettinato M. Conception, Pregnancy, and Birth Experiences of Male and Gender Variant Gestational Parents: It's How We Could Have a Family. *Journal of Midwifery & Women's Health*. 2015;60(1):62–69. doi:10.1111/jmwh.12213
13. LGBT Foundation. Trans and Non-Binary Experiences of Maternity Services: Survey Findings, Report and Recommendations. Published online 2022. Accessed August 2, 2022. https://lgbt.foundation/news/revealed-improving-trans-and-non-binary-experiences-of-maternity-services-items-report/475
14. Australian Institute of Health and Welfare. Stillbirths and Neonatal Deaths in Australia. Published online 2020. Accessed August 20, 2022. https://www.aihw.gov.au/reports/mothers-babies/stillbirths-and-neonatal-deaths-in-australia/contents/technical-notes/definitions-used-in-reporting
15. Zhu J, et al. Stillbirths in China: A Nationwide Survey. *BJOG*. 2021;128(1):67–76. doi:10.1111/1471-0528.16458

16. Ma R, Zou L. Stillbirth Trends by Maternal Sociodemographic Characteristics Among a Large Internal Migrant Population in Shenzhen, China, Over a 10-year Period: A Retrospective Study. *BMC Public Health*. 2022;22(325). doi:10.1186/s12889-022-12734-8

17. Qu Y, et al. Risk Factors of Stillbirth in Rural China: A National Cohort Study. *Scientific Reports*. 2019;9(365). doi:10.1038/s41598-018-35931-1

18. Murguía-Peniche T, et al. An Ecological Study of Stillbirths in Mexico from 2000 to 2013. *Bulletin of the World Health Organization*. 2016;94(5):322–330A. doi:10.2471/BLT.15.154922

19. UNICEF. Stillbirths. Published online 2020. Accessed August 20, 2022. https://data.unicef.org/topic/child-survival/stillbirths/

20. Fairbairn C. Registration of Stillbirth (Briefing paper Number 05595). Published online 2018. Accessed August 20, 2022. https://www.parliament.uk/globalassets/documents/commons-library/Registration-of-stillbirth-SN05595.pdf

21. American College of Obstetricians and Gynecologists. Management of Stillbirth: Obstetric Care Consensus No. 10. Published online 2020. Accessed August 20, 2022. https://www.acog.org/clinical/clinical-guidance/obstetric-care-consensus/articles/2020/03/management-of-stillbirth

22. World Health Organization (WHO). Making Every Baby Count: Audit and Review of Stillbirths. Published online 2016. Accessed August 20, 2022. https://apps.who.int/iris/rest/bitstreams/1060453/retrieve

23. Rose A, Oxlad M. The Lead Up To Loss: How Context Shapes LGBTQ+ Experiences of Pregnancy Loss. *LGBTQ+ Family: An Interdisciplinary Journal*. 2022;18(3):241–261. doi:10.1080/27703371.2022.2089308

24. Guyan K. *Queer Data: Using Gender, Sex and Sexuality Data for Action*. Bloomsbury; 2022.

25. National Institute for Health and Care Excellence (NICE). Ectopic Pregnancy and Miscarriage: Diagnosis and Initial Management. Published online 2019. Accessed July 25, 2022. https://www.nice.org.uk/guidance/ng126/resources/ectopic-pregnancy-and-miscarriage-diagnosis-and-initial-management-pdf-66141662244037

26. Earle S, Komaromy C, Layne LL. *Understanding Reproductive Loss: Perspectives on Life, Death and Fertility*. Routledge; 2012.

27. National Institute for Health and Care Excellence (NICE). NICE Style Guide. Published online 2023. Accessed March 9, 2023. https://www.nice.org.uk/corporate/ecd1/resources/nice-style-guide-pdf-1124007379909

28. UK Public General Acts. *Still-Birth (Definition) Act 1992 Section 1(1)*; 1992. https://www.legislation.gov.uk/ukpga/1992/29/section/1

29. UK Public General Acts. *Births and Deaths Registration Act 1953 Section 41*; 1953. https://www.legislation.gov.uk/ukpga/Eliz2/1-2/20/section/41

30. The Lancet. Miscarriage: Worldwide Reform of Care is Needed. *The Lancet*. 2021;397(10286):1597. doi:10.1016/s0140-6736(21)00954-5

31. Aminu M, van den Broek N. Stillbirth in Low- and Middle-Income Countries: Addressing the "Silent" Epidemic. *International Health*. 2019;11(4):237–239. doi:10.1093/inthealth/ihz015

32. DataBank. Health Nutrition and Population Statistics: Stillbirth Rate (Per 1,000 Births). Published online 2023. Accessed March 21, 2023. https://databank.worldbank.org/source/health-nutrition-and-population-statistics

33. Office for National Statistics (ONS). Births in England and Wales 2020. Published online 2021. Accessed August 2, 2022. https://www.ons.gov.uk/peoplepopulationandcomm unity/birthsdeathsandmarriages/livebirths/bulletins/birthsummarytablesenglandand wales/2020

34. Office for National Statistics (ONS). Deaths Registered in England and Wales. Published online 2021. Accessed August 2, 2022. https://www.ons.gov.uk/peoplepopulationand community/birthsdeathsandmarriages/deaths/datasets/deathsregisteredinenglandand walesseriesdrreferencetables

35. National Records of Scotland. Vital Events Reference Table 2020. Published online 2021. Accessed August 2, 2022. https://www.nrscotland.gov.uk/statistics-and-data/statistics/ statistics-by-theme/vital-events/general-publications/vital-events-reference-tables/2020

36. Northern Ireland Statistics and Research Agency (NISRA). Registrar General Annual Report 2020 Stillbirths and Infant Deaths. Published online 2021. Accessed August 2, 2022. https://www.nisra.gov.uk/publications/registrar-general-annual-report-2020-stillbirths- and-infant-deaths

37. Office for National Statistics (ONS). Births in England and Wales: 2021: Live Births, Stillbirths and the Intensity of Childbearing, Measured by the Total Fertility Rate. Published online 2022. Accessed August 20, 2022. http://www.ons.gov.uk/peoplepopula

38. Knight M, et al, eds. Saving Lives, Improving Mothers' Care: Lessons Learned to Inform Maternity Care from the UK and Ireland Confidential Enquiries into Maternal Deaths and Morbidity 2017–2019: MBRRACE-UK. Published online 2021.

39. Australian Psychological Society. Information Sheet: LGBT Pregnancy Loss. Published online n.d. Accessed July 27, 2022. https://psychology.org.au/getmedia/9ea8dd55-7c2b- 4653-8371-b1f732b70b58/lgbt_pregnancy_loss.pdf

40. Craven C, Peel E. Stories of Grief and Hope: Queer Experiences of Reproductive Loss. In: *Queering Maternity and Motherhood: Narrative and Theoretical Perspectives on Queer Conception, Birth and Parenting*. Demeter Press; 2014:97–110.

41. NHS. Causes: Miscarriage. Published online 2022. Accessed August 2, 2022. https://www. nhs.uk/conditions/miscarriage/causes/

42. Qu F, et al. The Association Between Psychological Stress and Miscarriage: A Systematic Review and Meta-Analysis. 2017;7(1):1731. doi:10.1038/s41598-017-01792-3

43. Everett BG, et al. Sexual Orientation Disparities in Pregnancy and Infant Outcomes. *Maternal and Child Health Journal*. 2019;23(1):72–81. doi:10.1007/s10995-018-2595-x

44. Malmquist A, et al. Minority Stress Adds an Additional Layer to Fear of Childbirth in Lesbian and Bisexual Women, and Transgender People. *Midwifery*. 2019;79:102551. doi:10.1016/j. midw.2019.102551

45. Malmquist A, et al. How Norms Concerning Maternity, Femininity and Cisgender Increase Stress Among Lesbians, Bisexual Women and Transgender People with a Fear of Child- birth. *Midwifery*. 2021;93:102888. doi:10.1016/j.midw.2020.102888

46. Everett B, et al. Sexual Identity Mobility and Depressive Symptoms: A Longitudinal Analysis of Moderating Factors Among Sexual Minority Women. *Archives of Sexual Behaviour*. 2016;45(7):1731–1744. doi:10.1007/s10508-016-0755-x

47. Quenby S, et al. Miscarriage Matters: The Epidemiological, Physical, Psychological, and Economic Costs of Early Pregnancy Loss. *The Lancet*. 2021;397(10302):1658–1667. doi:10. 1016/S0140-6736(21)00682-6

48. Tommy's. Devastating Impact of Miscarriage Laid Bare in New Research. https://www.tommys.org/about-us/news-views/devastating-impact-miscarriage-laid-bare-new-research. Published April 27, 2021. Accessed March 23, 2023.

49. Office for National Statistics (ONS). Birth Characteristics in England and Wales: 2021. Published online 2023. Accessed March 23, 2023. https://www.ons.gov.uk/people populationandcommunity/birthsdeathsandmarriages/livebirths/bulletins/birthcharacteri sticsinenglandandwales/2021

50. Rogers C, Greenfields M. Hidden Losses and 'Forgotten' Suffering: The Bereavement Experiences of British Romany Gypsies and Travellers. *Bereavement Care*. 2017;36(3):94–102. doi:10.1080/02682621.2017.1390281

51. Matthews R, et al. Understanding Ethnic Inequalities in Stillbirth Rates: A UK Population-Based Cohort Study. *BMJ Open*. 2022;12(2):e057412. doi:10.1136/bmjopen-2021-057412

52. Choudrey S. *Supporting Trans People of Colour: How to Make Your Practice Inclusive*. Jessica Kingsley; 2022.

53. Dissanayake MV, et al. Miscarriage Occurrence and Prevention Efforts by Disability Status and Type in the United States. *Journal of Women's Health*. 2020;29(3):345–352. doi:10.1089/jwh.2019.7880

54. Tarasoff LA, et al. Maternal Disability and Risk for Pregnancy, Delivery, and Postpartum Complications: A Systematic Review and Meta-Analysis. *American Journal of Obstetrics and Gynecology*. 2020;222(1):27.e1–28.e32. doi:10.1016/j.ajog.2019.07.015

55. McClelland A, et al. Seeking Safer Sexual Spaces: Queer and Trans Young People Labeled with Intellectual Disabilities and the Paradoxical Risks of Restriction. *Journal of Homosexuality*. 2012;59(6):808–819. doi:10.1080/00918369.2012.694760

56. Hodson K, Meads C, Bewley S. Lesbian and Bisexual Women's Likelihood of Becoming Pregnant: A Systematic Review and Meta-Analysis. *BJOG: An International Journal of Obstetrics and Gynaecology*. 2017;124(3):393–402. doi:10.1111/1471-0528.14449

57. Cioffi CC, Schweer-Collins ML, Leve LD. Pregnancy and Miscarriage Predict Suicide Attempts but not Substance Use Among Dual-Systems Involved Female Adolescents. *Children and Youth Services Review*. 2022;137:106494. doi:10.1016/j.childyouth.2022.106494

58. Hafeez H, et al. Health Care Disparities Among Lesbian, Gay, Bisexual, and Transgender Youth: A Literature Review. *Cureus*. 2017;9(4):e1184. doi:10.7759/cureus.1184

59. Gothwal S, et al. Effects of Substance Abuse During Pregnancy on Maternal and Fetal Health. *Perinatology*. 2023;23(3–4):153–160.

60. Olson-Chen C, Balaram K, Hackney DN. Chlamydia Trachomatis and Adverse Pregnancy Outcomes: Meta-Analysis of Patients With and Without Infection. *Maternal and Child Health Journal*. 2018;22(6):812–821. doi:10.1007/s10995-018-2451-z

61. Tang W, et al. Pregnancy and Fertility-Related Adverse Outcomes Associated with Chlamydia Trachomatis Infection: A Global Systematic Review and Meta-Analysis. *Sexually Transmitted Infections*. 2019;96(5):322–329. doi:10.1136/sextrans-2019-053999

62. Ban L, et al. Live and Non-Live Pregnancy Outcomes Among Women with Depression and Anxiety: A Population-Based Study. *PLoS One*. 2012;7(8):e43462. doi:10.1371/journal.pone.0043462

63. Kim M, et al. Pregnancy Prevalence and Outcomes in 3 United States Juvenile Residential Systems. *Journal of Pediatric and Adolescent Gynecology*. 2021;34(4):546–551. doi:10.1016/j.jpag.2021.01.005

64. Demakakos P, Linara-Demakakou E, Mishra GD. Adverse Childhood Experiences are Associated with Increased Risk of Miscarriage in a National Population-Based Cohort Study in England. *Human Reproduction*. 2020;35(6):1451–1460. doi:10.1093/humrep/deaa113

65. Zhong QY, et al. Adverse Obstetric Outcomes During Delivery Hospitalizations Complicated by Suicidal Behavior Among US Pregnant Women. *PLoS One*. 2018;13(2):e0192943. doi:10.1371/journal.pone.0192943

66. Boye K, Evertsson M. Who Gives Birth (First) in Female Same-Sex Couples in Sweden? *Journal of Marriage and Family*. 2021;83(4):925–941. doi:10.1111/jomf.12727

67. Office for National Statistics (ONS). Birth Characteristics in England and Wales: 2020. Published online 2021. Accessed August 29, 2022. https://www.ons.gov.uk/peoplepopulationand community/birthsdeathsandmarriages/livebirths/bulletins/birthcharacteristicsinengland andwales/2020

68. Martin JA, et al. Births: Final Data for 2021. *National Vital Statistics Report*. 2023;72(1): 1–53.

69. OECD. Age of Mothers at Childbirth and Age-Specific Fertility. Published online 2022. Accessed March 22, 2023. https://www.oecd.org/els/soc/SF_2_3_Age_mothers_childbirth. pdf

70. Liauw J, et al. Reproductive Healthcare in Prison: A Qualitative Study of Women's Experiences and Perspectives in Ontario, Canada. *PLoS One*. 2021;16(5):e0251853. doi:10.1371/journal.pone.0251853

71. Sufrin C, et al. Pregnancy Prevalence and Outcomes in U.S. Jails. *Obstetrics and Gynecology*. 2020;135(5):1177–1183. doi:10.1097/AOG.0000000000003834

72. Delap N. Pregnant Women in Custody. *British Journal of Midwifery*. 2022;30(4). Accessed July 25, 2022. https://www.britishjournalofmidwifery.com/content/charity-spotlight/pregnant-women-in-custody

73. Murray N, Summers H. Jailed Women in UK Five Times More Likely to Suffer Stillbirths, Data Shows. *The Observer*. https://www.theguardian.com/society/2021/dec/05/jailed-women-in-uk-five-times-more-likely-to-suffer-stillbirths-data-shows. Published December 5, 2021. Accessed August 25, 2022.

74. Prisons & Probation Ombudsman. Independent Investigation into the Death of Baby B at HMP&YOI Styal on 18 June 2020. Published online 2022. Accessed July 25, 2022. https://s3-eu-west-2.amazonaws.com/ppo-prod-storage-1g9rkhjhkjmgw/uploads/2022/01/F4376-20-Death-of-Baby-B-Styal-18-06-2020-NC-Under-18-0.pdf

75. Layne LL. *Motherhood Lost: A Feminist Account of Pregnancy Loss in America*. Routledge; 2014.

76. Kali KL. *Queer Conception: The Complete Fertility Guide for Queer and Trans Parents-to-Be*. Sasquatch Books; 2022.

77. Nadal KL, et al. Microaggressions towards Lesbian, Gay, Bisexual, Transgender, Queer, and Genderqueer People: A Review of the Literature. *Journal of Sex Research*. 2016;53(4–5):488–508. doi:10.1080/00224499.2016.1142495

78. Haines K, et al. "Not a Real Family": Microaggressions Directed toward LGBTQ Families. *Journal of Homosexuality*. 2018;65(9):1138–1151. doi:10.1080/00918369.2017.1406217

79. Perales F, et al. The Family Lives of Australian Lesbian, Gay and Bisexual People: A Review of the Literature and a Research Agenda. *Sex Research & Social Policy*. 2020;17(1):43–60. doi:10.1007/s13178-018-0367-4

80. Rose A, Oxlad M. LGBTQ+ Peoples' Experiences of Workplace Leave and Support Following Pregnancy Loss. *Community, Work and Family*. Published online 2022:1–17. doi:10.1080/13668803.2021.2020727

81. Riggs DW, Due C. Support for Family Diversity: A Three-Country Study. *Journal of Reproductive and Infant Psychology*. 2018;36(2):192–206. doi:10.1080/02646838.2018.1434491

82. Searle J, et al. Accessing New Understandings of Trauma-Informed Care with Queer Birthing Women in a Rural Context. *Journal of Clinical Nursing*. 2017;26(21–22):3576–3587. doi:10.1111/jocn.13727

83. Lacombe-Duncan A, et al. Minority Stress Theory Applied to Conception, Pregnancy, and Pregnancy Loss: A qualitative Study Examining LGBTQ+ People's Experiences. *PLoS One*. 2022;17(7):e0271945. doi:10.1371/journal.pone.0271945

84. Perlesz A, McNair R. Lesbian Parenting: Insiders' Voices. *Australian and New Zealand Journal of Family Therapy*. 2004;25(3):129–140. doi:10.1002/j.1467-8438.2004.tb00603.x

85. Andalibi N, et al. LGBTQ Persons' Use of Online Spaces to Navigate Conception, Pregnancy, and Pregnancy Loss: An Intersectional Approach. *ACM Transactions on Computer-Human Interaction*. 2022;29(1):2:1–2:46. doi:10.1145/3474362

86. Hagger-Holt S, Hagger-Holt R. *Pride and Joy: A Guide for Lesbian, Gay, Bisexual and Trans Parents*. Pinter and Martin; 2017.

87. Jaffe J. Detours on the Fertility Journey. *Psychotheraphy Networker, Washington*. 2020;44(4):20,22–27,54.

88. Gibson MF. *Queering Motherhood: Narrative and Theoretical Perspectives*. Demeter Press; 2014.

89. Perry Black B, Smith Fields W. Contexts of Reproductive Loss in Lesbian Couples. *MCN: The American Journal of Maternal/Child Nursing*. 2014;39(3):157–162. doi:10.1097/NMC.0000000000000032

90. Riggs DW, Due C, Power J. Gay Men's Experience of Surrogacy Clinics in India. *The Journal of Family Planning and Reproductive Health Care*. 2015;41(1):48–53. doi:10.1136/jfprhc-2013-100671

91. Rose A. *Adding More Layers to Loss: LGBTQ+ People's Experiences of Pregnancy Loss*. Bachelor of Psychological Science (Honours). The University of Adelaide; 2020.

92. Charter R, et al. The Transgender Parent: Experiences and Constructions of Pregnancy and Parenthood for Transgender Men in Australia. *International Journal of Transgenderism*. 2018;19(1):64–77. doi:10.1080/15532739.2017.1399496

93. Darwin Z, Greenfield M. Gestational and Non-Gestational Parents: Challenging Assumptions. *Journal of Reproductive and Infant Psychology*. 2022;40(1):1–2. doi:10.1080/02646838.2021.2020977

94. Abelsohn KA, Epstein R, Ross LE. Celebrating the "Other" Parent: Mental Health and Wellness of Expecting Lesbian, Bisexual, and Queer Non-Birth Parents. *Journal of Gay and Lesbian Mental Health*. 2013;17(4):387–405. doi:10.1080/19359705.2013.771808

95. Ross LE, et al. Perceptions of Partner Support Among Pregnant Plurisexual Women: A Qualitative Study. *Sexual and Relationship Therapy*. 2018;33(1–2):59–78. doi:10.1080/14681994.2017.1419562

96. Sullivan M. *The Family of Woman: Lesbian Mothers, Their Children, and the Undoing of Gender*. University of California Press; 2004.

97. Darwin Z, Greenfield M. Mothers and Others: The Invisibility of LGBTQ People in Reproductive and Infant Psychology. *Journal of Reproductive and Infant Psychology*. 2019;37(4):341–343. doi:10.1080/02646838.2019.1649919

98. NHS England. The NHS Long Term Plan. Published online 2019. Accessed August 29, 2022. https://www.longtermplan.nhs.uk/wp-content/uploads/2019/01/nhs-long-term-plan-june2019.pdf

99. Ratri A, et al. Fibrotic Changes in Transgender Ovaries due to Testosterone Exposure. *Cochrane Central Register of Controlled Trials*; *Fertility and Sterility*. 2020;(11):e528. doi:10.1016/j.fertnstert.2020.09.041

100. Moravek MB, et al. Impact of Exogenous Testosterone on Reproduction in Transgender Men. *Endocrinology*. 2020;161(3):bqaa014. doi:10.1210/endocr/bqaa014

101. Cheng PJ, et al. Fertility Concerns of the Transgender Patient. *Translational Andrology and Urology*. 2019;8(3):209–218. doi:10.21037/tau.2019.05.09

102. NHS. Testosterone and Pregnancy. Published online 2021. Accessed July 25, 2022. https://www.nhs.uk/pregnancy/having-a-baby-if-you-are-lgbt-plus/testosterone-and-pregnancy/

103. Hoffkling A, Obedin-Maliver J, Sevelius J. From Erasure to Opportunity: A Qualitative Study of the Experiences of Transgender Men Around Pregnancy and Recommendations for Providers. *BMC Pregnancy and Childbirth*. 2017;17(Suppl 2):332. doi:10.1186/s12884-017-1491-5

104. Kirubarajan A, et al. LGBTQ2S+ Childbearing Individuals and Perinatal Mental Health: A Systematic Review. *BJOG: An International Journal of Obstetrics and Gynaecology*. 2022; 00:1–14. doi:10.1111/1471-0528.17103

105. Stroumsa D, et al. The Power and Limits of Classification: A 32-year-old Man with Abdominal Pain. *The New England Journal of Medicine*. 2019;380:1885–1888. doi:10.1056/NEJMp1811491

Chapter 4

On abortion, sexual and gender minority pregnant people, and reproductive justice

A.J. Lowik

This chapter was written on the unceded territories of the xʷməθkʷəy̓əm (Musqueam), kwxwú7mesh (Squamish), and Səl̓ílwətaʔ (Tsleil-Watuth) peoples (a place colonially known as Vancouver, British Columbia). Forced sterilization, family break-up, and forced abortion are crimes that have been committed against Indigenous people since the arrival of my ancestors on these lands. These and other reproductive injustices have been integral elements of the egregious attempted genocide that was and is colonization.

INTRODUCTION

Abortion is an essential component of comprehensive health care, with around 73 million induced abortions occurring worldwide each year.[1, 2] The World Health Organization describes lack of access to safe, affordable, timely, and respectful abortion care as a "critical public health and human rights issue."[2] Abortion is also a cornerstone of reproductive justice, a term coined by Black feminists in the early 1990s to describe a series of interconnected human rights: the right to maintain bodily autonomy, the right to have children, the right not to have children, and the right to parent children in safe and sustainable communities.[3] Reproductive justice has always been an intersectional framework, a way of recognizing how systems of power and oppression operate to reify reproductive injustices, especially in the lives of the most precarious.[3] This chapter, then, is concerned with the abortion experiences of people who are precarious due to their being marginalized and minoritized based on their gender identities and/or sexualities. It is concerned with cisgender pregnant women who are queer, bisexual, pansexual, lesbian, or otherwise non-heterosexual (hereafter sexual minority), and with trans pregnant people of all gender identities and sexualities (hereafter gender minority).

DOI: 10.4324/9781003305446-5

Sexual and gender minority pregnant people are frequently erased from the abortion landscape – largely overlooked by researchers, regularly unconsidered by law, policy, and practice makers, and routinely removed from (or only peripherally included in) media coverage and activist efforts. This chapter will first consider what little is known about the abortion experiences of sexual and gender minority people, to inform clinical practice. It will then consider the various ways that abortion rights, queer rights, and trans rights are entangled. Sexual and gender minority people need and deserve access to safe, affordable, timely, and respectful abortion care; by considering the entanglement between abortion rights, trans rights, and queer rights, we can strategically work towards health, justice, and liberation for all.

THE EXPERIENTIAL

Sexual minority women and abortion

Sexual minority women need access to and have abortions – a fact that may seem paradoxical. Due to pervasive heteronormativity (the assumption that everyone is straight, and the treatment of heterosexuality as normal, natural, and more valuable than other sexualities), we have generally imagined the person accessing abortion to be a (cis) woman who has sexual and romantic relationships with (cis) men; and we have largely planned our research and service provision accordingly.[4, 5, 6, 7, 8, 9] Of course, the reality is much more complicated, and sexual minority women are involved in both intended and unintended (mistimed or unwanted) pregnancies. First, we must recall that the category of "sexual minority women" includes some women who have sexual and romantic relationships with (cis and trans) men, in ways that are compatible with their sexual identities or orientations (including, for example, bisexual, pansexual, and queer women, among others). Further, even among those sexual minority women whose sexual identity labels might signal an exclusive attraction to other women (eg, some lesbians), some women produce sperm (eg, some trans women). Therefore, it stands to reason that even in a relationship between two women, pregnancies can and do occur. Still other sexual minority women may have personal relationships exclusively with other women but engage in sex work with (cis) men clients.[10, 11, 12] Sexual minority women who are living in poverty, homeless or who have run away from their familial homes may engage in sex work, including survival sex and are at increased risk of being sexually exploited.[13] Finally, some sexual minority women may engage in "camouflage" sexual activities, that is, they may have sexual and romantic relationships with cis men to protect themselves against the potential discrimination and violence that can accompany being out as bisexual, lesbian, queer, etc.[14]

Given these facts, evidence suggests that sexual minority women experience intended, unintended and adolescent pregnancies at similar – and in some cases higher – rates than their straight counterparts. For instance, Bartelt et al.[5] found that bisexual women reported more incidences of unintended pregnancy and Everett et al.[15] found that all sexual minority women faced elevated risks of unintended pregnancy, in both cases as compared to straight women. Charlton et al.[16] found that all sexual minority women – except lesbians – were more likely to have ever been pregnant than their heterosexual peers. Among lesbian women, they were half as likely to have been pregnant as compared to heterosexual women.[16]

These incidences of pregnancy are attributed to a variety of factors, some of which parallel those impacting pregnancy prevalence among heterosexual women, and some of which are uniquely associated with the sexual identities, orientations, behaviours, and experiences of sexual minority women. For instance, cisgender, sexual minority girls report earlier average sexual initiation as compared to cisgender, heterosexual girls[16, 17] and sexual minority youth and adults generally have differences and gaps in their sexual health knowledge.[18, 19] Sexual minority women may also experience barriers to accessing and using contraceptive methods, including a lack of self-perception as someone who needs contraception, inconsistent or ineffective contraceptive use due to having the kinds of sex that may result in pregnancy infrequently, or due to past, actual and/or perceived discrimination in accessing sexual and reproductive health care services.[20, 21, 22] In order to make sense of pregnancy prevalence among sexual minority women, Everett et al.[15] highlights the importance of understanding sexual identity development over time, where someone may claim an identity today that stands in contrast to a previously held identity. It is also important to understand the difference between and to measure both sexual identity and sexual behaviour, where these are not always aligned in predictable ways.[15, 23]

Then, dishearteningly, sexual minority women experience sexual violence, rape, and reproductive coercion resulting in pregnancy, at increased rates compared to heterosexual women, including where the person's sexual minority identity is an aggravating or motivating factor in the assault.[13, 18, 24, 25] For instance, Jones, Jerman, and Charlton[26] found that one in ten pregnant lesbians reported that the pregnancy was the result of forced sex and were "18 times more likely than heterosexuals to report that the man involved in their pregnancy had sexually abused them." Forced sex and sexual violence during pregnancy were also reported at higher rates by bisexual women as compared to heterosexual women. Beyond pregnancies resulting from sexual intercourse (or sexual violence), sexual minority women may become intentionally pregnant via artificial reproductive technologies.

Some sexual minority women may endeavour to avoid pregnancy;[24] others may desire and actively seek out opportunities to become pregnant. These women will have a range of pregnancy intentions and by extension, a range of pregnancy outcomes, including where pregnancies are terminated for a variety of reasons. Sexual minority women may terminate their pregnancies for many of the same reasons as their heterosexual counterparts: due to relationship troubles, financial constraints, or medical concerns; because a pregnancy is mistimed; because of fetal anomalies; to reduce the number of fetuses they are carrying; or because they do not want any/any more children, etc.

Information regarding the prevalence of abortion among sexual minority women is scarce, and its reliability and validity are negatively impacted by a myriad of methodological challenges.[26] Notably, and for example, very few if any abortion providers collect patient sexual identities as a matter of practice. However, there is no doubt that sexual minority women have abortions, and at significant rates.[18] For instance, using data from the U.S. National Survey of Family Growth, Tornello et al.[27] estimated that bisexual youth were three times more likely to have had an abortion than heterosexual women – curiously, they found that no lesbian women reported past abortion experience. This stands in contrast to a 2004 study, which focused on the reproductive histories of 392 women who reported sexual activity with another woman in the last year.[28] Among the participants who identified as lesbian, one in five had been pregnant at least once, and 12% of those pregnancy-reporting lesbians indicating having had at least one induced abortion.[28] Januwalla et al.[29] found that sexual minority women in Toronto, Canada and Massachusetts, USA were more likely to report having terminated pregnancies as compared to heterosexual women, although the difference was not statistically significant.

Based on data from the Guttmacher Institute's 2014 Abortion Patient Survey, of abortion respondents who provided information about their sexuality, 94.5% identified as heterosexual, 4.1% identified as bisexual, 0.4% identified as lesbian, and a further 1.1% identified as something other than these three identities, most commonly as pansexual.[26] A systematic review examining the association of lesbian and bisexual women's identities and likelihood to become pregnant showed mixed results when it came to abortion incidences.[30] Across seven studies that reported induced abortion among lesbian and bisexual women, four showed lower rates and three showed higher rates in comparison with heterosexual women.[30] A study looking at the sexual and reproductive health of Kenyan women who have sex with women found that 13.2% of the 280 respondents reported having had at least one abortion, and whilst abortion was not related to age, level of education or employment status, it was related to income level and geographic region within the country.[31] The authors note that due to the widespread prevalence of unsafe abortions, and due to the barriers that sexual minority women face in accessing sexual and reproductive health care, sexual minority women in Kenya are at risk of developing post-abortion complications, including death.[31]

Where high rates of abortion are reported, this is likely due to higher incidences of unintended pregnancy among sexual minority women, rather than an indication of superior access to abortion care.[16] The factors impacting their decisions to terminate their pregnancies, some of which are itemized above, are as multifaceted as the factors influencing their becoming pregnant in the first place, and sexual minority women may experience substantial barriers to abortion care. Muzyczka et al.[32] found that sexual minority women contacted abortion providers sooner after discovering a pregnancy but reported longer temporal gaps between their initial contact and subsequent termination date as compared to heterosexual women. This means that sexual minority women were at the same average gestational stage of pregnancy at the time of their abortion as heterosexual women, despite having sought out abortion services sooner. Further, one participant in Carpenter et al.'s[24] study described how her sexual identity added an additional layer of difficulty in accessing abortion. Buffy, a 21-year-old pansexual woman from Salt Lake City described her identity as:

> "another layer of something that's already emotionally and financially and logistically difficult. And now it adds this whole other layer of something that is not quite what you identify with. Like if you don't really identify with wanting to have sex with people who could get you pregnant and then you do, it's another thing screwing up your life and you didn't even want the root of it."[24]

Not only may sexual minority women feel a sense of tension or incongruence between their identities, their sexual behaviours, and their subsequent need for abortion services, but abortion providers may inadvertently exasperate this tension. Abortion providers ought not assume that all patients will be heterosexual women[24, 26] and all sexual and reproductive health care providers ought not assume that sexual minority women should be precluded from sexual history taking, counselling, prescriptions, and referrals related to pregnancy and pregnancy prevention.[6, 8, 28] Erasure, in the form of heteronormativity, is manifest in explicit and implicit ways within abortion care settings, and abortion providers must work to acknowledge and plan for the arrival of sexual minority women.[6, 8]

Gender minority people and abortion

Gender minority people who were assigned female at birth need access to and have abortions. This includes people who identify as men, as nonbinary, as agender, or use a variety of other words to describe their gender identities, including some who claim "trans" as a component of their identities and others who do not. Gender minority people may engage in a range of sexual practices and identify with a range of sexual identity labels, ie, straight, gay, lesbian, queer, asexual, amongst others. Due to pervasive cisnormativity (the assumption that everyone is cisgender, and treatment of cisgender people as normal, natural, and more valuable than other gender modalities), researchers, clinicians and the general public alike, have generally imagined that the person accessing abortion services will be a (cis) woman, and abortion-related research and service provision have been designed and delivered accordingly.[5, 7, 24, 33] Of course, pregnancy is not contingent on gender identity, but is a phenomenon associated with sexed embodiment; where anyone assigned female at birth who has retained the anatomy and physiology of that sex assignment (and who has no others factors negatively impacting their fertility) can become pregnant and thus need abortion services.

In addition to cisnormativity, an interconnected framework called transnormativity is at play in our understanding of the sexual and reproductive lives of gender minority people. Transnormativity refers to a "specific ideological accountability structure to which transgender people's presentations and experiences of gender are held accountable."[34] Due to transnormativity, trans people are deemed more legitimate or authentic if they adhere to medicalized and binary narratives. For instance, a trans person is expected to reject their sexed body and its associated reproductive capacities as evidence of their gender identity, namely that they identify as the "opposite" gender to the one they were assigned.[35, 36, 37] As I have articulated in my previous work, "since men (cisnormatively speaking) do not have uteruses, vulvas, vaginas, do not get pregnant, do not give birth, do not lactate or nurse children, a transnormative ideology would reason that trans men, as men, should also not have these body parts, should not engage in these embodied, reproductive experiences."[35] The "right body" is framed as the cisgender one – to have been assigned female, and to identify as a woman, with a desire for gestational motherhood is framed as normal, natural and "right." The "wrong body," by contrast, is the trans person's body which stands in opposition to or is incongruous with their gender identity – a trans person is supposed to understand their sexed body as somehow "wrong" because it's not the body that (cisnormatively speaking) belongs to a person with their gender identity. To be a man, and have the capacity for pregnancy, is framed as having the "wrong" body. The "solution" (or "treatment") to having the "wrong body" is to reject that sexed body and to pursue social and medical means of transition – efforts to make one's body "right" – some of which will permanently foreclose the possibility of fertility and reproduction.[35]

While there are certainly some people whose personal experiences adhere to these narratives, there are many for whom this does not resonate. There are, for example, many trans people who do not seek out medical transition despite wanting to (eg, because they have health conditions that would be complicated by medical transition; because they cannot financially afford to transition; because access to medical transition is unavailable or heavily gatekept where they live; because they have concerns about hormonal or surgical outcome satisfaction). There are still others who have no desire to medically transition, and may experience their sexed body neutrally, or even positively.

When it comes to pregnancy, there are some trans people who cannot imagine the possibility of pregnancy, due to the potential dysphoria or distress it would induce.[38, 39] Others describe pregnancy as merely tolerable, where they have weighed the potential and actual embodied distress against their family forming plans and goals.[40] Still others experience no gender-specific dysphoria associated with pregnancy itself, although they may report distress associated with being misgendered, mistreated, and having to navigate legal and health care environments where they are unintelligible.[41] For some trans people, pregnancy is a positive experience – an opportunity to use their sex assigned bodies towards a desired goal. However, due to these transnormative logics, clinicians may find themselves surprised to learn that gender minority people use their genitals for the purposes of sexual pleasure and/or sexual reproduction.[42] The pregnancies of gender minority people are treated as exceptional, out of the ordinary and unexpected.[40, 43]

Evidence suggests that gender minority youth have the same rate of adolescent pregnancy (roughly 5%) as their cisgender counterparts.[44] Studies focusing on gender minority adults report pregnancy prevalence rates among the gender minority participants in their research projects, rather than comparing those rates to cisgender people. For instance, Stark et al.[45] identified a 5.3% pregnancy rate among trans adults aged 21–64 (with 3.3% ending in birth). Light et al.[46] indicated that 17% of the trans men aged 18+ who participated in their study reported one or more lifetime pregnancies – with 12% of the total reported pregnancies ending in abortion (as compared to the US abortion rate of 21% in 2011 and 19% in 2014). Finally, Moseson et al.[47] indicated that 12% of 1,694 gender minority survey respondents assigned female at birth had been pregnant at least once, reporting 433 pregnancies experienced by 210 individuals. Among those 210 individuals, 67 reported a total of 92 abortions, including 41 surgical abortions,[i] 23 medical abortions[ii] and 3 terminations by another method. Nearly 1/3 of the respondents indicated that their abortion(s) occurred at less than 9 weeks gestation. Across these three studies, gender minority people reported pregnancies that occurred while on testosterone, and after temporarily pausing or permanently stopping their use of testosterone.[45, 46, 47]

As with sexual minority women, there are a myriad of factors impacting intended and unintended pregnancy among gender minority people. These include a lack of comprehensive and inclusive sexual education (in school and clinical settings),[48, 49] barriers to accessing and using effective contraceptive methods,[33, 45] and misinformation about testosterone's effectiveness as a contraceptive.[39, 50] Gender minority youth and adults are also at increased risk of sexual violence, rape, and reproductive coercion,[51, 52] and some engage in sex work, including survival sex work.[4, 53] Again, gender minority people may also become intentionally pregnant including via sexual intercourse and/or artificial reproductive technologies. These people will have a range of pregnancy intentions and by extension, a range of pregnancy outcomes, including where pregnancies are terminated for a variety of reasons.

Research generated in the United States found that approximately 500 trans people obtained abortions in clinics in 2017.[54] This figure was based on provider reports, where providers were asked to calculate or estimate how many patients they had served who identified as transgender, gender nonbinary, or gender nonconforming. Importantly, many facilities responded in ways that indicated that since information about patients' gender identities was not routinely collected, no answer could be provided with any degree of certainty. Of the 1,069 non-hospital facilities providing abortion care, 85 reported having provided abortions to 230 trans people, with weighted estimates of between 462 and 530.[54] Importantly, it would not be unexpected for gender minority people to conceal their identities when accessing abortion, and most clinics do not collect patients' genders.[33, 55, 56] Therefore, this figure represents an underestimation. To gather more accurate data on the gender identities of abortion patients, Janiak et al.[56] conducted a large, multicenter patient survey in a single state of the USA. They found that 2.7% of the 1,553 participants who completed the survey identified as something other than female or woman. These 42 participants reported 14 different gender identities, including 11 (0.9%) who identified as a man, male, trans man or transmasculine person, 6 (0.4%) who identified as nonbinary, 6 (0.4%) identified as agender, 5 (0.3%) identified as Two-Spirit. Participants also reported their identities as gender nonconforming (n=3, 0.2%), gender fluid (n=3, 0.2%), genderqueer (n=2, 0.1%), gender expansive (n=1, 0.1%), bigender (n=1, 0.1%), boi (n=1, 0.1%), or another gender identity (n=3, 0.2%).[56]

Gender minority people's pregnancy termination decisions (including the type of abortion that they would prefer to access and/or do access) are impacted by concerns over privacy, autonomy, invasiveness, pain, certainty of success, and wanting to avoid or, alternatively, have access to health care providers.[57] Moseson et al.[58] found that some gender minority people have elected to attempt abortion without clinical supervision, including by means of herbs, vitamins, physical trauma, substance use, fasting, acupuncture, use of birth control or emergency contraception, and excessive physical activity. The reasons for attempting to end a pregnancy without supervision included barriers associated with cost, insurance, gestational limits, fear of partners finding out, as well as actual or perceived discrimination, misgendering, care denial, bias, and lack of trans competence on the part of abortion providers.[58] Gender minority youth experiencing homelessness and housing precarity may also attempt self-induced abortion outside of formal health care settings, due to lack of funds, and misinformation about abortion costs and steps needed to access abortion.[59]

Cisnormatively gendered reproductive health spaces, including abortion spaces, are replete with barriers for people who do not identify as women. These include all the same legal, logistical, financial, and emotional barriers experienced by cisgender, heterosexual and sexual minority women, as well as some barriers that are unique to gender minority people. For instance, gender minority people are frequently excluded from discussions about abortion – in schools, on television or in films, by news media, or around dinner tables – where this lack of representation affects abortion access.[4, 51] Additionally, abortion care is frequently delivered in ways that tether it specifically and exclusively to women, in ways that do not acknowledge the possibility of non-women abortion patients.[33] This is manifest in the use of gendered language to name and advertise clinical spaces, as well the language used during clinical encounters to talk about sexual partners, pregnancy risk and pregnancy prevention.[33, 56, 60, 61] Abortion staff may lack training in delivering trans culturally competent and gender-affirming care.[8, 55, 56, 60, 62] As a result, gender minority people may experience administrative violence (eg, inappropriate intake forms, issues with electronic medical records)[57, 60, 63] or misgendering and outing within abortion spaces.[47, 64] Some gender minority people also report having to engage with providers who espouse anti-trans sentiments,[4] being denied care due to provider "conscientious objection" and due to misunderstandings about the sexual and reproductive health care needs of gender minority people,[64] experiencing or witnessing discriminatory comments,[4, 61] and having their identities interrogated and/or invalidated by health care providers.[61, 64]

Abortion providers ought not assume that all patients will be women. Erasure, in the form of cisnormativity, is manifest in explicit and implicit ways within abortion care settings, and abortion providers must work to acknowledge and plan for the arrival of gender minority patients.

THE ENTANGLEMENT

Abortion rights are entangled with sexual and gender minority rights, because many sexual minority women and gender minority people of all genders have abortions.[65] As such, there are important opportunities for coalition and community building across activist and social justice movements, where cis and trans people of all genders and sexualities can work together to effectively secure, expand and safeguard abortion rights and access. Sexual and gender minority people have not sat idly by; they have actively contributed to the securement of abortion rights, despite attempts to render their activist contributions peripheral or controversial – this attempted erasure of trans and travesti[iii] abortion activists is notable in Argentina.[7, 67, 68] In this section, I will briefly itemize and explore the entanglement of queer, trans and abortion rights, in ways beyond the experiential.

Shared struggles, shared rights

We begin by acknowledging that sexual and gender minority people need abortions, and that as such, have stakes in all abortion rights efforts. Beyond that, however, many of the efforts to advance reproductive justice, and to advance the rights of sexual and gender minority people, as separate movements, evoke the same series of human rights – the right to privacy, bodily autonomy, dignity, etc. For example, it is frequently argued that abortion constitutes a private, medical decision, and as such ought to be protected due to the right to privacy guaranteed by many jurisdictions and constitutions.[69] At the same time, where the right to privacy includes the right to make decisions regarding one's marriage, family and children, there is some uncertainty as to whether this right is extended to sexual and gender minority people in the same way (eg, the United States Supreme Court refused to strike down the sodomy statute in Georgia, and argued that the right to privacy did not extend to private, consensual sexual conduct between people of the same gender. However, privacy state constitutions were used to invalidate sodomy laws in other states).[70] Further, Ashley[71] has effectively argued that the right to autonomy is central to ensuring that people below the age of majority can consent to health care that they want and need. This includes, for example, working to challenge jurisdictions that require parental consent for minors accessing abortion services *and* where minors require parental consent to access gender-affirming, medical transition interventions like hormones and surgery. Where efforts are made to curtail the rights of youth in either area of health care, youth rights in other areas of health care are similarly threatened. As such, Ashley[71] argues, we ought to be alarmed by efforts to limit youths' ability to consent to gender-affirming health care, because these limits would simultaneously undermine youths' ability to consent to abortion and vice versa – in each case, the right to bodily autonomy needs to be secured. By recognizing that all people ought to have bodily autotomy, the right to privacy, and other human rights, coalitions and alliances across social and reproductive justice movements can be forged.[7, 65]

Synchronicity of anti-attitudes, interconnected attacks?

Political commentators and politicians tend to assume that people who share a particular religious-based value that is anti-abortion, will similarly espouse anti-queer and anti-trans values, and vice versa.[72, 73] The assumed interconnectedness of these attitudes towards abortion and queer/trans people and rights is frequently evoked as evidence of a singular, unified, religious objection to both, such that particular candidates running for political office will be framed as ideal, based on their perceived willingness to work towards the eradication of these rights once in office, due to their "moral/family values." This synchrony of values is not supported by the evidence, however. Various factors impact whether people for whom religion is important, will also oppose abortion and/or same-sex marriage, and also impact whether or how they will vote.[72] When looking at national policies around abortion and gay rights, and country-level economic and cultural realities (eg, religiosity, fertility demands) it is ultimately how countries value *gender equality* that explains any potential correlation.[73] That is, where gender equality is valued, abortion legality and gay rights follow; securing abortion rights and advancing gay rights are possible, when a country values and works to achieve equality between (cis) men and women.[73] Importantly, recent, and ongoing attempts to restrict abortion in various Republican-dominated states in the United States of America, have been accompanied and preceded by a series of anti-trans bills.[74] In a kind of sad and infuriating irony, "protecting women and children" is evoked as a defense for anti-trans legislation, while the politicians who purport to want to protect women are working systematically to eliminate their ability to access abortion.[75]

Parallel pseudoscience

There are shocking parallels between the unvalidated and unvalidatable intervention that is "post-abortion grief counseling" and so-called "reparative or conversion therapies."[76] The former is the name given to typically religious-based, pseudoscientific "treatments" for people who are understood as necessarily experiencing grief following their having committed the "sin" of abortion. The latter is one of many names[iv] given to efforts to deny, suppress, repress or change the sexual identity, gender identity or gender expression of sexual and/or gender minority people. Each "therapy" relies on a series of unmeasurable and unvalidated assumptions which masquerade as science. Since 'post-abortion grief counseling' and 'reparative or conversion therapies' share similar ideological foundations and so-called "therapeutic" strategies, and since both occur in religious and purportedly therapeutic settings, there is an opportunity for coalition building among activists invested in their elimination. People working to eliminate pregnancy crisis centres,[77] and to discredit other proponents of 'post-abortion grief counseling' can learn from those working to eradicate sexual orientation and gender identity change efforts. These are two religious-based pseudosciences with similar goals and tactics; understanding their interconnectedness will only improve our efforts to ensure that all people's human rights are respected.

Sexuality- and trans-selective abortion?

Sex-selective abortion is the practice of terminating a pregnancy based on the predicted sex of the fetus, where there is a cultural or personal preference for children of a particular sex – typically male children, due to deep-rooted sexism and misogyny. Sex-selection abortion is practiced in certain regions of certain countries,[78, 79] although the exact prevalence is uncertain and, in some instances, its prevalence has been overstated.[80] A companion to sex-selective abortion, regardless of its prevalence, are concerns about sexuality and trans-selective abortion. In particular, there are fears that the search for genetic causes of sexual orientation could result in sexuality-selective abortion, where fetuses predicted to be something other than straight are aborted. There is a parallel fear that the search for genetic causes of non-cis gender modalities could result in trans-selective abortion, where fetuses predicted to be something other than cisgender are aborted.[81, 82] The likelihood of these possibilities is beyond the scope of this chapter. However, suffice to say that even the purely hypothetical potential for eugenics logics being used to abort fetuses that could grow into sexual and gender minority people is disturbing, and ought to be top of mind as genetic research and technology advances.

The role of stigma

Clearly, abortion remains highly stigmatized. People who access abortion care report the judgment of others, self-judgment, community condemnation and internally and externally imposed silence and isolation as sites of abortion stigma that they must navigate.[4, 8, 83] Similarly, abortion providers report having to navigate and manage stigma associated with their jobs, including by self-censorship, strategic identity concealment, and disavowal.[84] These are similar strategies undertaken by gender and sexual minority people, many of whom self-censor, and do not disclose their identities to health care providers, their employers, or others, for fear of the consequences.[85] Sexual and gender minority people who need access to abortion experience a double stigma, having to navigate stigmatized identities within stigmatized abortion care spaces.[84] Further, for individuals who are both abortion providers and sexual minorities, the stigma is also doubled with many reporting having to lie about, avoid, or hide one or both of their identities.[86] Efforts to destigmatize abortion, as well as gender and sexual minority identities would undoubtedly improve the health and wellbeing of all people who provide abortions, and all people who need them.

THE RECOMMENDATIONS

Based on what is known about the experiences of sexual minority women and gender minority people accessing abortion care, what follows is a brief list of recommendations for creating inclusive and affirming abortion care settings:

1. Plan for the arrival of sexual minority women and gender minority people, including by updating websites, intake forms, and language used to communicate about sex, pregnancy risk and pregnancy prevention.

These patients may access abortion for reasons that are entangled with and complicated by their sexual and/or gender identities, so providers need to be prepared to support these patients accordingly.

2.   Recognize the importance of asking abortion patients about their sexual orientations and gender identities (both as a matter of practice and for the purposes of research). Create climates that welcome and encourage patients and abortion providers to disclose these and other facets of their identities.

3.   Work to address barriers to care for sexual and gender minority youth, who may have particularly high rates of adolescent pregnancy, and particular barriers associated with accessing abortion care due to their ages.

4.   Abortion providers are well-positioned to offer gender-affirming care, and many non-hospital, free-standing abortion facilities (a clinic model that is used in some countries) are already providing trans-specific health care services.[54, 63, 81] Combining these services may be advantageous, but also logistically challenging. Be aware of the ways that gender minority people may experience abortion care spaces as de facto community clinics – including by alerting patients to the possibility of their having to navigate protestors.[84]

5.   Remember that sexual and gender minority people are already experiencing barriers to abortion, and that these barriers are exacerbated for folks who are also low income/living in poverty, racialized, disabled, etc.[65] Endeavour to create abortion spaces and services that are accessible for all.

THE MAIN LEARNING

1.   Sexual and gender minority people experience unintended, intended, and adolescent pregnancies, and as such need access to abortion services.

2.   The factors impacting sexual and gender minority people's pregnancy intentions and outcomes include legal, financial, logistical, and emotional factors that are not unique to them, as well as factors that are tied to their identities, expressions, experiences, and/or behaviours.

3.   Sexual and gender minority people experience barriers to abortion care, based on pervasive cisnormativity and heteronormativity, which position abortion as a health care need of primarily, if not exclusively, cisgender, heterosexual women.

4.   Abortion, queer and trans rights are entangled – not just because queer and trans people need abortions. These entanglements are opportunities to create coalition and community and stronger social and reproductive justice movements when we see our health and liberation as intertwined.

NOTES

i Also known as suction or vacuum aspiration abortion, surgical abortion is a minor surgical procedure, where tissue, products of conception or the fetus and placenta are removed from inside the uterus. Dilation and curettage (D&C) is a specific type of surgical procedure, where the cervix is widened and the contents of the uterus are removed using a surgical instrument called a curette. A D&C can be used to treat a variable of conditions, and sometimes the reason for this procedure is pregnancy termination.

ii Also known as medication abortion or abortion with pills, medical abortion is where a pregnancy is terminated using medications and without surgery.

iii While originally a pejorative, travesti has been reclaimed by Argentinian and Peruvian activists. It translates to "cross-dressing," and is used to refer to South American people who cross-genders, cross-sexes, and cross-dress. Peruvian performance artist and philosopher Giuseppe Campuzano has argued Spanish colonists were fixated on gender/sex binaries, including the "imperative to dress according to one's place within a rigid gender dichotomy,"[66] but that pre-Hispanic cultures did not treat gender as a binary. Travesti has thus been reclaimed and renamed as meaning "duality as power," and is seen by made as a political noun.[66]

iv The language of Sexual Orientation and Gender Identity Change Efforts (SOCIGE) has been recently adopted to more accurately describe these practices which have been scientifically discredited and denounced by many major mental health organizations. Both 'post-abortion grief counseling' and 'reparative or conversion therapies' are formatted in single quotes, to both use the language of the people who espouse these "treatments" and to cast this language into doubt.

REFERENCES

1. Perehudoff K, Pizzarossa LB, Stekelenburg J. Realising the Right to Sexual and Reproductive Health: Access to Essential Medicines for Medical Abortion as a Core Obligation. *BMC International Health and Human Rights*. 2018;18(1):1–7.

2. Abortion. World Health Organization. Accessed June 28, 2022. https://www.who.int/news-room/fact-sheets/detail/abortion. Published November 25, 2021.

3. Reproductive Justice. SisterSong: Women of Color Reproductive Justice Collective. (n.d.). Accessed June 28, 2022. https://www.sistersong.net/reproductive-justice.

4. Bartelet E. Sexual and Gender Minoritized Young Adult (14–26 Year Old) Abortion Experiences in the United States. [Dissertation]. Bloomington, IN: Indiana University; 2020.

5. Bartelet E, Fu T, Dodge B, Herbenick D. Lifetime Prevalence of Abortion Among Sexual Minority Populations in the United States. Oral presentation at: American Public Health Association Annual Meeting and Expo, November 2019; Philadelphia.

6. Everett BG, Sanders JN, Myers K, Giest C, Turok DK. One in Three: Challenging Heteronormative Assumptions in Family Planning Centers. *Contraception*. 2018;98(4):270–274.

7. Fernandez Romero F. 'We Can Conceive Another History': Trans Activism Around Abortion Rights in Argentina. *International Journal of Transgender Health*. 2020;22(1–2):126–140.

8. Gessner M, Bishop MD, Martos A, Wilson BDM, Russell ST. Sexual minority People's Perspectives of Sexual Health Care: Understanding Minority Stress in Sexual Health Settings. *Sexual Research and Social Policy*. 2019;17:607–618.

9. Sutton B, Borland E. Queering Abortion Rights: Notes from Argentina. *Culture, Health & Sexuality: An International Journal for Research, Intervention and Care*. 2018;20(12): 1378–1393.

10. Browne K, Cull M, Hubbard P. The Diverse Vulnerabilities of Lesbian, Gay, Bisexual and Trans Sex Workers in the UK. In: Hardy K, Kingston S, Sanders T, eds. *New Sociologies of Sex Work*. Routledge; 2010:197–212.

11. Lyons T, Kerr T, Puff P, Feng C, Shannon K. Youth, Violence and Non-Injection Drug Use: Nexus of Vulnerabilities Among Lesbian and Bisexual Sex Workers. *AIDS Care*. 2014; 26(9):1090–1094.

12. Shrage, LS. Do Lesbian Prostitutes Have Sex with their Clients: A Clintonesque Reply. *Sexualities*. 1999;2(2):259–261.

13. Robson R. Lesbians and Abortion. *NYI Review of Law & Social Change*. 2011;35: 247–279.

14. Saewyc EM, Poon CS, Homma Y, Skay CL. Stigma Management? The Links between Enacted Stigma and Teen Pregnancy Trends Among Gay, Lesbian and Bisexual Students in British Columbia. *Canadian Journal of Human Sexuality*. 2008;17(3):123–139.

15. Everett BG, McCabe KF, Hughes TL. Sexual Orientation Disparities in Mistimed and Unwanted Pregnancy Among Adult Women. *Perspectives on Sexual and Reproductive Health*. 2017;49(3):157–165.

16. Charlton BM, Everett BG, Light A, Jones RK, Janiak, E, Gaskins AJ, Chavarro JE, Moseson H, Sarda V, Austin SB. Sexual Orientation Differences in Pregnancy and Abortion Across the Lifecourse. *Women's Health Issues*. 2020;30(2):65–72.

17. Saewyc EM, Lin C, Santana Parrila J, Nath R, Ybarra M. First Time Sexual Experiences of Sexual Minority Girls in the United States. *Psychology & Sexuality*. 2022 [published online ahead of print].

18. Jerman J, Jones J, Onda T. Characteristics of US Abortion Patients in 2014 and Changes Since 2008. Guttmacher Institute. Accessed June 28, 2022. https://www.guttmacher.org/report/characteristics-us-abortion-patients-2014?TB_iframe=true&width=921.6&height=921.6

19. Paschen-Wolff MM, Greene MZ, Hughes, TL. Sexual Minority Women's Sexual and Reproductive Health Literacy: A Qualitative Descriptive Study. *Health Education Behavior*. 2020;47(5):728–739.

20. Bowling J, Simons M, Blekfeld-Sztraky D, Bartelet E, Dodge B, Vundarraman V, Lakshimi B, Herbenick D. 'It's a Walk of Shame': Experiences of Unintended Pregnancy and Abortion Among Sexual- and Gender-Minoritized Females in Urban India. *The Journal of Medicine Access @ Point of Care*. 2021;5:1–10.

21. Charlton BM, Janiak E, Gaskins AJ, DiVasta AD, Jones RK, Missmer SA, Chavarro JE, Sarda V, Rosario M, Austin SB. Contraceptive Use by Women Across Different Sexual Orientation Groups. *Contraception*. 2019;100(3):202–208.

22. Higgins JA, Carpenter E, Everett BG, Greene MZ, Haider S, Hendrick E. Sexual Minority Women and Contraceptive Use: Complex Pathways Between Sexual Orientation and Health Outcomes. *AJPH Perspectives*. 2019;109(12):1680–1686.

23. Hartnett CS, Lindley LL, Walsemann KM. Congruence Across Sexual Orientation Dimensions and Risk for Unintended Pregnancy Among Adult US Women. *Women's Health Issues*. 2016;27(2):145–151.
24. Carpenter E, Everett BG, Greene MZ, Haider S, Hendrick CE, Higgins JA. Pregnancy (Im)possibilities: Identifying Factors that Influence Sexual Minority Women's Pregnancy Desires. *Social Work in Health Care*. 2020;59(3):180–198.
25. Park J, Nordstrom SK, Weber KM, Irwin T. Reproductive Coercion: Uncloaking an Imbalance of Social Power. *American Journal of Obstetrics and Gynecology*. 2016;124(1):74–78.
26. Jones RK, Jerman J, Charlton BM. Sexual Orientation and Exposure to Violence Among U.S. Patients Undergoing Abortion. *Obstetrics and Gynecology*. 2018;132(3):605–611.
27. Tornello SL, Riskind RG, Patteron CJ. Sexual Orientation and Sexual Health and Reproductive Health Among Adolescent Young Women in the United States. *Journal of Adolescent Health*. 2014;54(2):1601–1668.
28. Marrazzo JM, Stine K. Reproductive Health History of Lesbians: Implications for Care. *American Journal of Obstetrics and Gynecology*. 2004;190(5):1298–1304.
29. Januwalla AA, Goldbert AE, Flanders CE, Yudin MH, Ross LE. Reproductive and Pregnancy Experiences of Diverse Sexual Minority Women: A Descriptive Exploratory Story. *Maternal and Child Health Journal*. 2019;23:1071–1078.
30. Hodson K, Meads C, Bewley S. Lesbian and Bisexual Women's Likelihood of Becoming Pregnant: A Systematic Review and Meta-Analysis. *BJOG: An International Journal of Obstetrics and Gynaecology*. 2016;124(3):393–402.
31. Zaid SS, Ocholla AM, Otieno RA, Sandfort TGM. Women Who Have Sex with Women in Kenya and their Sexual and Reproductive Health. *LGBT Health*. 2016;3(2):139–145.
32. Muzyczka Z, Brenner-Levoy J, Turner AN, Norris A, Bessett D. Timing is Everything: Differences in Timing of Abortion Care by Sexual Orientation. *Contraception*. 2021;104(4):454.
33. Fix L, Durden M, Obedin-Maliver J, Moseson H, Hastings J, Stoefflers A, Baum SE. Stakeholder Perceptions and Experiences Regarding Access to Contraception and Abortion for Transgender, Non-Binary and Gender-Expansive Individuals Assigned Female at Birth in the U.S. *Archives of Sexual Behavior*. 2020;49:2683–2702.
34. Johnson AH. Transnormativity: A New Concept and its Validation through Documentary Film About Transgender Men. *Sociological Inquiry*. 2016;86(4):465–491.
35. Lowik A.J. Betwixt, Between, Besides: Reflections on Moving Beyond the Binary in Reproductive Health Care. *Creative Nursing*. 2020;26(2):106–108.
36. Lowik, A.J. Reproducing Eugenics, Reproducing while Trans: The State Sterilization of Trans People. *The Journal of GLBT Family Studies*. 2018;14(5):425–445.
37. Verlinden J. Transgender Bodies and Male Pregnancy: The Ethics of Radical Self-Refashioning. In: Hampf HH, Snyder-Korber M, eds. *Machines: Bodies, Genders and Technologies*. Heidelberg; 2012:107–136.
38. Chen D, Matson M, Macapagal K, Johnson EK, Rosoklija I, Finlayson CA, Mustanski B. Attitudes Toward Fertility and Reproductive Health Among Transgender and Gender-Nonconforming Adolescents. *Journal of Adolescent Health*. 2018;63(1):62–68.
39. Kanj R, Conard L, Corathers SD, Trotman GE. Hormonal Contraceptive Choices in a Clinic-Based Series of Transgender Adolescents and Young Adults. *International Journal of Transgenderism*. 2019;20(4):413–420.

40. Lampe, NM, Carter, SK, Sumerau JE. Continuity and Change in Gender Frames: The Case of Transgender Reproduction. *Gender & Society*. 2019;33(6):865–887.

41. Malgaria A. Trans Men Giving Birth and Reflections on Fatherhood: What to Expect? *International Journal of Law, Policy and the Family*. 2020;34(3):225–246.

42. Cromwell J. Queering the Binaries: Transsituated Identities, Bodies and Sexualities. In: Stryker S, Whittle S, eds. *The Transgender Studies Reader*. Routledge; 2006:509–520.

43. Dietz E. Normal Parents: Trans Pregnancy and the Production of Reproducers. *International Journal of Transgender Health*. 2020;22(1–2):191–202.

44. Veale J, Watson RJ, Adjei J, Saewyc E. Prevalence of Pregnancy Involvement Among Transgender Youth and its Relation to Mental Health, Sexual Health, and Gender Identity. *International Journal of Transgenderism*. 2016;17(3–4):107–113.

45. Stark B, Hughto JMW, Charlton BM, Deutsch MB, Potter J, Reisner SL. The Contraceptive and Reproductive History and Planning Goals of Trans-Masculine Adults: A Mixed-Methods Study. *Contraception*. 2019;100(6):468–473.

46. Light, A, Wang, L, Zeymo, A & Gomez-Lobo, V. Family Planning and Contraception Use in Transgender Men. *Contraception*. 2018;98(4):266–269.

47. Moseson H, Fix L, Hastings J, Stoeffler A, Lunn MR, Flentje A, Lubensky ME, Capriotti MR, Ragosta A, Forsberg H, Obedin-Maliver J. Pregnancy Intentions and Outcomes Among Transgender, Nonbinary, and Gender-Expansive People Assigned Female or Intersex at Birth in the United States: Results from a National, Quantitative Survey. *International Journal of Transgender Health*. 2020;22(1–2):30–41.

48. Dodson NA, Langer M. The Reproductive Health Care of Transgender Young People: A Guide for Primary Care Providers. *Pediatric Annals*. 2019;48(2):64–70.

49. Rabbitte M. Sex Education in Schools, are Gender and Sexual Minority Youth Included: A Decade in Review. *American Journal of Sexuality Education*. 2020;15(4):530–542.

50. Gomez A, Walters PC, Dao LT. 'Testosterone in a Way is Birth Control:' Contraceptive Attitudes and Experiences Among Transmasculine and Genderqueer Young Adults. *Contraception*. 2016;94(4):422–423.

51. Charlton BM, Reynolds CA, Tabaac AR, Godwin EG, Porsch LM, Agenor M, Grimstad FW, Katz-Wise SL. Unintended and Teen Pregnancy Experiences of Trans Masculine People Living in the United States. *International Journal of Transgender Health*. 2021;22(1–2):65–76.

52. Du Mont J, Kosa SD, Solomon S, Macdonald S. Assessment of Nurses' Competence to Care for Sexually Assaulted Trans Persons: A Survey of Ontario's Sexual Assault/Domestic Violence Treatment Centres. *BMJ Open*. 2019;9:e023880.

53. Matthen P, Lyons T, Taylor M, Jennez J, Anderson S, Jollimore J, Shannon K. "I Walked into the Industry for Survival and Came Out of a Closet": How Gender and Sexual Identities Shape Sex Work Experiences Among Men, Two-Spirit and Trans People in Vancouver. *Men and Masculinities*. 2016;21(4):479–500.

54. Jones RK, Witwer E, Jerman J. Transgender Abortion Patients and the Provision of Transgender-Specific Care at Non-Hospital Facilities that Provide Abortions. *Contraception*. 2020;2:1–2.

55. Carpenter E. 'The Health System Just Wasn't Built for Us': Queer Cisgender Women and Gender Expansive Individuals' Strategies for Navigating Reproductive Health Care. *Women's Health Issues*. 2021;31(5):478–484.

56. Janiak E, Braaten KP, Cottrill AA, Fulcher IR, Goldberg AB, Agénor M. Gender Diversity Among Aspiration-Abortion Patients. *Contraception*. 2021;103(6):426–427.

57. Moseson H, Fix L, Ragosta S, Forsberg H, Hastings J, Stoeffler A, Lunn MR, Flentje A, Capriotti MR, Lubensky ME, Obedin-Maliver J. Abortion Experiences and Preferences of Transgender, Nonbinary and Gender-Expansive People in the United States. *American Journal of Obstetrics and Gynecology*. 2021;224(4):e76e1–e76e11.

58. Moseson H, Fix L, Gerdts C, Ragosta S, Hastings J, Stoeffler A, Goldberg EA, Lunn MR, Flentje A, Capriotti MR, Lubensky ME, Obedin-Maliver J. Abortion Attempts Without Clinical Supervision Among Transgender, Nonbinary and Gender-Expansive People in the United States. *BMJ Sexual & Reproductive Health*. 2022;48:22–30.

59. Begun S, Massey Combs K, Schwan K, Torrie M, Bender K. 'I Know They Would Kill Me': Abortion Attitudes and Experiences Among Youth Experiencing Homelessness. *Youth & Society*. 2018;52(8):1457–1478.

60. Pulice-Farrow L, Gonzalez KA, Lindley L. 'None of My Providers Have the Slightest Clue What to do With Me': Transmasculine Individuals' Experiences with Gynecological Health-care Providers. *International Journal of Transgender Health*. 2021;22(4):381–393.

61. Wingo E, Ingraham N, Roberts SCM. Reproductive Health Care Priorities and Barriers to Effective Care for LGBTQ People Assigned Female at Birth: A Qualitative Study. *Women's Health Issues*. 2018;28(4):350–357.

62. Lowik A.J. Trans-Inclusive Abortion Care: A Manual for Operationalizing Trans-Inclusive Policies and Practices in an Abortion Setting, United States. *PQPN, National Abortion Federation*. Accessed June 30, 2022. https://www.ajlowik.com/publications#/transinclusive-abortion

63. Ingraham N, Rodriguez I. Clinic Staff Perspectives on Barriers and Facilitators to Integrating Transgender Healthcare into Family Planning Clinics. *Transgender Health*. 2022;7(1): 36–42.

64. Mendieta A, Vidal-Ortiz S. Administering Gender: Trans Men's Sexual and Reproductive Challenges in Argentina. *International Journal of Transgender Health*. 2021;22(1-2):54–64.

65. Beaumonis Z, Bond-Theriault C. Queering Reproductive Justice: A Toolkit. *National LGBT Task Force*. Accessed June 30, 2022. https://www.thetaskforce.org/wp-content/uploads/2017/03/Queering-Reproductive-Justice-A-Toolkit-FINAL.pdf

66. Campuzano, G. Reclaiming Travesti Histories. *IDS Bulletin*. 2009;37(5):34–39.

67. Radi S. Reproductive Injustice, Trans Rights, and Eugenics. *Sexual and Reproductive Health Matters*. 2020;28(1):1–12.

68. Sutton B, Borland E. Queering Abortion Rights: Notes from Argentina. *Culture, Health & Sexuality: An International Journal for Research, Intervention and Care*. 2018;20(12): 1378–1393.

69. Magill S. The Right to Privacy and Access to Abortion in a Post-Puttaswamy World. *University of Oxford Human Rights Hub Journal*. 2020;3:160–194.

70. Strasser M. Sex, Law and the Sacred Precincts of the Marital Bedroom: On State and Federal Right to Privacy Jurisprudence. *Notre Dame Journal of Law, Ethics & Public Policy*. 2000;14:753.

71. Ashley F. Science, Abortion and the Effectiveness of Adolescent Medical Transition. [Video] Centre for Gender and Sexual Health Equity's YouTube. Accessed October 21, 2021.

https://www.youtube.com/watch?v=dy8mQHnw79s&ab_channel=CGSHE. Published October 21, 2021.

72. Dillon M. Asynchrony in Attitudes Towards Abortion and Gay Rights: The Challenge to Values Alignment. *Journal for the Scientific Study of Religion*. 2014;53(1):1–16.

73. Henry PJ, Steiger RL, Bellovary A. The Contribution of Gender Equality to the Coexistence of Progressive Abortion and Sexual Orientation Laws. *Sex Roles*. 2022;86:263–281.

74. The Associated Press. Arizona Governor Signs Bills Limiting Transgender Rights, Abortion. *NBC News*. 2022, March 30. https://www.nbcnews.com/nbc-out/out-politics-and-policy/arizona-governor-signs-bills-limiting-transgender-rights-abortion-rcna22286

75. American Civil Liberties Union. "Protecting Women and Children" is a Shield for Transphobia. At Liberty Podcast. 2022. Available at: https://www.aclu.org/podcast/protecting-women-and-children-is-a-shield-for-transphobia. Accessed June 30, 2022.

76. Panazzo D. Lessons from Reparative Therapy Applied to Post-Abortion Grief Counseling. *Journal of Homosexuality*. 2016;63(6):764–782.

77. Thomsen C, Morrison GT. Abortion as Gender Transgression: Reproductive Justice, Queer Theory, and Anti-Crisis Pregnancy Center Activism. *Signs: Journal of Women in Culture and Society*. 2020;45(3):703–730.

78. Channon MD, Puri M, Gietel-Basten S, Stone LW, Channon A. Prevalence and Correlates of Sex-Selective Abortions and Missing Girls in Nepal: Evidence from the 2011 Population Census and 2016 Demographic and Health Survey. *BMJ Open*. 2021;11(3):e042542.

79. Pörtner CC. Birth Spacing and Fertility in the Presence of Son Preference and Sex-Selective Abortions: India's Experience over Four Decades. *Demography*. 2022;59(1):61–88.

80. Abortion Rights Coalition of Canada. Position paper #24: Sex-Selection Abortions. 2020, November. Accessed October 30, 2022. https://www.arcc-cdac.ca/media/position-papers/24-Sex-Selection-Abortions.pdf

81. Murphy T. Abortion and the Ethics of Genetic Sexual Orientation Research. *Cambridge Quarterly of Healthcare Ethics*. 1995;4(3):340–350.

82. McChesney C. Abortion, Eugenics, and a Threat to Diversity. *The Modern American*. 2006;2(1):16–20.

83. Corckrill K, Upadhyay UD, Turan J, Foster DG. The Stigma of Having an Abortion: Development of a Scale and Characteristics of Women Experiencing Abortion Stigma. *Perspectives on Sexual and Reproductive Health*. 2013;45(2):79–88.

84. Ingraham N, Hann L. 'Stigma R Us': Stigma Management at the Intersection of Abortion Care and Transgender Care in Family Planning Clinics. *SSM: Qualitative Research in Health*. 2022;2:100043.

85. White Hughto JM, Reisner SL, Pachankis JE. Transgender Stigma and Health: A Critical Review of Stigma Determinants, Mechanisms, and Interventions. *Social Science & Medicine*. 2015;147:222–231.

86. Youatt E, Debbink M, Martin L, Eagen-Torkko M., Hassinger J, Harris L. 'Can't Talk about Work, Can't Talk about My Relationship': Sexual Minority Abortion Providers Cope with Stigma and Identity Disclosure. *Contraception*. 2012;86(3):28.

Chapter 5

Antenatal education

Kayleah Logan and Slade Riverfield

INTRODUCTION

In many societies globally and throughout time, there was no requirement for formalised education regarding birth and childcare.[1] In different times and cultures birth would often be supported at home by birth attendants who were members of the community and friends and family members, birth was a community event.[2,3] As a consequence it may have been more common for a person to have attended a birth prior to having their own baby and so learning about what to expect during labour would be through observation.[4] Additionally, education surrounding birth would have been accessible through oral histories from loved ones who had given birth or through trusted community members who assisted births.[4] Additionally, in a more communal way of living, new parents would have been supported by members of their family in the care of their newborn. Therefore, by the time you came to look after your own newborn you may have had practical experience in the care of a baby through helping family members care for their children.

However, in modern Western society birth is often relocated to hospitals and birth centres in which only one or two birth partners may attend. This removes birth from the attention of the community and decreases the exposure of the general public to the actualities and physiology of birth. As a consequence, first time parents in modern Western society are not as likely to have gained the same rich observational learning experiences as would have been accessible when birth was more likely to occur at home. Additionally, prenatal care now often happens in hospitals, birth centres and medical facilities and midwives and doctors are not as present in the community reducing the opportunities for first time parents to learn about birth through storytelling and the lived experiences of birth attendants.

DOI: 10.4324/9781003305446-6

As they are not able to gain information surrounding birth from traditional modalities, it has been increasingly noted that first time parents in modern Western society are drawing their knowledge from mediums that are more accessible to them – mostly from the media. This can come in a variety of formats: television, movies, books, and social media. The intention of media is to captivate and compel an audience and perhaps to generate income, which can be easily done with stories surrounding birth as it is an incredibly emotive topic. It is identified that in media birth can often be represented as dramatic, painful and of high risk[5] thus generating tension to grasp the attention of an audience. However, the repeated internalisation of these tense stories can invoke anxiety in first time parents who have no other modalities of gaining insight into the realities of birth.[6, 7]

In this chapter we will begin by considering the purpose of general antenatal education, how LGBTQ+ people's experiences may be different to cisheterosexual participants, and what educators can do in order to better meet these needs. We will then examine some current LGBTQ+ specific antenatal education provision.

BENEFITS OF ANTENATAL EDUCATION

Many expectant parents report seeking antenatal education to increase their knowledge of childbirth, infant care, feeding or to reduce anxiety around birth.[2, 8]

Those attending antenatal classes identified the following topics as those they wished to cover:

1)   physical and physiological changes during pregnancy
2)   what happens physiologically during labour
3)   care options from health care professionals
4)   self-care during pregnancy, labour, and the postpartum period
5)   possible complications
6)   caring for newborns[9]

This could imply that expectant parents in modern western society identify within themselves a lack of knowledge surrounding the realities of childbirth, neonatal care, and the postnatal period. This lack of knowledge could therefore be eliciting a feeling of anxiety. Additionally, the knowledge they have already gained through media could lead them to expect a poor outcome for themselves or their babies and this could also contribute to feelings of anxiety surrounding birth.

Regarding the actual benefits of antenatal education, research reports a variety of benefits including:

- reduced use of epidural analgesia
- reduced occurrence of caesarean section
- increased levels of self-efficacy[10]
- fewer admissions in early labour
- increased partner involvement
- reduced stress or anxiety in the gestational parent[11]

Conversely, literature also reports that gestational parents who attended antenatal education experienced the opposite effects with increased intervention, induction of labour and epidural use reported, alongside findings no differences in outcome of mode of birth, obstetric outcomes or psychosocial outcomes when compared to those who did not attend antenatal education.[11, 12]

It is apparent that the literature is not in agreement with itself regarding what the benefits are of antenatal education, and in some circumstances, if there are actually benefits at all. Antenatal education is incredibly diverse in its nature, as a consequence there are a number of variables that are difficult to control or take into account when considering conducting high quality research into the benefits. These variables include:

- The modality of the education
- The content of the education
- The ethos and approach of the modality
- The practical delivery (eg, online, small group, larger group, a lecture/ conference style)
- The demographics of the parents attending
- The delivery of the facilitator
- The environment of the classes

To conduct good quality research into the benefits of antenatal education it would be important to control for each different variable to observe the maximum benefits on different demographics of participants, however, that is a complex practicality due to the rich nature of antenatal education.

CORE CONTENT OF GENERAL ANTENATAL EDUCATION

There is little research and no national guidance in the UK regarding necessary content for practitioners to cover when they are developing or delivering antenatal education, making it difficult to decipher what best practice would be regarding the delivery of antenatal education.[13] Consequently, antenatal education differs depending on cultural and social norms, meaning the content and curriculum can vary drastically depending on a range of factors including the lived experiences and beliefs of the person writing the content and the perceived wants and needs of whichever demographic the creator anticipates it will attract.[14]

For example, if the content creator personally had a home birth themselves and personally believes that a birth involving a lesser level of intervention is more beneficial or a "better" experience, this may inherently sway their content in favour of birth that promotes a lesser level of intervention. Their respective approach may also attract a demographic of parent who shares a similar ethos. Similarly, if a content creator considers birth as risky then their content may centre risk, being aware of risk, risk avoidance and so forth and this would attract parents who also share the same perceptions of birth being of high risk and who value education on how to manage, avoid or negate risk. Consequently, there can be significant differences in the curriculum of antenatal education that is often influenced by the ethos, values and aims of the organisation that delivers it.[14]

There is little further research on how the personal beliefs of content creators affect the goals of the different modalities of antenatal education and how these goals align with the personal goals of the parents. Additionally, there is no standardisation of what the common goals or best practice in antenatal education should be and consequently how to achieve these goals.[15, 16] In the absence of this information there exists significant variation of opinions on how best to educate parents and deliver the information that is desired, which contributes to the wide variety of approaches that can be seen in the field of parent education.

LGBTQ+ PARTICIPANTS ANTENATAL EDUCATION NEEDS

Becoming a parent is an experience that affects many aspects of life; physical, emotional, mental, financial, social and for some religious, spiritual or ritual.[17] Antenatal education can address many of these topics, however being an LGBTQ+ person can also affect many of these aspects of life.[18] LGBTQ+ people and cisgender, heterosexual people may experience these transitions differently, and may have different wants and needs with regards to antenatal education. As there is currently no standardisation or core curriculum in antenatal education and this in turn results in little research regarding LGBTQ+ parents experiences of antenatal education.[16] Therefore, research regarding the experiences of LGBTQ+ parents and people beyond antenatal education will be used and applied to antenatal education to examine what is being done and what can be done better. Broadly, current research shows that LGBTQ+ people who access antenatal education need the same things as cisheterosexual people, but have additional needs too. Those additional needs can be divided into two groups; inclusion, and specific content. We will examine each of these separately.

Inclusion

In the UK currently, there is an increase in hostility towards LGBTQ+ people, with hate crimes trebling from 2013 to 2020.[19, 20] A key consideration for LGBTQ+ families when they are navigating in wider society is safety. In the context of antenatal education, safety would include physical safety, emotional safety, and mental safety.

With regards to physical safety, expectant parents need to know they can attend antenatal education without threats of violence or intimidation. Whilst the likelihood of threats of violence may be low in such settings, concern about such incidents can be very real to some LGBTQ+ people.[22] In order to instil confidence, providers of antenatal education could consider including a statement on how they would manage such issues within their policies. Additionally, the location of the antenatal classes may have an influence on the physical safety of LGBTQ+ people, for example if the area has a high rate of hate crimes. Hate crimes towards the LGBTQ+ community can be influenced by the political leaning of geographic areas and so it could be possible that LGBTQ+ people would need to travel further or look for tailored courses in order to feel safe which could limit access.

In the context of the mental and emotional safety of LGBTQ+ parents there are a number of influences that could be considered to not only ensure safety but promote wellbeing amongst LGBTQ+ parents. One such example can be found in language. Language regarding pregnancy, birth and families tends to be very gendered and this can greatly impact individuals' experiences of their reproductive journey.[23] This occurs from the very first interaction with a service. For example, the interaction may start with accessing a website to find more information, then completing a form to register interest, followed by a review of the educational content, and careful consideration of the language used by teachers. If language is used that is very gendered and does not align with their personal feeling and does not represent their family, LGBTQ+ people may experience a range of negative experiences and consequently may disengage from the service. Gendered language can range from being jarring to harmful to LGBTQ+ parents, both gestational and non-gestational.[24, 25] However, if language is used that aligns with their feelings of themselves and their families, LGBTQ+ people may feel validated and confident with the service and choose to engage with confidence.

For trans men and non-binary gestational parents, language that is gendered differently to their own identity can influence emotional, mental and psychological harm with feelings of hurt, upset, disgust, anger, rejection or dysphoria.[26, 27] This can also hinder their access to information that may be important for them to receive, resulting in a future negative impact on their physical outcomes too.[24] The first UK National Health Trust to acknowledge the impact of language on non-binary and transgender pregnant people was Brighton and Sussex University Hospitals, who created a policy to guide the use of language, which includes using "chestfeeding" in conjunction with "breastfeeding" and the use of terms such as "perinatal care". Their examples can be usefully extrapolated and applied to practise within antenatal education.[28]

Non-gestational parents who are women can find the heterosexist assumption that all non-gestational parents will be men damaging to their sense of identity as a parent, whilst non-gestational parents who do not identify as men but are socially read as men can find this misgendering causes sadness, grief, hurt, frustration, invalidation.[29] Simple changes to language can help to avoid eliciting negative feelings and validate LGBTQ+ parents' identities. Table 5.1 demonstrates gendered

Table 5.1 Examples of gender-neutral language that can be used in addition to gendered language regarding families and pregnancy

Gendered term that might appear in antenatal education	Non-gendered term that could be substituted or added
Mum	Gestational parent, birthing parent, pregnant parent (in policies) "Name" when speaking to a person
Woman/Pregnant woman	Person/pregnant person
Mums	Those who are pregnant
Dad (referring to the non-gestational parent)	Non-gestational parent, non-birthing parent- (in policies) "Name" when speaking to a person
Dads (referring to the non-gestational parent)	Those who aren't pregnant
Breast/breast feeding	Chest/Chest feeding, feeding from your body
Cervix, Uterus	Cervix, Uterus nb: Biological language is non-gendered

words that are commonly used in antenatal education and provides additional gender-neutral terms that can be used in addition to or instead of gendered terms. It is important to acknowledge that language adaptations can be used as additive language, where the original term is kept and non-gendered language is added, to respect the identity of those who identify with the gendered and non-gendered terms alike.

To explore this further, we suggest completing the exercise below:

EXERCISE 1

Find an informative article where the target audience is pregnant people and highlight in it all of the words that presumes the gender of someone who is pregnant.

In terms of emotional safety, it has been identified that 25% of LGBTQ+ people experienced what they call "inappropriate curiosity".[30] Inappropriate curiosity refers to situations where questions posed to an LGBTQ+ person which are not necessary within the context of the situation. It is important to note that transgender and non-binary people experience a higher prevalence of inappropriate questioning at 48% and 36% respectively than cisgender LGBQ+ people. Inappropriate curiosity can occur with well-meaning individuals, thus can feel invasive and unsettling regardless of the intentions of the people using the language. Application within antenatal education make it important for the class leaders to be aware of their own conduct as well as to anticipate how they may navigate a situation in which they witness another attendee asking inappropriate and potentially personal questions. Figure 5.1 displays some peoples' experience with inappropriate curiosity within antenatal education.

Another potential difficulty for LGBTQ+ parents in antenatal care is cisheteronormativity (operating under the assumption that the people you meet are cisgender and heterosexual without much consideration of the possibility that people you interact with may be of a different gender identity or sexual orientation).[29, 31] As mentioned previously the content of antenatal education will often be influenced by the writer of the curriculum. If that person is a cisgender heterosexual person then content and information is likely to be filtered through that lens – meaning that there would be little consideration for experiencing pregnancy in any other way. Cisheteronormativity might mean that assuming all

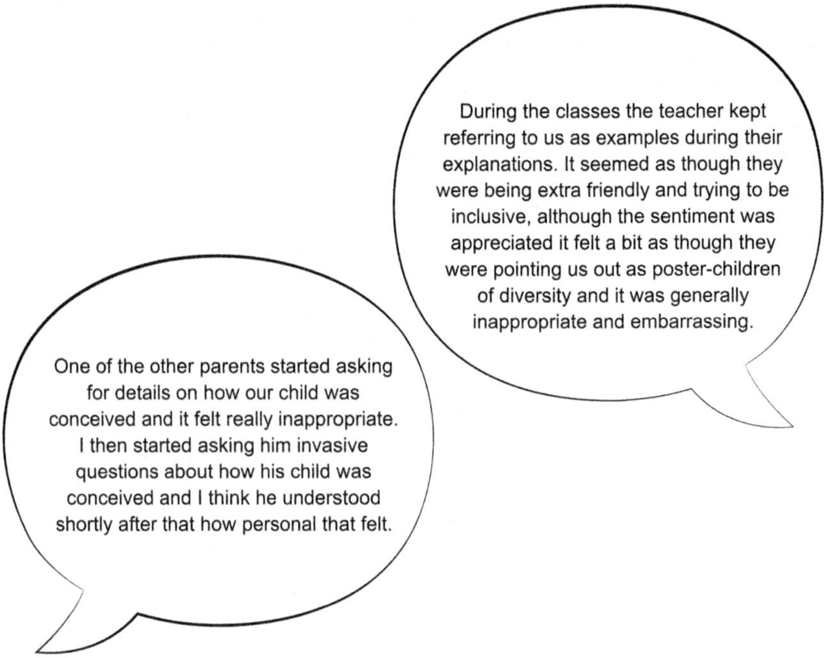

During the classes the teacher kept referring to us as examples during their explanations. It seemed as though they were being extra friendly and trying to be inclusive, although the sentiment was appreciated it felt a bit as though they were pointing us out as poster-children of diversity and it was generally inappropriate and embarrassing.

One of the other parents started asking for details on how our child was conceived and it felt really inappropriate. I then started asking him invasive questions about how his child was conceived and I think he understood shortly after that how personal that felt.

Figure 5.1 Reports from LGBT families regarding their experiences with inappropriate curiosity.

the pregnant people within the sessions would identify as women and the people that were with them as their romantic partners would identify as men and fathers. These assumptions may be problematic in a number of ways for LGBTQ+ parents.

A common assumption within a cisheteronormative view of parenting is that the non-gestational parent is known as a "dad" and is often assumed to have less of a role in the care of a newborn – they are often disregarded or regarded as secondary or of less importance than the gestational parent.[32] However, gender roles within LGBTQ+ families often differ drastically regarding both childcare and the division of domestic labour.[33] Research shows that many LGBTQ+ families find it important that professionals regard the non-gestational parent as having equal importance to the gestational parent.[34] Therefore, if an antenatal education curriculum is written through a cisheteronormative lens, content may neglect the non-gestational parents' experience during pregnancy, labour, birth and postpartum, and fail to provide information on how to care for them during a time of great change. This could result in invalidation of the non-gestational parents' experiences in becoming a parent, causing distress. Similarly, information can be provided with biases that may not take into account some of the lived experiences of LGBTQ+ parents, as the example in Case Study 1 shows.

CASE STUDY 1—LUCI AND IONNA

Luci and Ionna are a lesbian couple attending antenatal education at 37 weeks. The instructor is talking about caring for the new baby and asks the group to separate into mums and dads. Ionna feels uncomfortable because she is a mum but she is put into the dads' group because she is not the pregnant one. The instructor makes some jokes about how dads don't know how to change a nappy and how for breastfeeding mums it is so annoying watching dads snore while they are up all night feeding and changing the baby. The instructor urges the dads to do the dishes in the early weeks because mum will be so tired. Ionna is a nursery nurse and "can change a nappy blindfolded", she "does the dishes better than Luci" and as a couple they consider themselves equal parents and plan to split care tasks 50/50 like they do with their other domestic tasks. Ionna feels invalidated as a future mother through having been categorised in the dads' group and deeply hurt that the assumption that she would be an inadequate caregiver to her partner and baby.

Specific content

LGBTQ+ families are not homogenous – they have many different possible formations. Genetic, gestational, legal, and social parenting roles are likely to be more complex than they are in cisheterosexual families. Conceptions may have happened within clinic or home settings, may include egg and/or sperm donations, or working with surrogates, in turn affecting who holds parental responsibility and at which point this is gained. The reproductive history of the family may not be catered for in terms of the language currently used in antenatal education, for example a person's first physical pregnancy may not be their first child.

In some families no parent may have the physical ability to chest- or breastfeed, in some families more than one parent may have this ability. Therefore, some LGBTQ+ participants might need information about inducing lactation in a non-gestational mother, who might be cisgender or transgender, whilst other families might need information about chestfeeding, ranging from the physical possibilities of chestfeeding after chest masculinisation surgery and/or testosterone therapy to the psychological impact of chestfeeding on gender dysphoria.

Perinatal mental health may also be different for LGBTQ+ participants in a multitude of ways, including:

—   Gender dysphoria as a perinatal mental health condition
—   Secondary tokophobia in primiparous pregnancies[35]
—   Less visible experiences of reproductive losses[36]

The content needed in the specific presentation will depend on the audience; not all participants will need access to all information. However, most general antenatal education courses do not currently include this kind of specific content even if participants require it. [37] Ensuring that antenatal educators can provide access to this kind of information should a participant require it is necessary if antenatal education is to meet the needs of LGBTQ+ people, as Case Study 2 shows.

CASE STUDY 2—KAI

Kai is a transgender man who is 36 weeks pregnant and attending an antenatal education class with his girlfriend. In this session the instructor is discussing infant feeding. She is discussing the benefits of breastfeeding. Kai is interested. The instructor talks about how hormones after pregnancy make breastfeeding a normal and natural act, and proceeds to say that breastfeeding is the way to give your baby the best start in life and the best way to bond with the baby.

Kai has dysphoria with regards to his chest. During the pregnancy he has a bit more fatty tissue in his chest than he had pre-pregnancy and it causes him distress. He feels uncomfortable in his body and the idea of anyone touching his chest makes his skin crawl. He is very keen to be able to resume taking testosterone after the birth, and to be able to bind his chest again. The instructor does not mention whether either of these are safe to do whilst breastfeeding, so he assumes they are not.

He listens to what the instructor says. He wants to give his baby the best start, can he grit his teeth, continue to not take testosterone and bind his chest, and also tolerate that amount of interaction with his chest? If he can't, does that make him a bad parent? Will he be able to bond with his baby if he doesn't chestfeed? Will he be able to if he does?

Kai's girlfriend also listens to the instructor. She would really like to breastfeed their baby, but as the instructor focuses on the relationship between pregnancy and breastfeeding she assumes it isn't possible for her. She wants her baby to have the best start in life so hopes Kai will be able to chestfeed, but leaves worried that she won't be able to bond with her baby in the same way if Kai is chestfeeding and she isn't.

THE IMPACT OF LGBTQ+ PEOPLE'S EXPERIENCES OF HEALTH CARE

Antenatal education does not happen in a vacuum. People's previous life experiences interact with the content provided by the educator to create positive and negative results. One area of previous experiences that is likely to have an influence on the effect of antenatal education is previous experiences of health care. Research shows that 13% of LGBT+ people have experienced unequal treatment from health care staff as a result of being LGBTQ+ and 23% of LGBTQ+ people have witnessed negative remarks from health care staff about those in the LGBTQ+ community.[30] A distinct theme highlighted in this research was that some LGBTQ+ people will delay or avoid accessing care due to fear of discrimination.

This may specifically interact with content presented about health care professionals in antenatal education. Some antenatal education has been identified as presenting bias regarding different choices in relation to birth and childcare depending on the approach adopted by the respective provider. For example, if it is the intention or claim of the education provider to reduce the rate of intervention then there may be a bias presented against care providers who are perceived as likely to recommend intervention. However, it is important to bear in mind that LGBTQ+ people's previous experiences of homophobia, transphobia, and consequent poor care may already have disrupted their trust in health care providers. Consequently, it could be hypothesised that presenting a bias against health care providers who are more likely to offer intervention may negatively affect LGBTQ+ parents' already less trusting relationship with health care providers. Further studies found that 30% of transgender or non-binary pregnant people did not access any perinatal care during their pregnancy. Of those who chose not to access perinatal care, 80% said they were not confident to access the services even if they really needed to.[38]

This may leave antenatal educators with a difficult balance – perinatal services in the UK do not currently always respect autonomy and informed decision making.

Antenatal education plays an important role in promoting these, but when working with LGBTQ+ clients additional care is needed to avoid eliciting fear or negatively impacting relationships with support services. One solution might be for antenatal classes to invite local services in, acting as an intervention to build positive relationships with local care providers, enabling LGBTQ+ families to feel more comfortable accessing support if they would like to, and beginning to repair the fearful relationships as represented in the statistics above. To do this successfully, local services must first ensure that they are able to offer inclusive services with staff who are comfortable and confident in working with LGBTQ+ people, or further damage may be caused.

IMPROVING LGBTQ+ INCLUSIVITY IN GENERAL ANTENATAL EDUCATION

Within the current environment in which LGBTQ+ people regularly face prejudice within health care systems, and often report being fearful, distrusting, and reluctant to access perinatal care. It can make parents hypervigilant about which spaces may be safe or unsafe. Cisheteronormativity can be interpreted as an indicator of a space that is not as inclusive or welcoming as it has not been updated with the idea in mind that it is a possibility that LGBTQ+ people may utilise the service.

When evaluating whether an existing service is cisheteronormative, two questions can be asked. First, how prepared is the service for a member of the LGBTQ+ community right now? Secondly, how does the service demonstrate its acceptance and warm welcome to the LGBTQ+ community prior to the family making first contact? With regards to the former question, it can be advisable to do a theoretical walkthrough of the service through the perspective of an LGBTQ+ person. Figure 5.2 demonstrates chronological points of contact LGBTQ+ families might have with antenatal education and what the potential consequences of both good and bad interactions are at each step. This illustrates some of the theoretical ideas mentioned above in practice for an LGBTQ+ person who wants to participate in an antenatal education course.

Examples of good practice with regards to LGBTQ+ participants can be found within some general antenatal education within the UK. Within the NHS, Chesterfield Royal Hospital NHS Foundation Trust has appointed an Infant Feeding Lead Midwife who can offer lactation support to all parents with a desire to breastfeed, including intended parents via surrogacy, trans women, and non-gestational parents. Best Beginnings, who provide antenatal education via a

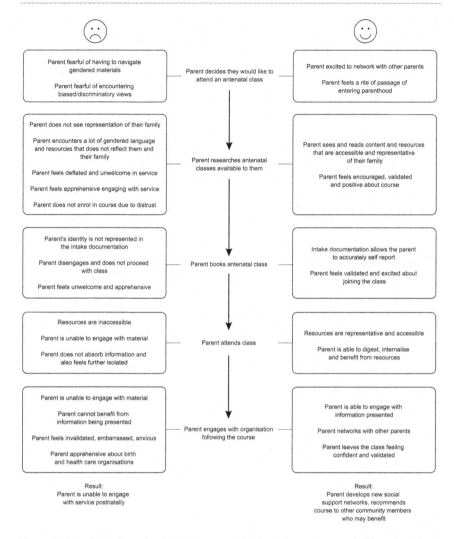

Figure 5.2 An illustration of and LGBTQ+ parents' potential experiences at different points of contact with antenatal education.

free app called Baby Buddy, have a specific pathway for non-gestational mums (although not currently for gestational parents who aren't women), and have recently commissioned research to improve their LGBTQ+ inclusivity. Lamaze International's style guide now requires the use of "birth parent" and "chest/breastfeeding" in all their materials and courses, in line with organisational inclusion standards. La Leche League produce factsheets on induced lactation for non-gestational mothers and on chestfeeding for trans men and non-binary people, and has a specific international section for LGBTQI families.

Researching and sharing good practice about how antenatal education providers include LGBTQ+ participants better could help to improve the antenatal education offered.

LGBTQ+ LED ANTENATAL EDUCATION

In addition to general antenatal education providers who have made improvements to their LGBTQ+ inclusivity, there are a number of antenatal education providers in the UK which are led by LGBTQ+ people, and which aim to improve LGBTQ+ antenatal education. Some of these organisations provide antenatal education directly to participants, whilst others offer training to health care professionals, including antenatal educators. Below are listed a selection of these organisations.

Queer Birth Club

The Queer Birth Club is an organisation that is pioneered by an LGBTQ+ birth worker that aims to educate perinatal care providers and practitioners with regards to the needs of LGBTQ+ families. It is a practitioner facing service that provides competency training that aims to ensure practitioners feel confident in providing good and culturally relevant care to LGBTQ+ families in any aspect of the perinatal journey.

The Queer Birth Club offers a range of services including competency training entitled "LGBTQ+ competency in birth and beyond", "LGBTQ+ competency in lactation", sensitivity checks with regards to language, speaking and writing. The Queer Birth club has the potential to greatly impact LGBTQ+ families' access needs in a range of perinatal education settings by acting as a bridge between LGBT+ parents and service providers.

The Queer Parenting Partnership

The Queer Parenting Partnership is a community interest company run by a queer doula and a queer former midwife. They provide antenatal education for LGBTQ+ families, networking opportunities for families to connect and resources for LGBTQ+ parents regarding many aspects of pregnancy and birth. The philosophy of their classes is to provide non-judgemental, evidence-based information regarding pregnancy, birth and care of the family in the postpartum period in a safe and culturally relevant environment free from cis heteronormativity.

One particularly unique aspect of the Queer Parenting Partnership is the focus on networking opportunities for families. All sessions are conducted online to enable access for LGBT+ families across the country. Additionally, they provide many accessible resources, not only for pregnant women and people but also practitioners that work with LGBTQ+ families.

Kinhood Collective

Kinhood Collective offer a non-judgemental space for LGBTQ+ pregnant people, parents, and kin. They exist to support LGBTQIA+ folks navigating family building and reproductive experiences; conception, adoption, pregnancy, birth, abortion, loss, postpartum, and more. This broad spectrum and focus on a variety of aspects of the reproductive experience allows LGBTQ+ people to access specific targeted support on matters that are most relevant to them.

Queer Birth Project

The Queer Birth Project is an American-based organisation that hosts antenatal education, networking opportunities for parents and practitioner training. They also host an online directory of practitioners. Within their networking parent groups they also run focused sessions for new/prospective parents, non-gestational parents, trying to conceive and pregnancy loss.

Braw Birth

Braw Birth is an organisation run by a doula based in Scotland. They offer antenatal education, workshops aimed at parents and training for practitioners. They offer doula services for the LGBTQ+ community during fertility treatments and pregnancy and many of their workshops centre advocacy during fertility treatments. They offer their services online which allows LGBTQ+ families to access them from around the country.

The practitioner training they conduct offers a unique perspective on preconception care and support, an area that is often under-represented. They offer an intersectional approach that opens conversations regarding fatness and chronic illness and demonstrate a representation of many different family types, abilities, and races.

Pride in Birth podcast

In each episode of this free podcast, a different academic researcher discusses the findings of their research about LGBTQ+ conception, pregnancy, or parenthood with the host.

KEY LEARNING POINTS

In this chapter, we have covered the following:

- Research on antenatal education is divided on benefits, outcomes, and drawbacks with the exception of it needing to be evidence-based and patient-centred.
- There are currently no bodies that regulate or govern antenatal education providers in the UK.
- There are currently no guidelines that set out standardised best practise in antenatal education in the UK.
- There is little research about LGBTQ+ parents' experiences and needs with regard to antenatal education.
- There is even less research detailing what constitutes best practice in antenatal education for LGBTQ+ parents.
- LGBTQ+ participants need to be included in antenatal education in ways that account for their physical and emotional safety.
- LGBTQ+ participants may need access to antenatal education that is not routinely provided to cisheterosexual participants.
- Without both inclusion and access to LGBTQ+ content, antenatal education is unlikely to meet the needs of LGBTQ+ participants.
- There are a variety of ways that existing antenatal education may be adapted and modified to cater to the needs of LGBT+ families.
- Good practice examples of inclusion exist in general antenatal education providers, which could be shared and implemented more widely.

There are a number of LGBTQ+ led antenatal education organisations who can provide education and training for LGBTQ+ expectant parents and/or health care professionals.

If you are a midwife, obstetrician, or other health care practitioner who provides intrapartum care, it may be helpful to bear in mind that LGBTQ+ people may not have accessed antenatal education for some of the reasons mentioned in this chapter. If your role includes antenatal education, and you would like to improve the relevance of your content for LGBTQ+ parents, the rest of this book covers important topics for your review, and this chapter has given you relevant information to consider in the delivery of your education.

REFERENCES

1. Renkert S and Nutbeam D. Opportunities to Improve Maternal Health Literacy through Antenatal Education: An Exploratory Study. *Health Promotion International*. 2001;16(1): 381–388.

2. Gagnon AJ, Sandall J. Individual or Group Antenatal Education for Childbirth or Parenthood, or Both. *Cochrane Database Syst Rev*. 2007;3. https://pubmed.ncbi.nlm.nih.gov/17636711/

3. Cutajar L, Miu M, Fleet J, et al. Antenatal Education for Childbirth: Labour and Birth. *European Journal of Midwifery*. 2020;4.:11.

4. Leister N, Riesco MLG. Childbirth Care: The Oral History of Women who Gave Birth from the 1940s to 1980s. *Enferm*. 2013;22(1). https://www.scielo.br/j/tce/a/j3x6K34kgCjtKcfxj36W8Cz/?lang=en

5. Kennedy HP, Nardini K, McLeod-Waldo R, Ennis L. Top-Selling Childbirth Advice Books: A Discourse Analysis. *Birth*. 2009;36(4):318–324.

6. Luce A, Cash M, Hundley V et al. "Is it Realistic? The Portrayal of Pregnancy and Childbirth in the Media. *BMC Pregnancy Childbirth*. 2016;16(40). https://doi.org/10.1186/s12884-016-0827-x

7. Sayakhot P, Carolan-Olah M. Internet Use by Pregnant Women Seeking Pregnancy-Related Information: A Systematic Review. *BMC Pregnancy and Childbirth*. 2016;16(65):65.

8. Ricchi A, La Corte S, Molinazzi MT et al. Study of Childbirth Education Classes and Evaluation of their Effectiveness. *Clinical Therapeutics*. 2020;170(1):78–86.

9. Sullivan PL. Felt Learning Needs of Pregnant Women. *Canadian Nurse*. 1993;89(1):42–45.

10. Hong K, Hwang H, Han H, Chase J et al. Perspectives on Antenatal Education Associated with Pregnancy Outcomes: Systematic Review and Meta-Analysis. *Women Birth*. 2021; 34(3):219–230.

11. Ferguson S, Davis D, Browne J. Does Antenatal Education Affect Labour and Birth? A Structured Review of the Literature. *Women and Birth*. 26(1):5–8

12. Brixval V, Axelsen S et al. The Effect of Antenatal Education in Small Classes on Obstetric and Psycho-Social Outcomes—A Systematic Review. *Systematic Reviews*. 2015;20. https://doi.org/10.1186/s13643-015-0010-x

13. O'Meara, CM. Childbirth and Parenting Education—The Provider's Viewpoint. *Midwifery*. 1993;9:76–84.

14. Coast E, Jones E, Portela A et al. Maternity Care Services and Culture: A Systematic Global Mapping of Interventions. *PLoS One*. 2014;9(9). https://www.ncbi.nlm.nih.gov/pmc/articles/PMC4182435/

15. Katona C. Approaches to Antenatal Education. *Social Science and Medicine. Part A: Medical Psychology and Medical Sociology*. 1981;15(1):25–33.

16. Griggs B. Antenatal Education Service Development. *National Institute of Clinical Excellence*. https://www.nice.org.uk/sharedlearning/antenatal-education-service-development

17. Svensson J, Barclay L, Cooke, M. Randomised-Controlled Trial of Two Antenatal Education Programmes. *Midwifery*. 2009;25(2):114–125.

18. Goldberg A. LGBTQ-Parent Families: Diversity, Intersectionality and Social Context. *Current opinion in Psychology*. 2023;49. https://www.sciencedirect.com/science/article/abs/pii/S2352250X2200238X

19. Hunte B. 'I Thought I was Going to Die' in a Homophobic Attack. *BBC*. 2020. https://www.bbc.co.uk/news/uk-54470077

20. Hubbard L. The Hate Crime Report 2021: Supporting LGBT+ Victims of Hate Crime. *GALOP*. 2021. https://galop.org.uk/wp-content/uploads/2021/06/Galop-Hate-Crime-Report-2021-1.pdf

22. Maine A. Perceptions of Violence and the Self-Regulation of Identity for LGBTQ People in the UK. *The Journal of Criminal Law*. 2022;86(2):60–74.

23. Fischer, O. Non-Binary Reproduction: Stories of Conception, Pregnancy and Birth. *International Journal of Transgender Health*. 2021;22(1):77–88.

24. Obedin-Maliver J, Makadon HJ. Transgender Men in Pregnancy. *Obstetric Medicine*. 2016; 9(1):4–8.

25. Malmquist A. "But Wait where Should I Be, Am I a Mum or a Dad?" Lesbian Couples Reflect on Heteronormativity in Regular Antenatal Education and the Benefits of LGBTQ+ Certified Options. *DiVA*. 2016;3(3):7–10.

26. Kerr L, Jones T, Fischer CM. Alleviating Gender Dysphoria: A Qualitative Study of Perspective of Gender Diverse People. *Journal of Health Services, Research and Policy*. 2022;27(1)4–13.

27. Paz GM, Pulice-Farrow L, Lindley L. "Every Time I Get Gendered Male, I Feel a Pain in My Chest": Understanding the Social Context for Gender Dysphoria. *Stigma and Health*. 2020;5(2):109–208.

28. Green H, Riddington A. Perinatal Care for Trans and Non-Binary People. *Brighton and Sussex University Hospital*. 2020. https://www.bsuh.nhs.uk/maternity/wp-content/uploads/sites/7/2021/01/MP005-Perinatal-Care-for-Trans-and-Non-Binary-People.pdf

29. Bachmann CL, Gooch B. LGBT in Britain: Health Report. *Stonewall*. 2018. https://www.stonewall.org.uk/system/files/lgbt_in_britain_health.pdf

30. Charguit J, Burns J, Pettle S, Tasker F. Lesbian Co-Mothers' Experiences of Maternity Health Care Services. *Journal of Advanced Nursing*. 2013;69(6);1269–1278.

31. Malmquist A, Klittmark S. Heteronormative Obstacles in Regular Antenatal Education and the Benefits of LGBTQ+ Certified Options. *Contemporary Issues in Perinatal Education*. 2022. 1st Ed.

32. Pezaro DS, Crowther R, Pearce G et al. Perinatal Care for Trans and Non-Binary People Birthing in Heteronormative "Maternity" Services: Experiences and Educational Needs of Professionals. *Gender and Society*. 2022. https://pure.coventry.ac.uk/ws/files/57778004/Published.pdf

33. May C, Fletcher R. Preparing Fathers for the Transition to Parenthood: Recommendations for the Content of Antenatal Education. *Midwifery*. 2013;29(5):474–478.

34. Kurdek LA. The Allocation of Household Labour in Gay, Lesbian and Heterosexual Married Couples. *Journal of Social Issues*. 1993;49(3):127–139.

35. Greenfield M, Darwin Z. Trans and non-Binary Pregnancy, Traumatic Birth, and Perinatal Mental Health: A Scoping Review. *Int J Transgend Health*. 2021 Nov. 19;22(1–2):203–216.

36. Craven C. *Reproductive Losses: Challenges to LGBTQ+ Family Making*. Routledge. 2019. 1

37. Malmquist A, Klittmark S. Heteronormative Obstacles in Regular Antenatal Education, and the Benefit of LGBT Certified Options. *Contemporary Issues in Perinatal Education*. 2022. 1

38. LGBT Foundation. Trans and Non-Binary Experiences of Maternity Services: Survey Findings, Reports and Recommendations. *LGBT Foundation*. 2022. https://dxfy8lrzbpywr.cloudfront.net/Files/97ecdaea-833d-4ea5-a891-c59f0ea429fb/ITEMS%2520report%2520final.pdf

Chapter 6

Navigating choices in pregnancy and birth

El Molloy and Kate Luxion

INTRODUCTION

When considering choice in antenatal care, it is important to understand the historical and cultural approaches and philosophies that underpin contemporary reproductive health systems. While this can vary by geographic context, there are patterns that repeat themselves, as with the push to medicalise birth in the global south, despite attempts to address and reduce the over-medicalisation of birth in the global north. These patterns lead to similarities in care developing, despite different contexts, over time. Conversely, despite centuries of co-developing knowledge in midwifery and obstetrics and gynaecology, there are still differences in their philosophies of care and what that can mean for decision making, autonomy, control, and the idea of choice during pregnancy and wider reproductive health care. The reasons behind the philosophical divide, and how this influences antenatal care, lays the groundwork for better understanding the environment LGBTQ+ people have to navigate while accessing antenatal care. Similarly, understanding how policies, procedures, and administrative and legal systems can impact choice, and who is able to make which choices, helps frame what is important for providing affirming and inclusive health care.

HOW REPRODUCTIVE HEALTH CARE HISTORY SHAPES CONTEMPORARY CHOICE

Starting with early evidence around pregnancy and birth, from which medicalised knowledge stems, it was believed that the uterus was merely a vessel with sperm providing all the necessary biological material for procreation.[1] Later conceptions of science continued these traditions through asserting that to understand nature it must be dominated and dissected.[2] These hypotheses, combined with the limitation of the professions of science and medicine to men, meant that theories and conceptualisations of reproductive health knowledge within obstetrics were

DOI: 10.4324/9781003305446-7

produced without direct involvement of those who gave birth. This contributed to the framing of pregnancy as a condition requiring treatment, rather than a physiological process that could unfold without unnecessary intervention. While there have been efforts to improve this framing, these stances still shape the dichotomies present between the philosophies in obstetrics and midwifery.[1, i] Being aware of the dichotomies is necessary if we are to implement change and acknowledge if/when progress towards more equitable models of care has been achieved. In juxtaposition to the academic discipline of obstetrics, the model of care within midwifery stemmed from community-based knowledge passed down through generations of healers, before being removed and reframed within an academic context, and consequently subject to licensing and policy,[3] while ensuring a hierarchy in which midwives generally report or defer to obstetricians.[4]

Beyond the underlying principles of each care model, access to choice is also shaped by the social and medical contexts where the reproductive care is being received. For the UK and Ireland, this has meant a formal prioritising of clinical, and at times pseudo,[5] midwifery care, positioning the "ideal" place of birth as being away from the home care that was previously more common in lower class homes,[4–6] while stigmatising that which was accessible. Within the United States, it has meant sanctioning "granny midwives," typically older women of colour and/or lower social class who provided health care and midwifery, removing their ability to practise through licensure laws requiring those practicing midwifery to access to Higher Education, which in turn was segregated by race.[3] Despite adequate evidence to the benefits of the midwifery care model,[7] the choices of care available have become limited by the letter of the law; though not everyone has always abided by the law. Midwifery has in fact continued in some places despite being illegal, due to the need for midwives, and midwifery has frequently eventually been reintegrated as a legal care option.[3] However, licensure-based limitations result in a narrowed scope of practice for midwives, which directly correlates with the choices that they are able to offer and facilitate for antenatal service users.

While there has been some progress in complementary care models, historically obstetric medicine was presented as a means of overcoming the "witchcraft" of midwifery and health care outside of the clinical model or academy.[8, 9] Traditional and oral knowledge that had been passed down by midwives and healers was meant to be superseded by "science" as defined by the educated, ruling classes across various cultures.[3, 8] This is relevant here due to the way in which it has shaped the models of choice that are available during care, as well as the urgency with which those choices must be made. For midwifery, knowledge has historically tended to be inclusive of the variations of experience, while using proactive observation to address potential concerns.[10] Clinical medicine more often encourages decisions made based on averages, with a focus on reducing risks through interventions,[11] though some progress has been made in stepping back on measures if aligned with patient wishes. While it is becoming more common to see discussion about informed choice and true consent, these efforts stem more from influence of midwifery models of care helping to shape and facilitate the low-to-no intervention approach (ie, physiological birth) within obstetrics.[12]

Another historical layer of choice in pregnancy care, which is especially relevant to LGBTQ+ pregnant parents and their partners, are stigmas and assumptions made within clinical spaces. If and when choices are offered can depend on whether expectant parents hold enough social power to be "heard" within the space of perinatal care. For parents of colour, this lack of power can be seen in the failure to treat pain and concern as valid, with racist and inaccurate medical education leading to higher risks and lower quality in care.[13, 14] Similarly, assumptions made about LGBTQ+ people impact both how they are seen and heard in health care,[15] as well contributing to the invisibilising of their partners.[16] For example, concerns around the quality of health care they will receive can keep some bisexual and lesbian mothers from sharing their sexual orientation and partnership status private.[17, 18]

A lack of choice may be due to assumptions about what is possible, rather than actualities, as well as limitations based on what clinical services can be provided locally. In both instances, minoritised groups face double jeopardy (ie, higher risk of mistreatment, which may result in poorer outcomes, but also results in increased minority stress, which itself may result in poorer outcomes) and therefore a higher prevalence of preventable suboptimal outcomes. Across multiple geographic contexts, patterns of systemic racism lead to higher maternal mortality rates failing to reduce preventable deaths due to a myriad of reasons.[13, 19, 20] While little is known about the direct impacts of stigma on birth outcomes for LGBTQ+ people, early research suggests a higher likelihood of having to navigate choices and interventions based on differences in birth outcomes when compared to cisgender, heterosexual peers.[21]

From inadequate medical education materials,[22] to outdated assumptions around race and pain tolerance that result in harm,[23] to unethical management of clinical services along racial lines, we can see a pattern of institutional racism embedded into health care services. This is especially unfortunate when considered alongside the simultaneous push towards more medicalised perinatal care within the global majority,[24] despite evidence in support of the midwifery care model and decolonising reproductive health care.[25, 26] A lack of empirical evidence at the intersections of race, gender, and sexual orientation is in itself a demarcation of the need for improvements that acknowledge the diversity of people navigating pregnancy and reproductive health spaces.

CONTEMPORARY BARRIERS AND FACILITATORS OF CHOICE

For choice to be supported within the context of antenatal care, it is important to know who is expected to access care provisions. If heterosexual families are assumed to be the primary service user, this shapes everything from the intake forms to the discharge form, and every process in between. Awareness of LGBTQIA+ families needs to start at the policy and planning stages to reduce limited pathways. Meaning that there are "on the rails"[ii] experiences that low-risk pregnant people might experience, which limits the choices available to them, rather than providing patient-led care. An example of good practice, as supported by NICE guidelines,[27] includes access to elective caesarean section to help mitigate fear and/or dysphoria related to vaginal birth.

THE ROLE OF POLICY

Policies within reproductive health services come from a variety of sources, including governmental policies alongside guidance and policies from professional organisations, the latter of which can operate both globally and at various levels in specific countries. Local departmental-level and/or private practice policies may clarify or augment these policies. However, the existence of policies does not ensure the enactment of the approaches and solutions provided within them, particularly if and when there are policy recommendations that are at odds with each other, as well as at odds with the desires of the service users whose choices and actions are restricted by them. In part, this can be a result of "doing the document,"[28] where so many resources are used to create the guidance that they are exhausted, leaving no resources left to provide the education and support necessary to act on recommendations within the context of care provision. This can result in people receiving care either strictly to guidelines, despite irrelevance, and/or subjected to additional questions and stigmas because they are "off guidelines" for reasons not all members of the care team may agree upon.

In some cases, how care recommendations are interpreted is influenced by what is possible within existing systems of care. Local availability may then affect what different expectant parents are told a policy or guideline means. An example of this is the different interpretations of UK continuity of carer guidance, which ideally should be read as a consistent single provider meeting with the same services users,[29] but has also been interpreted by some as a restriction to a limited number of providers,[30] even if it does not have a tangible change to the care team that service users are working with (ie, always meeting with a new provider).[31] This is due to "the system" being the documents and policies that are separate from the people that may enact them, including how limited those implementations might be. In other words, health care administration and policies can limit even the most educated and altruistic health care professionals, keeping them from making spaces inclusive and welcoming of LGBTQ+ families.

While these limitations extend to the general provision of perinatal care, they are not insurmountable. As a health care professional, there is a responsibility to be familiar with all levels of guidance, from local policies to national recommendations from governmental institutions and professional organisations. In instances of private and/or insured care, there may also be a requirement to be familiar with the restrictions placed on health care professionals, as well as there being additional bureaucratic barriers in clinical spaces due to insurance policies.[32] Understandably this can complicate the ability to provide health services for midwives and other health care professionals.[33] In part, this is due to the organisational culture created through policy and strictness within the implementation of those policies,[iii] alongside the culture of inclusive care that is enabled, or hindered, as a result. Thus, policies impact the interactions possible between service user and health care professional, requiring awareness from the health care professional about how the adoption, and implementation, of policy can limit parents' choices through limiting acknowledgement of who is present within family constellations.

Maternity and reproductive health care operates in a field of exclusively gendered language which predominantly refers to mothers *versus* fathers which inherently diminishes choice through policy. There has, historically and currently, been a lack of acceptance that asking about gender and sexuality within perinatal care could be necessary; because of the assumptions about parenting and gender being fixed and binary. The only exception to this rule in UK society currently would be same-sex couples who adopt, as same-sex adoption is more visible in society. However, these families are not expected to need access to perinatal care as this is almost unconsciously viewed by mainstream society as a form of asexual reproduction. For LGBTQ+ families, this cisheteronormativity embedded into perinatal care can mean diminished quality of care, as well as creating extra work by making it necessary for them to actively seek out more supportive health care institutions and professionals.[34]

NAVIGATING PROVIDER ASSUMPTIONS AND EXPECTATIONS

When, after making a series of choices leading to their pregnancy (as discussed in the previous chapters), LGBTQ+ families access perinatal care, they continue to have to navigate a limited array of options due to heteronormative assumptions and the limitations that they place on service options and quality. While there may be time in some instances to challenge and change exclusionary policies, not all LGBTQ+ people will be able to do this. This could be because they are accessing care in an emergency or high stress circumstances, or it could be because the pregnant LGBTQ+ person does not feel entitled to insist that the correct pronouns are used, or that their same-sex partner is allowed to accompany them. In all instances, it is imperative that health care professionals, and supporting administrative staff, be mindful of inclusive practice to ensure that all documentation and paperwork is clear and avoid confusion and delay, and avoid adding extra minority stressors.

One of the first instances where this is relevant is the collection of data at the start of care provision (ie, booking appointment). Due to policy-based assumptions, how data is collected about parents and parents-to-be as they begin their maternity journey is constrained by the facility which health care providers have to capture such information. Within the UK paper-based notes held by the pregnant parent throughout their maternity journey are commonly used. These notes which capture information about both this pregnancy, social and health factors, and reproductive history. In their present state, there is no facility to capture information which sits outside of cisgendered, heteronormative assumptions. Even where questions asking about partners' details are not specifically gendered, the assumptions which are made by others about relationships may impact how care is delivered. The potential for discriminatory care may result in some same-gender couples reconsidering how they present to perinatal services where the non-birthing parent is a trans woman. A trans woman listed with her chosen name on her partner's green notes may be less likely to be seen as a parent in her own right, even if she is the biological parent to their child. Completing the form using her deadname[iv] is untrue to herself and may contribute to or retrigger gender dysphoria, but may result in her being viewed as a legitimate parent to their baby. Thus, even the decision making about how forms are filled in has the potential to cause harm, whichever choice the couple makes.

An exemplar of good practice here is the data capture used in the Brighton and Sussex maternity notes[35] which have been specifically designed to incorporate the use of additive language alongside gendered language.[v] This neither diminishes the language of maternity or that which relates to women, nor excludes those who do not identify as women, or whose families sit outside the assumed heteronormative configurations. However, the forms themselves do not automatically result in good experiences for LGBTQ+ parents. This is dependent upon the proper application and recording of the questions—with comfort level on the part of the health care provider influencing whether or not a question is asked properly, or even at all. In some cases, the assumptions of health care providers may be recorded as answers in place of service user answers. There may also be a choice made by the pregnant parent to not disclose their gender and/or sexual orientation at this first meeting, especially if it seems that disclosing that information will place them at risk of receiving lower quality care and support. This may however be a decision that could limit the ability for a partner to make choices in their care in emergency circumstances in the future. It is therefore important that health care providers recognise that this is key data which should be recorded accurately at the start of care, with information provided by the service user, as it will determine what care pathways and what services will be made available to the pregnant parent.

Once booked, pregnant parents, along with their partners, will face decisions around testing, health care, and interventions throughout their pregnancy. For all parents, these choices rely on having a health care professional that they trust, who is able to provide them with information about options in a way that facilitates informed consent and shared decision making.[36] Exploratory research suggests that sexual and gender minority parents may be offered more interventions due to higher risks of complications for some forms of assisted conception. They may therefore need to make more decisions about health care during pregnancy. Adding to this additional stress, finding a supportive health care provider may not be as straightforward for LGBTQ+ parents as it is for their cisgender heterosexual peers due to homophobia and transphobia. LGBTQ+ expectant parents who have used assisted conception may have had to interact with more health care providers from a wider range of disciplines than the average cisgender heterosexual expectant parent, thereby increasing the opportunities for them to experience not being supported in the choices they wish to make. They may also have encountered stigmatising policies and heterosexist assumptions around infertility.[34, 37] While LGBTQ+ people's existence may be increasingly supported within the general population, this is not always mirrored within reproductive health spaces.[38–40] LGBTQ+ people may therefore face additional pressure to avoid, or be hesitant to select certain options within health services due to additional layers of stigma (ie, IVF, birthing outside the hospital, elective C-section, etc.).

To summarise, not all service users experience pregnancy care in the same way. Restrictions to the care it is possible to choose is heavily dependent on the thoroughness with which a person can navigate those spaces as themselves (ie, being freely non-cisheteronormative in a presumptively cisheteronormative space). Additionally, for high quality shared decision making to be feasible, there must be a trusting relationship with a health care provider who is aware of this and adopts inclusive practices. Similarly, informed consent is only possible when inclusive documentation and data collection is present.

LEGAL RECOGNITION OF CO-PARENTS

In the UK, parental responsibility is automatically granted to the birthing parent, who is assumed to be the mother of the infant.[41] The second parent is assumed societally to be the male partner and therefore father of the baby. A father usually either assumes automatic parental responsibility by being married to the birthing mother, or by being listed on the birth certificate if the parents are not married prior to birth.[41] This joint registration means the father must be present at registration. The UK Government website states that:

> "same-sex partners will both have parental responsibility if they were civil partners at the time of the treatment, e.g., donor insemination or fertility treatment. Where same-sex partners are not civil partners, the second parent can get parental responsibility by applying for parental responsibility if a parental agreement was made, or becoming a civil partner of the other parent and making a parental responsibility agreement or jointly registering the birth."[42]

Already we see a discrepancy between registration requirements, where requirements for joint registration apply to unmarried heterosexual couples, but also to same-sex couples who **are** in a civil partnership. Alternatively, same-sex couples may make a parental responsibility agreement which must be signed and witnessed at the local court and accompanied by a copy of the child's birth certificate. Currently the wording on the gov.uk site identifies the routes for fathers and step-parents to acquire parental responsibility. There is no further specific reference to parents who do not conform to these heteronormative assumptions of family make up. The heterosexist assumptions behind these routes also do not recognise situations common amongst LGBTQ+ families, such as where the second parent may be the biological parent (in that their gametes may have been used) but not the birthing parent. This also means that the egg providing parent is the biological parent but, because they are not the birth parent, they may have no parental rights in law without a parental responsibility agreement, which the birthing parent could choose not to sign. Depending on how the baby was conceived, the biological but non-birthing parent could also require the consent of the biological father to gain parental responsibility.

Decisions about becoming parents and also decisions about who will be the gestational parent also come from within this understanding of the framework of legal assumptions about who will be the legal parent. Sometimes, these legal complexities are misunderstood or not fully understood by LGBTQ+ people prior to becoming parents. Navigating these legal complexities also influences the way in which co-parents in LGBTQ+ families share control and decision making.

EXPERIENCES OF CHOICE AND SOURCES OF COERCION

In both the global north and global south, heteronormative assumptions about relationships and family make-up influence who is seen as a valid parent. This occurs on societal, legal, and clinical levels. LGBTQ+ families often have relationships with their children which are more legally complex than relationships between heterosexual couples and their children. Historically, genetic links to children have predominantly been seen as the defining feature of parenthood, but many LGBTQ+ parents do not have genetic links to their children. For some parents in various forms of LGBTQ+ families, fertility and conception are hampered by lack of gametes.[43] For example, a cis woman may be partnered with another cis woman or a trans man, and therefore experience social infertility because there is no source of sperm within the partnership. Equally the person who wants to become pregnant may be a trans man partnered with a cis woman, where assumptions may be initially made about who the pregnant parent is, as well as the conception journey. Cis men who are partnered with other cis men or trans women experience social infertility because there is no source of ova within the relationship, and no person capable of carrying a pregnancy.

Decision making about birth options for LGBTQ+ parents will therefore be made within the context of having navigated a potentially complex and expensive conception process (see chapter 2).

Point for reflection on practice: Being aware of the complexity of parents' experiences of conception will allow for greater insight into their decision making around birth choices and also enable appropriate support to be put in place

---

How control is divided between the co-parents

We have already seen that LGBTQ+ families will have been navigating multiple decisions about becoming parents and also decisions about who will be the gestational parent also come from within the framework of legal assumptions of who will be the legal parent(s). Whilst decisions around bodily autonomy for the pregnant parent may legally lie solely with the pregnant parent, there is evidence that decision making about birth choices and place of birth may be ceded by the pregnant parent to the non-pregnant parent, to compensate for the marginalisation of their parenting role imposed by the complexities of the legal frameworks around who the legal parents of the infant are.[34]

These complexities around sharing of control and decision making may simultaneously be perceived as, and/or mask, control and coercion within couple relationships. Nursing staff and maternity staff have been identified as having low comfort levels with asking questions around domestic abuse (DA).[44] There are multiple barriers to disclosure of DA which have been identified.[45, 46] These include a lack of recognition that some non-violent experiences are abusive, disclosure of histories of DA which are met with disbelief, victim blaming, and critical judgement.[45]

Historically, DA has been viewed through a heteronormative lens, and predominantly framed within a gendered paradigm, in which men are usually the perpetrators. DA has therefore been considered to be how men act to gain and retain control and domination over those around them, which is reinforced and informed by patriarchal expectations.[47] This means it may be less likely for some health care professionals consider LGBTQ+ relationships as containing the same risk factors for DA as heterosexual relationships. The bi-directional body of research around DA ie, female partner on male partner, and that which is within LGBTQ+ partner relationships is sparse but increasing.[47] One systematic literature review, by Otero et al. found that most studies related to DA in LGBTQ+ partnerships conceptualised relationships with at least one trans partner as a homosexual relationship.[48] This review found that the prevalence of DA ranged from 18% to 80% in relationships between transgender, transsexual, and intersex couples.

Choices around birth

Where both partners have the potential to carry a pregnancy, dynamics may also be different regarding choices in birth depending on the obstetric history of the couple, rather than just the obstetric history of the pregnant person. The choice about who gives birth may be related to gender identity and previous exposure to stigma and prejudice in the health care system. Decisions may also depend on any previous births and any trauma which may have been experienced by either partner. Even within cishet couples there is an element of expectation around who gets to choose birthplace and type, again informed by patriarchal structures of society. Choices around place of birth for cishet women are informed by perceptions of risk, risk management, and social narratives around the "blame" for poor outcomes during birth.[49] Perception of the safe birth sits on one end of a continuum which positions hospital and obstetric medical models of birth at one end and freebirthing with no birth attendants at the opposite end. For LGBTQ+ families this risk perception is likely to sit in opposition to heteronormative perceptions of safety and care because of their previous or current interactions with health care providers, in this or previous pregnancies.[50] This is backed up by studies showing that pregnant trans men and sexual minority women in the UK are more likely to either have or seriously consider freebirth than pregnant heterosexual women.[51,52]

LGBTQ+ individuals are at higher risk of having experienced sexual trauma and abuse over their lifetime and this itself may also influence the choices made about pregnancy and birth, the decision making about conception, and the choices made about decisions during labour and birth.

Point for reflection on practice: Staff need to not just be thinking about individual needs of the couple in front of them, but potentially the wider implications of what a person's gender or sexuality may also mean. This relates to their health and reproductive journey to have got to this point, and any barriers and restrictions they may have already encountered, or barriers they may face in the future in negotiating reproductive health care as part of a non-hetero, and/or gender binary conforming couple.

Autonomy and risk management

. Vulnerability for all pregnant people during pregnancy and postpartum health care is due to personal risk management involved in navigating antenatal care and organisational policies.[53] It is also about the ability to make choices and the perception of autonomy within their health care and subsequent decision making. For LGBTQIA+ individuals, this can include the choice to disclose their gender and/or sexual orientation, or to keep that information private so as to reduce the risk of maltreatment.[54] For all pregnant people, each choice, or loss of choice, can add together, with additional, preventable stresses occurring when people are made to justify all their health care related choices (ie, preferring a dimly lit birth environment or declining a particular invention). For LGBTQIA+ individuals who do disclose their gender and/or sexual orientation, an additional risk is created, as stigma and prejudice may skew their health care team's opinion of their choices and preferences.[54,55]

Compounding this is the common assumption that all forms of supported conception, including IUI, IVF and, in some cases, home donor insemination are inherently more precarious and therefore higher risk. This assumption comes from statistics from fertility clinics, which fail to separate out results based on social infertility versus medical infertility, which are then translated into clinical guidance.[56] In such situations the pregnancy is often more closely monitored and there are further restrictions placed around what are considered medically safe options for birth (ie, at term but not at 42 weeks). This is another way in which minority stress is present in reproductive health care spaces, and in a way that explicitly shapes choice for LGBTQIA+ pregnant people.

LGBTQ+ pregnant people may therefore face barriers to asserting autonomy from both a health care system and potentially from coercive relationships with partner(s) or family member(s) that are leading to the way that choices are made during care. Similarly, it could be that because of the way in which non-gestational parents are frequently delegitimised as parents both socially and legally, within the couple relationship the birthing parent chooses to devolve much of the decision making to their partner to allow them to feel more involved in the process and as an equal contributor to the pregnancy and birth than may otherwise happen within current socio-legal and medical frameworks.

Birth Plans

One of the main ways that choice is laid out in a shareable format is as a Birth Plan. This document is meant to be a statement of the pregnant person's, and potentially couple's, preferences during childbirth. Motivation for creating these types of plans is to address potentialities in a way that allows for a process of informed decision making by the pregnant person, both individually and in collaboration with their partner(s). It is particularly valuable in cases where the pregnant person might have to rely on a partner and/or doula to advocate for them. For LGBTQIA+ individuals, this plan might include not only their preferences for care, but also information about their pronouns, gender, and/or sexual orientation as a means of introducing themselves to the care team that will be assisting them during childbirth. However, when providers are dismissive of these documents, it undermines choice on more than one level. Dismissal of a Birth Plan, or shaming of service users for providing them, one way that service users have reported loss of choice/autonomy in care. This is a form of coercive health care which diminishes both medical and personal choices, thus directly impacting health care needs. In the case of LGBTQIA+ people, it may also contribute to the erosion of identity through the removal of care options that are protective against minority stressors.

Informed consent/choice

While informed consent is often framed as an "in the moment" activity, there is a benefit to starting the discussion early by exploring all of the possibilities and the person's preference (ie, informed decision making). This is because it is important to establish trust and rapport between provider and service user as a routine part of the decision-making process. Additionally, creating a longer discussion, facilitated through continuity of carer, allows for there to be more than one option presented at the time of need. This means that there is time for all of the possibilities to be explored and understood by the pregnant person (and their partner where relevant). Having a better understanding of what may or may not happen and the risks of the choices available is a key tenet of informed choice, which should be considered the ideal form of choice in any scenario. For LGBTQIA+ parents, it is extremely important to understand their individual desires for their pregnancies and childbirth, as these will be unique to each person that is supported. It is paramount that previous caregiving experiences with other LGBTQIA+ families not inadvertently limit the choices and possibilities offered, or be used to pressure the pregnant person into certain "usual" options due to assumptions. Additionally, it is important to consider if professional and professional biases, in place of evidence-based approaches, are playing a role in the care provisions being offered to pregnant people.

RECOMMENDATIONS FOR IMPROVING CHOICE IN PERINATAL CARE PATHWAYS FOR LGBTQ+ PARENTS

Recent efforts in reproductive health care have shown progress towards making inclusive spaces for more diverse family and parenting constellations. In an effort to continue that momentum the following recommendations seek to improve how, who, and when choice is possible within the space of antenatal care, though these recommendations are also relevant to other facets of reproductive health care as well.

Professional and organisation guidelines

Present professional organisational guidance on shared decision making and informed consent focus on the general population,[57, 58] without mention of the importance of nuance that may be present within marginalised groups.

An example would be to include guidance on how to build trust and communicate with various groups within the communities served, including recommendations around language use to improve policies and documentations locally. As well as momentum and awareness that can help to improve having supportive and community-centred policies. As discussed earlier within the chapter, the guidelines at Brighton and Sussex Hospital[35] help to clarify and improve concurrent policies to make sure that there is a welcoming context for LGBTQIA+ parents, as well as more active implementation of professional guidance at an organisational level.

Legal and policy recommendations

As health care professionals, it is important to be aware of and advocate for the parents that are under your care. For LGBTQIA+ parents, this includes helping to expand governmental documentation that allows for the accurate recording of parent's lived experiences and relationships with their child(ren). As government documentation is often a key means of determining what care pathways people are able to access, it is important to ensure that they are able to choose the proper pathway for their experiences within reproductive health care. For example, there needs to be a clear pathway that supports the option for trans women to store and retrieve their gametes, and for a father who has given birth to have the right to be listed as father on their child's birth certificate. These legal decisions have direct implications to LGBTQIA+ health care choices, so should be improved and supported going forward.

Training which prepares

As exemplified within this text, training and health care professional curricula need to expand to include knowledge about LGBTQIA+ people. This can be done through the addition of diverse case studies, as well as in-depth discussions on the importance of cultural humility. The latter recommendation speaks to the importance of viewing knowledge about patient populations as being an on-going learning process. The more knowledgeable a provider is, the more prepared they can be to offer appropriate options, while understanding that service user's needs are not homogenous, which helps to build trusting relationships and open communication. In addition to active engagement with the literature, it is also recommended that health care professionals and organisations connect with their local communities to ensure that their needs are being met and that all relevant options are made available for when it comes time for parents to choose the best pathways for their care.

KEY LEARNING POINTS

Not all choices in reproductive care are equally available to everyone. Within the role of health care professional, it will be imperative that you translate information and ensure that it is inclusive and accessible to make sure that the people you are caring for are able to make the right decisions for themselves, as well as being able to provide informed consent in relation to those decisions.

- Trust and communication are key facets of facilitating shared decision making.
- LGBTQIA+ pregnant parents may have to make more decisions, while also facing lower levels of representation within the informational materials.
- The health care professional is responsible for being aware of all possible options and to provide them with cultural humility.

NOTES

i   The etymology of the words midwife and obstetrician can sometimes help to elucidate the expectations of the clinician roles historically, including acknowledging the professional tension between said roles.

ii   "On the rails" is used to describe experiences that are fixed pathways with no room for change or personalisation.

iii This phenomenon of "doing the document" in place of facilitating equity can be further explored within Sarah Ahmed's work to aid in understanding barriers and working to improve policy and implementation.[28]

iv   This may be a person's former and/or legal name in place of the name that they are known. Using a person's deadname is disrespectful and may contribute to misgendering alongside misuse of pronouns based on the gendered expectations some names carry.

v   This practice is becoming more common at Hospital Trusts due to local efforts. At the time of publication, the statement by Green and Riddington was the most public example within the UK as well as being a gold standard in guidance for Trusts.

REFERENCES

1. Aristoteles, Peck AL. *Aristotle. 13: Generation of Animals / with an Engl. transl. by A. L. Peck*. Repr. Harvard Univ. Press; 2007.
2. Bacon F. *New Atlantis*. (Smith GCM, ed.). Cambridge University Press; 2014.
3. Schwartz MJ. *Birthing a Slave: Motherhood and Medicine in the Antebellum South*. Harvard University Press; 2006.
4. McIntosh T. *A Social History of Maternity and Childbirth: Key Themes in Maternity Care*. 1st ed. Routledge; 2013. doi:10.4324/9780203124222

5. Bergen JA. Birth and Death in Nineteenth-Century Dublin's Lying-In Hospitals. In: Farrell E, ed. *'She Said She Was in the Family Way': Pregnancy and Infancy in Modern Ireland.* Institute of Historical Research; 2012. doi:10.14296/117.9771909646476

6. O'Toole E. Medicinal Care in the Eighteenth- and Early Nineteenth-Century Irish Home. In: Farrell E, ed. *'She Said She Was in the Family Way': Pregnancy and Infancy in Modern Ireland.* Institute of Historical Research; 2012. doi:10.14296/117.9771909646476

7. Sutcliffe K, Caird J, Kavanagh J, et al. Comparing Midwife-Led and Doctor-Led Maternity Care: A Systematic Review of Reviews. *J Adv Nurs.* 2012;68(11):2376–2386. doi:10.1111/j.1365-2648.2012.05998.x

8. Ehrenreich B, English D. *Witches, Midwives, and Nurses: A History of Women Healers.* 2nd ed. Feminist Press at the City University of New York; 2010.

9. Chamberlain G. *From Witchcraft to Wisdom: A History of Obstetrics & Gynaecology in the British Isles.* RCOG Press; 2007.

10. Towler J, Bramall J. *Midwives in History and Society.* 1st ed. Routledge; 2022. doi:10.4324/9781003378105

11. Healy S, Humphreys E, Kennedy C. Midwives' and Obstetricians' Perceptions of Risk and its Impact on Clinical Practice and Decision-Making in Labour: An Integrative Review. *Women Birth.* 2016;29(2):107–116. doi:10.1016/j.wombi.2015.08.010

12. Owens K. When Less is More: Shifting Risk Management in American Childbirth. In: *Advances in Medical Sociology.* Emerald Publishing Limited; 2019:45–62. doi:10.1108/S1057-629020190000020008

13. on behalf of MBRRACE-UK. *Saving Lives, Improving Mothers' Care Core Report –Lessons Learned to Inform Maternity Care from the UK and Ireland Confidential Enquiries into Maternal Deaths and Morbidity 2018-20.* (Marian Knight, Kathryn Bunch, Roshni Patel, et al., eds.). National Perinatal Epidemiology Unit, University of Oxford; 2022. Accessed April 16, 2023. https://www.npeu.ox.ac.uk/assets/downloads/mbrrace-uk/reports/maternal-report-2022/MBRRACE-UK_Maternal_MAIN_Report_2022_v10.pdf

14. Hailu EM, Maddali SR, Snowden JM, Carmichael SL, Mujahid MS. Structural Racism and Adverse Maternal Health Outcomes: A Systematic Review. *Health Place.* 2022;78:102923. doi:10.1016/j.healthplace.2022.102923

15. Casanova-Perez R, Apodaca C, Bascom E, et al. Broken Down by Bias: Healthcare Biases Experienced by BIPOC and LGBTQ+ Patients. *AMIA Annu Symp Proc AMIA Symp.* 2021; 2021:275–284.

16. Mitchell LA, Jacobs C, McEwen A. (In)visibility of LGBTQIA+ People and Relationships in Healthcare: A Scoping Review. *Patient Educ Couns.* 2023;114:107828. doi:10.1016/j.pec.2023.107828

17. Wilton T, Kaufmann T. Lesbian Mothers' Experiences of Maternity Care in the UK. *Midwifery.* 2001;17(3):203–211. doi:10.1054/midw.2001.0261

18. Röndahl G, Bruhner E, Lindhe J. Heteronormative Communication with Lesbian Families in Antenatal Care, Childbirth and Postnatal Care. *J Adv Nurs.* 2009;65(11):2337–2344. doi:10.1111/j.1365-2648.2009.05092.x

19. Ujah IAO, Aisien OA, Mutihir JT, Vanderjagt DJ, Glew RH, Uguru VE. Factors Contributing to Maternal Mortality in North-Central Nigeria: A Seventeen-Year Review. *Afr J Reprod Health.* 2005;9(3):27. doi:10.2307/3583409

20. Fleszar LG, Bryant AS, Johnson CO, et al. Trends in State-Level Maternal Mortality by Racial and Ethnic Group in the United States. *JAMA*. 2023;330(1):52. doi:10.1001/jama.2023.9043

21. Luxion K. Serving LGBT+ Parents: How Patient Experiences Influence Birth Outcomes. In: Southeastern Women's Studies Association; 2018.

22. Louie P, Wilkes R. Representations of Race and Skin Tone in Medical Textbook Imagery. *Soc Sci Med*. 2018;202:38–42. doi:10.1016/j.socscimed.2018.02.023

23. Amutah C, Greenidge K, Mante A, et al. Misrepresenting Race — The Role of Medical Schools in Propagating Physician Bias. Malina D, ed. *N Engl J Med*. 2021;384(9):872–878. doi:10.1056/NEJMms2025768

24. Miani C, Wandschneider L, Batram-Zantvoort S, et al. Individual and Country-Level Variables Associated with the Medicalization of Birth: Multilevel Analyses of IMAgiNE EURO Data from 15 Countries in the WHO European Region. *Int J Gynecol Obstet*. 2022; 159(S1):9–21. doi:10.1002/ijgo.14459

25. Oladapo O, Tunçalp Ö, Bonet M, et al. WHO Model of Intrapartum Care for a Positive Childbirth Experience: Transforming Care of Women and Babies for Improved Health and Wellbeing. *BJOG Int J Obstet Gynaecol*. 2018;125(8):918–922. doi:10.1111/1471-0528. 15237

26. Lokugamage AU, Robinson N, Pathberiya SDC, Wong S, Douglass C. Respectful Maternity Care in the UK Using a Decolonial Lens. *SN Soc Sci*. 2022;2(12):267. doi:10.1007/s43545-022-00576-5

27. Royal College of Obstetricians & Gynaecologists. *Considering a Caesarean Birth*. Royal College of Obstetricians & Gynaecologists; 2022. Accessed December 17, 2023. https://www.rcog.org.uk/for-the-public/browse-our-patient-information/considering-a-caesarean-birth/

28. Ahmed S. 'You End up Doing the Document Rather than Doing the Doing': Diversity, Race Equality and the Politics of Documentation. *Ethn Racial Stud*. 2007;30(4):590–609. doi:10. 1080/01419870701356015

29. Sandall J, Soltani H, Gates S, Shennan A, Devane D. Midwife-Led Continuity Models Versus Other Models of Care for Childbearing Women. Cochrane Pregnancy and Childbirth Group, ed. *Cochrane Database Syst Rev*. 2016;2016(4). doi:10.1002/14651858.CD004667. pub5

30. National Institute of Clinical Excellence. Antenatal Care Quality Standard [QS22: Quality Statement 3, Continuity of Carer. Published online 2012. https://www.nice.org.uk/guidance/QS22/chapter/quality-statement-3-continuity-of-carer

31. NHS England. *Maternity Transformation Programme, Implementing Better Births: Continuity of Carer*; 2021. https://www.england.nhs.uk/mat-transformation/implementing-better-births/continuity-of-carer/

32. Thompson E, Lewis P. Midwifery Independence – Past, Present and Future. *Br J Midwifery*. 2013;21(10):732–735. doi:10.12968/bjom.2013.21.10.732

33. Feeley C. *Supporting Physiological Birth Choices in Midwifery Practice: The Role of Workplace Culture, Politics and Ethics*. (First Edition). Routledge; 2023. doi:10.4324/97810 03265443

34. Greenfield M. *LGBTQ+ Mums Research*. Best Beginnings; 2023. doi: 10.5281/zenodo. 8326480

35. Green H, Riddington A. Gender Inclusive Language and Perinatal Services: Mission Statement and Rationale. Published online December 2020. https://www.bsuh.nhs.uk/maternity/wp-content/uploads/sites/7/2021/01/Gender-inclusive-language-in-perinatal-services.pdf

36. O'Brien D, Butler MM, Casey M. A Participatory Action Research Study Exploring Women's Understandings of the Concept of Informed Choice During Pregnancy and Childbirth in Ireland. *Midwifery*. 2017;46:1–7. doi:10.1016/j.midw.2017.01.002

37. Priddle H. How Well are Lesbians Treated in UK Fertility Clinics? *Hum Fertil*. 2015;18(3):194–199. doi:10.3109/14647273.2015.1043654

38. Wingo E, Ingraham N, Roberts SCM. Reproductive Health Care Priorities and Barriers to Effective Care for LGBTQ People Assigned Female at Birth: A Qualitative Study. *Womens Health Issues*. 2018;28(4):350–357. doi:10.1016/j.whi.2018.03.002

39. Kohli M, Reeves I, Waters L. Homophobia in the Provision of Sexual Health Care in the UK. *Lancet HIV*. 2024;11(2):e125–e130. doi:10.1016/S2352-3018(23)00302-8

40. Sbragia JD, Vottero B. Experiences of Transgender Men in Seeking Gynecological and Reproductive Health Care: A Qualitative Systematic Review. *JBI Evid Synth*. 2020;18(9):1870–1931. doi:10.11124/JBISRIR-D-19-00347

41. Foster D. *Parental Responsibility in England and Wales*. House of Commons Library; 2023. Accessed June 24, 2024. https://researchbriefings.files.parliament.uk/documents/CBP-8760/CBP-8760.pdf

42. UK Government. *Parental Rights and Responsibilities*; 2024. Accessed June 24, 2024. https://www.gov.uk/parental-rights-responsibilities/who-has-parental-responsibility

43. Lo W, Campo-Engelstein L. Expanding the Clinical Definition of Infertility to Include Socially Infertile Individuals and Couples. In: Campo-Engelstein L, Burcher P, eds. *Reproductive Ethics II*. Springer International Publishing; 2018:71–83. doi:10.1007/978-3-319-89429-4_6

44. Bradbury-Jones C, Molloy E, Clark M, Ward N. Gender, Sexual Diversity and Professional Practice Learning: Findings from a Systematic Search and Review. *Stud High Educ*. 2020;45(8):1618–1636. doi:10.1080/03075079.2018.1564264

45. Warman J. Testimonial Smothering and Domestic Violence Disclosure in Clinical Contexts. *Episteme*. 2023;20(1):107–124. doi:10.1017/epi.2021.3

46. Heron RL, Eisma MC. Barriers and Facilitators of Disclosing Domestic Violence to the Healthcare Service: A Systematic Review of Qualitative Research. *Health Soc Care Community*. 2021;29(3):612–630. doi:10.1111/hsc.13282

47. Hine B, Noku L, Bates EA, Jayes K. But, Who Is the Victim Here? Exploring Judgments Toward Hypothetical Bidirectional Domestic Violence Scenarios. *J Interpers Violence*. 2022;37(7-8):NP5495–NP5516. doi:10.1177/0886260520917508

48. Otero LMR, Carrera Fernández MV, Lameiras Fernández M, Rodríguez Castro Y. Violencia en parejas transexuales, transgénero e intersexuales: una revisión bibliográfica. *Saúde E Soc*. 2015;24(3):914–935. doi:10.1590/S0104-12902015134224

49. Coxon K, Sandall J, Fulop NJ. To What Extent are Women Free to Choose Where to Give Birth? How Discourses of Risk, Blame and Responsibility Influence Birth Place Decisions. *Health Risk Soc*. 2014;16(1):51–67. doi:10.1080/13698575.2013.859231

50. Martos AJ, Wilson PA, Gordon AR, Lightfoot M, Meyer IH. "Like Finding a Unicorn": Healthcare Preferences Among Lesbian, Gay, and Bisexual People in the United States. *Soc Sci Med*. 2018;208:126–133. doi:10.1016/j.socscimed.2018.05.020

51. LGBT Foundation. *Improving Trans and Non-Binary Experiences of Maternity Services (ITEMS) Report*; 2022:63. Accessed December 6, 2023. https://dxfy8lrzbpywr.cloudfront.net/Files/97ecdaea-833d-4ea5-a891-c59f0ea429fb/ITEMS%2520report%2520final.pdf

52. Greenfield M, Payne-Gifford S, McKenzie G. Between a Rock and a Hard Place: Considering "Freebirth" During Covid-19. *Front Glob Womens Health*. 2021;2. doi:10.3389/fgwh.2021.603744

53. Briscoe L, Lavender T, McGowan L. A Concept Analysis of Women's Vulnerability During Pregnancy, Birth and the Postnatal Period. *J Adv Nurs*. 2016;72(10):2330–2345. doi:https://doi.org/10.1111/jan.13017

54. Greenfield M, Darwin Z. Trans and Non-Binary Pregnancy, Traumatic Birth, and Perinatal Mental Health: A Scoping Review. *Int J Transgender Health*. 2021;22(1–2):203–216. doi:10.1080/26895269.2020.1841057

55. Stewart M. Lesbian Parents Talk about their Birth Experiences. *Br J Midwifery*. 1999;7(2):96–101. doi:10.12968/bjom.1999.7.2.8377

56. Meads C, Thorogood LR, Lindemann K, Bewley S. Why Are the Proportions of In-Vitro Fertilisation Interventions for Same Sex Female Couples Increasing? *Healthcare*. 2021;9(12):1657. doi:10.3390/healthcare9121657

57. American College of Obstetricians and Gynecologists. Informed Consent and Shared Decision Making in Obstetrics and Gynecology. Published online 2021.

58. Royal College of Obstetricians & Gynaecologists. Obtaining Valid Consent: Clinical Governance Advice No. 6. Published online 2015. Accessed December 17, 2023. https://www.rcog.org.uk/media/pndfv5qf/cga6.pdf

Chapter 7

Birthing in the context of minority stress, fear of childbirth, and birth trauma

*Sofia Klittmark, Hanna Grundström,
Katri Nieminen, Josephine Lindén Åsell,
and Anna Malmquist*

INTRODUCTION

There is comprehensive evidence that a positive birth experience can contribute to increased long-term health. In contrast, a negative experience increases the risk of mental illness in the postpartum period[1-5] and in the long term. In addition, it can also negatively affect the child's start in life.[6] Care during birth and the relations to health care professionals (HCPs) are significant for both birth outcomes and birth experiences, and being able to have continuous support during birth reduces the risk of complications as well as negative birth experiences.[7, 8]

To some extent, LGBTQ+ families have the same needs as everyone else when becoming a parent, but they also have specific needs concerning pregnancy and birthing and may enter reproductive care carrying minority stress. Reproductive care, like society in general, is characterised by cisheteronormative structures and attitudes which may negatively affect the treatment of LGBTQ+ people within health care. Deficiencies in care and minority stress may also affect the ability to trust the caregiver.[9]

Fear of childbirth (FOC) and negative birth expectations also increase the risk of having a negative or traumatic childbirth experience.[3] Fear of childbirth, both before and during pregnancy, as well as postpartum, is associated with anxiety and depression in general.[1, 3, 4] As the prevalence of mental illness in general is increased among lesbian, gay, bisexual, transgender, and queer (LGBTQ+) people,[9]

DOI: 10.4324/9781003305446-8

the risk of FOC and birth trauma may also be increased.[10] Therefore, awareness of FOC and birth trauma among LGBTQ+ people is important.

Increased knowledge of the impact of cisheteronormativity and minority stress experiences during pregnancy and childbirth is crucial for HCPs to develop adjusted interventions to meet the needs of gestational and non-gestational LGBTQ+ prospective parents. Adequate support before, during and after birth is a key factor for increasing the long-term reproductive health of LGBTQ+ people and may lower minority stress, FOC, negative birth experiences, birth trauma, postpartum depression, postpartum PTSD, and secondary fear of childbirth.

In this chapter, we discuss FOC and birth trauma in an LGBTQ+ context and share experiences from lesbian, bisexual, trans and queer gestational and non-gestational parents, taking part in our interview and survey studies, as well as clinical experiences from Sweden,[10–12, 14–20] followed by key points for HCPs on how to provide competent and well-adjusted care for LGBTQ+ parents during birth.

FEAR OF CHILDBIRTH IN AN LGBTQ+ CONTEXT

FOC can vary from disturbing thoughts to paralysing fear.[21] The fear is commonly focused around one or more specific aspects of giving birth, such as fear of pain, injury, loss of control, or death. FOC can be oriented towards one's own potential or up-coming birth, as well as the partner's birth.[22] FOC have a negative impact on life during pregnancy for the one who is pregnant and also for non-pregnant partners with FOC, and can predispose both a pregnant and non-pregnant person to experience birth as a traumatic event.[21] Severe FOC increases the risk of prolonged labour, instrumental and caesarean births.[23]

FOC is generally focused on specific aspects of childbirth, but it must be contextualised and understood in relation to broader experiences of social and/or psychological vulnerability, including a person's identity and self-image. Mental illness, such as anxiety disorders and depression, are vulnerability factors predisposing individuals to severe FOC.[1, 3, 4, 24] People with previous experiences of sexual or physical abuse are more prone to develop severe FOC, as well as those with previous experiences of other trauma.[1, 20, 25] Furthermore, FOC has been shown to have increased prevalence in specific groups such as Black and minority ethnic women,[26] women with socioeconomic vulnerability and those who lack social support in their personal network or from a partner.[1]

Increased prevalence among pregnant LGBTQ+ people

FOC has mainly been studied in Western countries, among cisgender heterosexual women and – to some degree – their partners.[21, 22] A meta-analysis of FOC in the general pregnant population worldwide showed a prevalence of 14%, including both nulliparous and multiparous pregnant people.[27] In our survey study of 80 pregnant LGBTQ+ individuals, the prevalence of severe FOC was 20%,[10] which is considerably higher than previously measured worldwide prevalence. The prevalence of severe FOC among participants with clinical symptoms of general anxiety or depression in our study was high (46%). This indicates that LGBTQ+ people with these conditions are at higher risk of FOC, which can be addressed through adequate and competent professional support.

It is further worth noting that the prevalence of FOC among LGBTQ+ identified partners was low (9%) compared to the pregnant respondents. This is also slightly lower than the previously reported prevalence of FOC in cisgender male partners of pregnant heterosexual women in Sweden (11–14%).[28, 29]

Negotiating who gives birth and the influence of fear of childbirth

Deciding who will be the gestational parent, when more than one person in a family has the potential to carry a child, is an important decision that can affect parenting roles for many years ahead. FOC has been shown to contribute to the decision in couples where both partners have child-bearing capacities. In one of our studies with lesbian, bisexual and transgender individuals with a pronounced FOC, the fear was negotiated as one of many aspects that contributed to deciding who would be the one giving birth.[16] Several participants chose to become pregnant despite their fears, due to a desire to be the genetic parent and/or have the social role as the biological mother in the family. Other participants decided to refrain from pregnancy due to FOC and were delighted that their partner would give birth. Jeanette had a FOC and her partner did not. Her partner was the one who gave birth and Jeanette explained her reasons like this:

> *"Well, the biggest reason [for me not to become pregnant] is that I've always had a phobic fear of childbirth and haven't had the desire or any longing to get pregnant, so I was hugely relieved that she wanted to do it."*
>
> *(Jeanette, non-gestational parent)*

In other couples, one partner feared childbirth, while the other partner had other medical, social, or personal reasons for not being willing to get pregnant.

The couples explained that they negotiated around who could be considered to be the least vulnerable person, which led some of them to become pregnant despite FOC, if their partner was considered more vulnerable for other reasons. Emelie, who was pregnant with her first child at the time of the interview, had decided with her partner, a transgender man, that she was least vulnerable in relation to childbearing. She described their considerations as:

> *"He is, you know, non-white, like, non-cis (laughs), and like, he has quite a few factors. [...] Umm, he has previously come up against quite a lot of structural discrimination, umm, and maybe that was why we thought that it would be too much, like."*
>
> *(Emelie, pregnant)*

Thus, it is important to acknowledge that either or both partners in an LGBTQ+ couple may suffer from severe FOC, which may affect family planning even before pregnancy. It is also important to view FOC from an intersectional perspective, as structural discrimination in many forms may impact on the choice to become pregnant or not, as well as on the fears during pregnancy.

How norms and ideals interact with fear of childbirth

Gender dysphoria among transgender and genderqueer people often increases during pregnancy[30, 31] and may also increase FOC. Maternity, pregnancy, and childbirth are surrounded by strong cultural norms and expectations[32, 33] and in addition to transgender and genderqueer people, also lesbian and bisexual women can be bothered by such norms. In our study, LGBTQ+ individuals described how these types of norms and ideals contributed to their FOC and added extra dimensions to their fears.[15] Participants experienced stress related to an idealisation of "natural" births and a strong "primal woman" giving birth without much pain, or without complaints. Further, a cisnormative society will expect pregnant people to be women and feminine, and pregnant bodies are expected to fulfil female gender ideals. Emelie, a self-identified woman with an androgynous gender expression, feared that her pregnancy would be a dysphoric experience for her because of bodily changes which she expected would give her a more feminine body:

> *"Even if I'm, like, not trans or nonbinary, I can imagine that it will, definitely, be quite an, umm, physical and maybe dysphoric experience for me [being pregnant]. I'm like used to being a very androgynous body, um, and always have been."*
>
> *(Emelie, pregnant)*

Studies of transmasculine people's experiences of pregnancy and childbirth report feelings of exclusion, isolation, and loneliness[31, 34, 35] Our interviewees with an androgynous or masculine gender expression or gender identity described how the norms surrounding pregnancies made them uncomfortable, and that it contributed to their FOC. They feared that their pregnancies would increase body dysphoria and that they would feel uncomfortable being perceived as feminine and/or as women. Jonathan, a transgender man, shared in his interview a fear of becoming pregnant, because he feared being disrespectfully treated as a man giving birth.

> *"I want it [birth giving] to, like, be a nice memory even if it won't, like, be fantastic all the way through probably, but. And it feels like it could potentially be a situation where you instead come up against ignorance or discrimination or incorrect care or yes, that sort of thing."*
>
> *(Jonathan, has no children)*

Cisnormativity and femininity norms with its messages around who and how a person giving birth should be, identify as, behave, feel, or dress, could be identified as stressors for some participants.[15] This can be understood as minority stress affecting those who break norms around feminine body ideals or feminine gender expressions during pregnancy and childbirth.

Minority stress adds an additional layer to fear of childbirth

Minority stress offers an explanation for the increased prevalence of FOC in LGBTQ+ people. In our study of LGBTQ+ people with a pronounced FOC,[14] participants described fears similar to those previously described in the literature on FOC, eg, unbearable pain, being injured or losing control[1, 21, 27] But in addition to those fears, our participants added that they feared being deficiently treated because of their sexual orientation and/or gender identities.[14] In that way, fear of insufficient or prejudicial treatment in health care became part of the FOC. Experiences of cisheteronormativity together with fearing hatred of LGBTQ+ people added an additional layer to their fear of childbirth. Petra experienced her birth as traumatic, and explained how her level of stress increased as the midwife assumed her wife to be her sister:

> *"I feel, instead of assuming a relationship, she could have just asked, "What is your relationship?" it doesn't take long. And that was really important because, amidst all the traumatic stuff, it was just another thing that was difficult too, "Don't assume that we are sisters, you idiot" [...] It's more humiliating to say the wrong thing than to ask."*
>
> *(Petra, gestational parent)*

Other participants explained how erroneous or tactless assumptions and questions had made them feel offended, invisible, and stressed. Some of them pointed out that they often handle cisheteronormative assumptions in their everyday life, but during labour and birth, they were particularly vulnerable and already stressed due to FOC – therefore, dealing with cisheteronormativity became particularly stressful.

The exposure to minority stress led some LGBTQ+ people to develop hypervigilance. Previous experiences of diminished quality of health care led to expectations of homo-, bi-, or transphobia in future HCP interactions, causing lower trust in HCPs. This is important as hypervigilance and low trust will affect the possibility of reaching out to a person and successfully treating FOC. Furthermore, lack of a trusting relationship with HCPs is an additional risk factor for a traumatic birth.[8, 36]

Cisheteronormative ideas and negative attitudes about LGBTQ+ people can also be incorporated into one's self-image, leading to internalised homo-, bi-, or transphobia. Stina, a lesbian participant, provided an example of how internalised homophobia affected her FOC. She suffered from severe FOC and described that good support from her partner during birth would be particularly important for her to feel safe. However, her partner was uncomfortable with disclosing their intimate relation to others, which made it difficult for her partner to provide the kind of support she wanted:

> "The few times we've held each other's hand or, like, shown in public that we're a couple and if someone has said something, then it affects her experience massively, and she feels that she has done something wrong and, she doesn't want to subject herself, or me, to get negative feelings linked to our relationship or to me, and to everything. So that's why, so, it will be present ahead of delivery, because she, I think that she thinks that if she acts like she is my partner, holds my hand or kisses me or something, she risks being met by homophobia, which will cause her to get a huge amount of negative emotions and she doesn't want that, at that time, so she doesn't do it."
>
> (Stina, non-gestational parent planning to become pregnant)

Low or negative expectations of health care and HCPs were common among LGBTQ+ participants in our interview studies.[11, 12, 14–19] Helen, who was the pregnant partner in a lesbian couple, described how the midwife's heteronormative treatment during antenatal appointments affected her ability to talk about FOC and ask for help.[11] She avoided telling the midwife about her FOC, despite wanting and needing support:

> "I felt very odd as a lesbian to go there (the prenatal clinic), and I think that was a reason, I felt like I turned things off and did not want to talk to her about other things that I find difficult and so on, because I felt that there is no point in bringing things up. So even fear of childbirth and like my thoughts about it, I felt like I could not bring up in that environment, or what to say. And it would certainly have been better to do it earlier, but well, I couldn't do it."
>
> *(Helen, gestational parent)*

Several non-gestational parents also described a lack of attention from HCPs about their fear of childbirth, or mental wellbeing generally, during their partner's pregnancy. Exploring and treating a non-gestational parent's FOC gives better conditions for the gestational parent to be supported by their partner during birth, and reduces the risk of birth trauma.

The importance of building trust

Midwives supporting pregnant people with FOC need to be competent, sensitive, and professional when addressing the fears.[37] Working to build trust is a prerequisite to being able to treat FOC. When a parent-to-be is not feeling safe in health care appointments, it becomes complicated to build a trusting relationship, which increases the risk that care needs are not noticed or met. LGBTQ+ people with severe FOC can be seen as a particularly vulnerable group of patients whose care needs sometimes are not addressed in health care. The cisheteronormative structures and attitudes existing in pregnancy care, together with the consequences of minority stress, might make LGBTQ+ people hesitant to even seek care or open up to HCPs. Therefore, HCPs need to learn how to build trust in relation to LGBTQ+ people, to be able to explore and reduce FOC.

Key points

FOC treatments and interventions for LGBTQ+ people must be designed to acknowledge the importance of:

- Building trust in the caring relationship by being flexible and responsive to the wishes and needs of LGBTQ+ people.
- Carefully exploring previous negative experiences of health care and experiences of homo, bi-, or transphobic hatred.

- Acknowledging and validating previous negative experiences in health care.
- Not forgetting to investigate fears and expectations around giving birth related to a person's gender identity, sexuality, and family constellation.
- Addressing how norms concerning assumptions around gender and femininity affect the individual's comfort with being pregnant and how that influences the FOC.
- Investigating whether and how FOC influenced the decision of who is giving birth (in case there is more than one prospective parent who can become pregnant) to be able to provide adequate support to both gestational and non-gestational parents before, during and after birth.
- Addressing both gestational and non-gestational prospective parents' expectancies of childbirth and offering treatment when *any partner* fears childbirth.
- Exploring earlier birthing experiences of *any partner* if they have given birth before.

BIRTH TRAUMA IN AN LGBTQ+ CONTEXT

Giving birth may be a traumatic event for the person giving birth, as well as for a partner/co-parent witnessing the birth.[22, 28] Birth trauma is influenced by several factors, both predisposing factors before birth and by factors during birth.[5, 38] Two predisposing risk factors are FOC and/or previous mental illness, which puts LGBTQ+ people at elevated risk for both birth trauma and postpartum FOC, as traumatic birth experiences, in turn, increase FOC in subsequent pregnancies.[39] In terms of factors during birth, subjective negative experiences of care are one of the most significant factors for birth trauma and the development of postpartum PTSD.[40, 41] Lack of information and support during birth increases the risk of trauma in both gestational and non-gestational parents.[42-44] Negative interactions with HCPs, such as disrespectful treatment, threats and violation of integrity, or HCPs failing to obtain informed consent to interventions increase the risk of a traumatic experience. Other risk factors are experiencing feelings of powerlessness, loss of control, lack of trust or experiencing stigma.[7, 36, 45, 46]

Mental illness before and/or during pregnancy increases the risk of obstetric complications, such as emergency caesarean, instrumental birth, major haemorrhage, and perineal lacerations.[47] Births without complications requiring obstetric interventions may be experienced as traumatic,[38] but experiencing complications increases the risk.[48, 49] When unexpected obstetrical interventions arise, care experiences often deteriorate.[36, 50] However, birthing people often do not identify the intervention in itself as traumatic, but rather *how* the interventions were performed, making the interactions significant for the traumatic experience.[45, 51]

Adequate treatment for FOC and mental illness during pregnancy is one important factor for optimising the conditions for a positive birth experience and lowering the risk for birth trauma.[52] Among LGBTQ+ people, the impact of minority stress creates other risk factors that elevate the risk of negative birth experiences. In one of our studies, LGBTQ+ gestational and non-gestational participants shared their experiences of birth trauma and experiencing complications at birth.[11, 12, 18, 19] Heteronormative structures within both pregnancy and birthing care and heteronormative treatment from HCPs during both pregnancy and birthing were central to their subjective trauma experiences. Even prior to attending antenatal care, the participants feared that they would be treated cisheteronormatively. Unfortunately, these fears were realised for many participants, which in turn added feelings of stress, frustration, and anxiety. Experiencing a lack of support during pregnancy meant that participants approached birth with high levels of minority stress, being hypervigilant and having low trust in HCPs, which in turn contributed to negative and traumatic birth experiences. Thus, interventions by HCPs to lower minority stress and build trustful caring relationships need to begin during pregnancy.

Addressing risk factors during pregnancy

Some of our participants described that information provided around birth and parenting during pregnancy was not adjusted to their family situation, which created knowledge gaps.[11, 12] Information directed to non-gestational parents was missing, for example about the social role of becoming a non-gestational mother, or witnessing birth in the context of having planned to give birth in the future, or with previous own childbirth experience(s). This lack of thorough information contributed to stress and anxiety before and during childbirth and in the early stages of parenthood. Feelings of confusion around one's parenting role may add stress before the upcoming birth and aggravate a traumatic experience. HCPs should enable preparation for childbirth by providing LGBTQ+ families with adapted information about the transition to parenthood and parental roles. Patient information needs to be inclusive of all parents, regardless of their gender, parenting roles, and biological connection(s).

LGBTQ+ families in our study described lack of inclusion of the non-gestational parent as a risk factor for a negative birth experience.[11, 12] This also negatively affected the pregnant participants, as they felt a responsibility for the inclusion of the partner, an effort taking focus from preparing for birthing. Lovisa, a gestational parent, described that the exclusion of her partner was stressful for her:

> *"They almost never included her, really. Which she also told me some time, that she thought it was very... it was sad, that they did not do that, like, ever. If she was in the room, of course, they said hello and so, but it was not the case that they were very inviting, so that she would be involved in any way."*
>
> *(Lovisa, gestational parent)*

Non-gestational parents need to be supported in their own transition to parenthood. This support will also help them to be able to give optimal support to the gestational parent during birth. There is a risk that a non-gestational parent carries difficult experiences of a previous birth that can negatively affect the upcoming experience. It is essential that HCPs offer support to process previous negative birth experiences, regardless of whether a person was the gestational parent or not, and also help prepare for how a partner's birth may affect a non-gestational person's own future thoughts about pregnancy and childbirth.

Key points

It is important to address LGBTQ+ specific risk factors for birth trauma during pregnancy by:

- Using inclusive language, correct pronouns, and adequate parental terms in relation to the parents-to-be.
- Providing sufficient and adapted LGBTQ+ specific information about childbirth in combination with general information about births.
- Offering information about the transition to parenthood and parental roles, especially for non-gestational mothers, non-genetic parents, and/or parents with trans identities.
- Including non-gestational parents-to-be in care meetings.
- Supporting non-gestational parents in their supportive role of the gestational parent.
- Acknowledging non-genetic/non-gestational parents as equal parents.
- Giving all prospective parents possibilities to process previous negative birth experiences (as a gestational or non-gestational parent).
- Helping non-gestational parents prepare for how their partner's birth may affect their own future thoughts and feelings about pregnancy and childbirth.

EXPERIENCING BIRTH TRAUMA

Both gestational and non-gestational LGBTQ+ parents in our studies describe how HCPs' treatment and actions had affected their subjective experience of the birth and contributed to the experience of trauma when obstetrical and/or neonatal complications occurred.[11, 12, 19] An important part of their trauma experiences were that they had been separated from their child and/or partner during or immediately after birth, experiencing being left alone and/or experiencing a lack of inclusion. Support from family and loved ones is a strong protective factor against trauma and important when healing from trauma.[53] Complications leading to separation of the family are particularly stressful for many LGBTQ+ families. The complications led to an increase in the number of HCPs and wards caring for our study participants, and these new meetings created additional situations with incorrect cisheteronormative assumptions and/or confusion around the family members. When the family members were separated, they were no longer visible as LGBTQ+ people, which in turn created the need to come out and inform HCPs about their LGBTQ+ identity, at the same time as the participants went through frightening emergency situations. In addition, as many non-gestational parents are not their children's genetic and/or legal parents, they may carry minority stress around not being recognised as a parent or accepted as a family member by HCPs and the health care system. Therefore, inclusion and validation of the family as a family and of all parents as parents are of particular importance.

Gestational parents' trauma experiences

Several gestational parents had experienced disrespectful treatment from HCPs that violated their bodily or personal integrity, which became part of the traumatic birth experience. These participants described negative, punitive, and threatening comments and/or actions directed towards them from HCPs and explained that such treatment made them feel bad at birthing, that they did the wrong thing, or were a disappointment to the HCPs.[19] The parents expressed various types of strong stress reactions during birth, where intense fear and loss of control were central.[12] They described feelings of not being the owner of their own body and of not being involved in decisions about their body, their birth, and their unborn baby. They also expressed a lack of communication and information both during the complicated birthing situations and afterwards – where HCPs could have provided the information that the person did not get in the emergency situation earlier.

In general, our participants described birthing care as burdened with stress and a lack of resources, explaining how these deficiencies had become part of the trauma. They emphasised that the stress they felt and saw amongst HCPs affected them negatively. The gestational LGBTQ+ parents' experiences of birth trauma are similar to those of heterosexual women as described in previous literature,[38, 42, 43] but the LGBTQ+ identity sometimes added an additional dimension to the trauma experience, as the HCPs they met at the birthing ward were burdened with stress and had not been able to provide care adapted to the specific needs of an LGBTQ+ person.

Some gestational parents talked about how the separation from their partner that happened due to the obstetrical complications became part of the trauma. Veronica, a gestational parent with FOC, explained that her imagined "worst nightmare" came true when she got a major tear that needed surgery. She explained how the separation affected her:

> *"I had to go away after that [the birth] and get stitches at surgery, so I was parted from both my wife and my child, barely afterwards, and it was also something that I thought was very traumatic as well, for me, because I was terrified of getting a tear, so well, that was it, I was not afraid of the birth itself, I was terrified of getting some kind of injury from the birth."*
> *(Veronica, gestational parent with birth trauma)*

When separation from her partner was added to the situation, support from the partner was out of reach. In that way, being left alone augmented the risk of trauma.

Non-gestational parents' trauma experiences

Non-gestational parents with a childbearing capacity enter birth with a unique perspective, which may influence their experience. They may have given birth before, and if so, those experiences may impact how they react to witnessing the partner giving birth. For non-gestational parents who have previously undergone a traumatic birth, FOC can be aroused during the partner's pregnancy, and the person may re-experience painful memories during the partner's birth, which may be re-traumatising. In addition, some non-gestational parents have plans or will make plans to give birth in the future. Such plans may also affect how the partner's birth is experienced.[14, 16] Stina, a non-gestational mother, explained how she had been shocked by witnessing her wife giving birth:

> *"It was absolutely shocking to understand how bad it hurt. I had never imagined that. It was really then [I became afraid to give birth], because already then we had plans to have siblings, and that I would carry that baby, and then I thought, "so I will never be able to do it". [...] Standing beside,*

seeing everything, and then knowing that "I will do this too", probably, and I, so "How will I make it?" Yes, I was not prepared that it would hit me so hard."

(Stina, non-gestational mother)

This experience can serve as an example of how plans for future children and pregnancies may change due to birth trauma.

Non-gestational parents in our studies described deficiencies in care during birth regarding lack of information.[12, 19] Furthermore, non-gestational parents who had given birth previously or planned to become pregnant in the future described lack of support for them in witnessing their partner giving birth. Non-gestational parents described how their feelings and reactions during birth were not considered important and were given little or no attention, which made it impossible for them to "take up any space" with their feelings, despite experiences of panic or breaking down. Frida, a non-gestational mother who had previous difficult birth experiences, shared how she panicked during her partner's birth:

"It was when we came in that it became difficult, because then all my birth memories came back, and then it became, it became like, it surprised me in some way both in terms of scents, just the smell of the laughing gas, so everything became so incredibly noticeable somehow, and standing there in my own fear of childbirth and at the same time supporting my partner, it was awful indeed."

(Frida, first gestational and now non-gestational parent)

At one point during the birth, she needed to leave the room and sat in the corridor and cried. No HCP stopped to ask how she was feeling, and no one had asked about her mood after returning home when she suffered from postpartum depression.

Another non-gestational parent, Cornelia, described how the separation from her partner during the birth affected her. She experienced the birth as traumatic and believed that this feeling was reinforced by being left alone twice, first when her partner underwent an emergency caesarean and then afterwards, when she sat with her new-born child in the ward and no one cared for her. She shared how no HCP took the time to talk to or support her in the extremely stressful situation where she thought she might lose her partner and child. Instead, she overheard the HCPs talking about her partner's belly being a bit small:

"I heard them talking about her, and I felt like I was left there. [...] Yes, it was very hard then, or, like, I thought I would lose, part of me thought I would lose my partner and child, like, it was very tough, and that it went so fast

like, also like this, also to see blood and that I just saw, because it's quite special, so when they put someone to sleep, it looks a bit like someone disappears."

(Cornelia, non-gestational mother)

Lack of support postpartum

Both gestational and non-gestational LGBTQ+ parents described a lack of support postpartum. They expressed a need for an LGBTQ+ safe place after their complicated births, where they would not need to handle cisheteronormativity, homo- bi- or transphobia, but instead could focus on healing after a difficult birth and on the transition to parenthood.[12, 18, 19] In general, they wished that supportive conversations had been a more prominent and important part of the care during, as well as directly after their traumatic birth experiences. They believed this could have made the experience easier to handle. Most participants mentioned not receiving sufficient psychological support from HCPs after a difficult birth experience, and talked about a lack of systematic follow up on mental health prior to being discharged. Some were offered support that was not carried through, and the participants then felt uncertain of where to turn for help. Some had been struggling for months to get some kind of follow-up around their birth trauma. This made participants feel neglected by health care and it affected their overall postpartum experience negatively. Some perceived this neglect from health care as a prolonged birth trauma.[18]

Gestational parents' postpartum experiences

Some gestational parents described how HCPs focused only on their physical health but did not ask questions about their mental health. Other gestational parents described a lack of information about their physical health as well. Alma asked for information about her birth injuries after being operated on:

"I had to ask what had happened, and she [the midwife] says to me, this is the same day as it happened, she says "You can read about it in your chart", and I just say, "My chart?!" I didn't say anything; I just started crying [...] I didn't know then that they had sutured me, I didn't know they had put a tamponade in me, which is, well, meter after meter of fabric that you push in to stop the bleeding, I found out about that later, about one day later when they came to pull it out of me, which was an extremely unpleasant feeling, when someone just drags a lot of fabric out of you."

(Alma, gestational mother)

Asking for information is also asking for support and validation, something that cannot be found in one's chart. In this situation, Alma was left without information about her health status, not knowing what interventions had been done to the most intimate parts of her body, and without support for the traumatic experience.[19]

Non-gestational parents' postpartum experiences

It is common that the non-gestational parent's birth experience is not explored by HCPs postpartum.[54] In the case of complicated births, the gestational parent in our studies was often offered psychological support postpartum, while the non-gestational parent often was not. In general, non-gestational partners in our studies have not been given the chance to process the trauma in an adequate way. Many of them expressed feelings of not being important, and those feelings were reinforced when they were not given attention after the birth, in particular if they were left alone with the new-born child while the gestational parent required treatment in an operating theatre in a separate ward. They might have been promised a sandwich, someone to talk to, or instructions about caretaking of the baby, but in the end, no one attended to them. They described how they did not receive any attention or help from HCPs to handle their reactions, making the situation extra difficult. This can become a contributing factor to trauma as well as to the development of subsequent mental illness in non-gestational parents.[12]

Some non-gestational participants described how they were traumatised from a birth with no complications requiring obstetric interventions, while their partners who gave birth had gained a positive birth experience. In such cases, the non-gestational parents' experiences were not addressed in the birthing ward, and they were not able to raise it themselves. One of these participants, Frida, described having experienced a lack of support around the role of the non-gestational mother already during pregnancy, for example information about co-nursing. She found it difficult to handle the situation during postpartum care when the gestational mother was starting to breastfeed their new-born child. She began questioning her parental role and wondered: "Is there room for two mothers?"

> "I ended up like feeling left out again, somehow, all focus was only on [gestational parent] and the breastfeeding, [...] and it was such incredible power in this, because then I lost like my partner at this point, like, what was ours, this focus that we had had somehow, for so many years, disappeared, and I remember at that night I stood there on my own and gazed out the hospital window and thought "I'm going to jump, I can't stand it", it was so enlarged."
>
> (Frida, first gestational and now non-gestational parent)

Monica, another non-gestational mother, expressed that she would have liked more targeted support and questions about her birth experience because of her unique position as a potential gestational mother in the future. She wanted the opportunity to process the negative experience so that any future birth(s) could be as good as possible:

> "It is special that I could potentially carry a child and give birth to a child, and I would like maybe that they were a little alert on those signals [...] that they would ask a little more concrete questions about my birth experience."
> (Monica, non-gestational parent)

Key points

Essential interventions during birth for LGBTQ+ parents to lower the risk of experiencing birth trauma and/or to create optimal conditions for starting to process birth trauma postpartum:

- Individualised, respectful birthing care. Optimal staff resources on each birthing ward.
- Strive for zero separation. Keeping the family together during all stages of birth is a protective factor, especially in cases where either partner has severe FOC and/or complications have arisen.
- Separating the family in the event of obstetrical and/or neonatal complications may reinforce trauma.
- If separation is needed:
    - validate the LGBTQ+ family by using inclusive and adequate language
    - enable contact or mediate information continuously
    - acknowledge to each parent that you see them as a parent and as part of the family
    - reunite the family as soon as possible
- Explore all parents' birth experiences postpartum, especially when a partner has a childbearing capacity, as a non-gestational partner may have planned to give birth in the future
- Non-gestational parents who have witnessed a partner giving birth may have experienced birth trauma and may be at risk of developing FOC postpartum, PPD and postpartum PTSD
- Treatment should be offered to *any* parent with a traumatic experience

THE IMPORTANCE OF THE CARING RELATIONSHIP

A trusting caring relationship is central to reducing the risk of experiencing birth trauma. A caring relationship can be described as an empowering partnership or alliance where the patient can experience respect, safety, and trust.[55] Experiencing support from HCPs when giving birth is, in general, protective against negative experiences,[2, 7, 56] also when obstetrical and/or neonatal complications arise. Cisheteronormativity can disrupt the trust in the caring relationship despite good intentions from HCPs, creating deteriorating conditions for HCPs to build safety in the birthing situation. Indelicate questions or cisheteronormative assumptions, as well as direct homo-, bi-, or transphobia, add considerable extra stress to vulnerable life situations. Therefore, it is essential that HCPs cultivate awareness of the consequences of their own attitudes and language.

Strive for continuity of carer

One way of working with the caring relationship is striving for continuity of carer. Lack of continuity among HCPs can be especially hard for LGBTQ+ families, and several of our participants expressed great satisfaction with care forms that give continuity of carer and minimise the number of different HCPs, for example, midwifery-led case-loading models of care. Some of our interviewees said they did not tell new HCPs about their needs or feelings because they did not have the strength to establish a new relationship. This can be understood as a consequence of minority stress and/or earlier negative experiences. Continuity of care and carer create optimal conditions for good care by creating the possibility of feeling safe and being open with needs and wishes. Alma, a gestational mother with FOC, emphasised the importance of continuity of carer during pregnancy and at birth:

> *"We had a really great contact with our midwife and, so all like visits and meetings that were connected to the midwife [...] was very very good, and to build a relationship and meet the same person was a huge relief."*
>
> *(Alma, gestational parent)*

Building a respectful and trustful caring relationship does not always have to take a long time. Monica, a non-gestational parent, described a few seconds that became very important to her when her partner was taken away for emergency surgery:

> *"A very lovely and significant thing that happened was that he who was to operate on [gestational partner], that is, he who was the doctor in charge of the ward, looked at me and he saw that I became very sad, and kind of broke down there, when [gestational parent] was rolled out and then he took the seconds he could afford, to put a hand on my shoulder and say, "You know what, I know this looks scary, and we'll do everything we can", so there, and it was one thing that was very, I carried that with me then, so it felt very important."*
>
> *(Monica, non-gestational parent)*

In the traumatic event of seeing her partner being moved to the operating theatre in a separate ward, the physician's quick and gentle acknowledgement of her feelings and of her as part of the family had been of importance for her.[19]

Key points

LGBTQ+ parents can benefit from changes in pregnancy and birthing care on structural levels, as well as individual HCPs working on relationship building and safety in care appointments:

- Acknowledge the importance of the caring relationship.
- Work on awareness of the consequences of one's own attitudes and language.
- Strive for continuity of carer.
- Recommend care models like midwifery-led case-loading, or models where HCPs follow the family from pregnancy to birthing ward, and where the number of new HCPs is reduced to a minimum.
- Facilitate unavoidable transitions between health care wards or changes in HCPs, especially if obstetrical and/or neonatal complications have arisen.
- Document and/or transfer information verbally (always in agreement with the family) to reduce normative assumptions and the need for "coming out". This may include explanations of the family constellation, gender identities, pronouns, preferred labels, or other specific needs the family has shared.

REFERENCES

1. Saisto T, Halmesmäki E. Fear of Childbirth: A Neglected Dilemma. *Acta Obstet Gynecol Scand*. 2003;82(3):201–208.doi.org/10.1034/j.1600-0412.2003.00114.x
2. *WHO Recommendations: Intrapartum Care for a Positive Childbirth Experience*. Geneva: World Health Organization; 2018. Available from: https://www.ncbi.nlm.nih.gov/books/NBK513809/
3. Söderquist J, Wijma B, Thorbert G, Wijma K. Risk Factors in Pregnancy for Post-Traumatic Stress and Depression after Childbirth. *BJOG*. 2009;116(5):672–680. doi:10.1111/j.1471-0528.2008.02083.x
4. Rouhe H, Salmela-Aro K, Gissler M, Halmesmäki E, Saisto T. Mental Health Problems Common in Women with Fear of Childbirth. *BJOG*. 2011;118(9):1104–1111. doi:10.1111/j.1471-0528.2011.02967.x
5. Garthus-Niegel S, von Soest T, Vollrath ME, Eberhard-Gran M. The Impact of Subjective Birth Experiences on Post-Traumatic Stress Symptoms: A Longitudinal Study. *Arch Women's Ment Health*. 2013 Feb;16(1):1–10. doi:10.1007/s00737-012-0301-3. Epub 2012 Sep 1. PMID: 22940723.

6. Seefeld, L., Weise, V., Kopp, M., Knappe, S., & Garthus-Niegel, S. (2022). Birth Experience Mediates the Association Between Fear of Childbirth and Mother-Child-Bonding up to 14 Months Postpartum: Findings from the Prospective Cohort Study DREAM. *Frontiers in Psychiatry*. 12:2567. doi:10.3389/fpsyt.2021.776922

7. Bohren, M. A., Hofmeyr, G. J., Sakala, C., Fukuzawa, R. K., & Cuthbert, A. (2017). Continuous Support for Women during Childbirth. The Cochrane Database of Systematic Reviews, 7(7), CD003766. doi:10.1002/14651858.CD003766.pub6

8. Elmir R, Schmied V, Wilkes L, Jackson D. Women's Perceptions and Experiences of a Traumatic Birth: A Meta-Ethnography. *J Adv Nurs*. 2010;66(10):2142–2153. doi:10.1111/j.1365-2648.2010.05391.x

9. Bränström R. Minority Stress Factors as Mediators of Sexual Orientation Disparities in Mental Health Treatment: A Longitudinal Population-Based Study. *J Epidemiol Community Health*. 2017;71(5):446–452. doi:10.1136/jech-2016-207943

10. Hallström S, Grundström H, Malmquist A, Eklind M, Nieminen K. Fear of Childbirth and Mental Health Among Lesbian, Bisexual, Transgender and Queer People: A Cross-Sectional Study [published online ahead of print, 2022 Jun 24]. *J Psychosom Obstet Gynaecol*. 2022; 1–6. doi:10.1080/0167482X.2022.2089555

11. Karlsson G, Ulfsdotter, A. *"It Felt Like I did Wrong and was Wrong in Different Ways" – LBTQ-People with Difficult Experiences of Childbirth and Perceived Treatment in Reproductive Healthcare*. 2022. Linköping University: Master thesis.

12. Lindén Åsell, J. *När barnafödandet blir ett Trauma Hbtq-personers erfarenheter av trau-matiska Förlossningsupplevelser [When Childbirth becomes a Trauma Experiences of Traumatic Childbirth Among Hbtq-People]*. 2013. Linköping University: Master thesis.

13. Malmquist A, Jonsson L, Wikström J, Nieminen K. Minority Stress Adds an Additional Layer to Fear of Childbirth in Lesbian and Bisexual Women, and Transgender People. *Midwifery*. 2019;79:102551. doi:10.1016/j.midw.2019.102551

14. Malmquist A, Wikström J, Jonsson L, Nieminen K. How Norms Concerning Maternity, Femininity and Cisgender Increase Stress Among Lesbians, Bisexual Women and Transgender People with a Fear of Childbirth. *Midwifery*. 2021;93:102888. doi:10.1016/j.midw.2020.102888

15. Malmquist A, Nieminen K. Negotiating who Gives Birth and the Influence of Fear of Childbirth: Lesbians, Bisexual Women and Transgender People in Parenting Relationships. *Women Birth*. 2021;34(3):271–278. doi:10.1016/j.wombi.2020.04.005

16. RFSL/Swedish Federation for Lesbian, Gay, Bisexual, Transgender, Queer and Intersex Rights. *Hbtq-kompetens – för dig som arbetar med blivande och nyblivna föräldrar*. [LGBTQ Competence – for You who Work with Expectant and New Parents]. 2021, accessible online. Stockholm: RFSL.

17. Nerström, E. & Niit, J. *LBTQ Parents' Experiences and Needs Following a Difficult Birth: A Qualitative Analysis*. 2022. Karolinska Institute: Master thesis.

18. Klittmark, S., Malmquist, A. Karlsson, G., Ulfsdotter, A., Grundström, H. & Nieminen, K. When Complications Arise During Birth: LBTQ People's Experiences of Care. *Midwifery*, 2023;121;103649. doi.org/10.1016/j.midw.2023.103649.

19. Grundström, H., Malmquist, A., Karlsson, A. & Nieminen, K. Previous Trauma Exposure and Its Associations with Fear of Childbirth and Quality of Life among Pregnant Lesbian, Bisexual,

Transgender, and Queer People and Their Partners, *LGBTQ+ Family: An Interdisciplinary Journal*, 2023,19:2, 175–185. doi:10.1080/27703371.2023.2167760

20. Wijma K, Wijma B. A Woman Afraid to Deliver: How to Manage Childbirth Anxiety. In: *Bio-Psycho-Social Obstetrics and Gynecology*. Cham: Springer International Publishing; 2017:3–31. doi.org/10.1007/978-3-319-40404-2_1

21. Hanson S, Hunter LP, Bormann JR, Sobo EJ. Paternal Fears of Childbirth: A Literature Review. *J Perinat Educ*. 2009;18(4):12–20. doi:10.1624/105812409X474672

22. Sydsjö G, Bladh M, Lilliecreutz C, Persson AM, Vyöni H, Josefsson A. Obstetric Outcomes for Nulliparous Women who Received Routine Individualised Treatment for Severe Fear of Childbirth – A Retrospective Case Control Study. *BMC Pregnancy Childbirth*. 2014;14:126. doi:10.1186/1471-2393-14-126

23. Lukasse M, Schei B, Ryding EL; Bidens Study Group. Prevalence and Associated Factors of Fear of Childbirth in Six European Countries. *Sex Reprod Healthc*. 2014;5(3):99–106. doi:10.1016/j.srhc.2014.06.007

24. Lukasse M, Vangen S, Øian P, et al. Childhood Abuse and Fear of Childbirth—A Population-Based Study. *Birth*. 2010;37(4):267–274. doi:10.1111/j.1523-536X.2010.00420.x

25. Redshaw M, Heikkilä K. Ethnic Differences in Women's Worries about Labour and Birth. *Ethn Health*. 2011;16(3):213–223. doi:10.1080/13557858.2011.561302

26. O'Connell MA, Leahy-Warren P, Khashan AS, Kenny LC, O'Neill SM. Worldwide Prevalence of Tocophobia in Pregnant Women: Systematic Review and Meta-Analysis. *Acta Obstet Gynecol Scand*. 2017;96(8):907–920. doi:10.1111/aogs.13138

27. Bergström M, Rudman A, Waldenström U, Kieler H. Fear of Childbirth in Expectant Fathers, Subsequent Childbirth Experience and Impact of Antenatal Education: Subanalysis of Results from a Randomised Controlled Trial. *Acta Obstet Gynecol Scand*. 2013;92(8):967–973. doi:10.1111/aogs.12147

28. Hildingsson I, Johansson M, Fenwick J, Haines H, Rubertsson C. Childbirth Fear in Expectant Fathers: Findings from a Regional Swedish Cohort Study. *Midwifery*. 2014;30(2):242–247. doi:10.1016/j.midw.2013.01.001

29. Ryan M. The Gender of Pregnancy: Masculine Lesbians Talk about Reproduction. *J Lesbian Stud*. 2013;17(2):119–133. doi:10.1080/10894160.2012.653766

30. Ellis SA, Wojnar DM, Pettinato M. Conception, Pregnancy, and Birth Experiences of Male and Gender Variant Gestational Parents: It's How we Could Have a Family. *J Midwifery Women's Health*. 2015;60(1):62–69. doi:10.1111/jmwh.12213

31. Miller T. Is This What Motherhood is all About?: Weaving Experiences and Discourse Through Transition to First-Time Motherhood. *Gender Soc*. 2007;21(3):337–358. doi:10.1177/0891243207300561

32. Símonardóttir S, Rúdólfsdóttir AG. The "Good" Epidural: Women's Use of Epidurals in Relation to Dominant Discourses on "Natural" Birth. *Feminism & Psychology*. 2021;31(2):212–230. doi:10.1177/0959353520944808

33. Charter R, Ussher J M, Perz J, Robinson K. The Transgender Parent: Experiences and Constructions of Pregnancy and Parenthood for Transgender Men in Australia. *Int. J. Transgenderism*. 2018,19(1):64–77. doi:10.1080/15532739.2017.1399496

34. Falck F, Frisén L, Dhejne C, Armuand G. Undergoing Pregnancy and Childbirth as Trans Masculine in Sweden: Experiencing and Dealing with Structural Discrimination, Gender

Norms and Microaggressions in Antenatal Care, Delivery and Gender Clinics. *Int J Transgend Health*. 2021;22(1–2):42–53. doi:10.1080/26895269.2020.1845905

35. Bohren MA, Vogel JP, Hunter EC, et al. The Mistreatment of Women during Childbirth in Health Facilities Globally: A Mixed-Methods Systematic Review. *PLoS Med*. 2015;12(6): e1001847. Published 2015 Jun 30. doi:10.1371/journal.pmed.1001847

36. Striebich S, Mattern E, Ayerle GM. Support for Pregnant Women Identified with Fear of Childbirth (FOC)/Tokophobia – A Systematic Review of Approaches and Interventions. *Midwifery*. 2018;61:97–115. doi:10.1016/j.midw.2018.02.013

37. Sun X, Fan X, Cong S, Wang R, Sha L, Xie H, Han J, Zhu Z, Zhang A. Psychological Birth Trauma: A Concept Analysis. *Front Psychol*. 2023 Jan 13;13:1065612. doi:10.3389/fpsyg. 2022.1065612.

38. Sydsjö G, Angerbjörn L, Palmquist S, Bladh M, Sydsjö A, Josefsson A. Secondary Fear of Childbirth Prolongs the Time to Subsequent Delivery. *Acta Obstet Gynecol Scand*. 2013; 92(2):210–214. doi:10.1111/aogs.12034

39. Patterson J, Hollins Martin C, Karatzias T. PTSD Post-Childbirth: A Systematic Review of Women's and Midwives' Subjective Experiences of Care Provider Interaction. *J Reprod Infant Psychol*. 2019;37(1):56–83. doi:10.1080/02646838.2018.1504285

40. Andersen LB, Melvaer LB, Videbech P, Lamont RF, Joergensen JS. Risk Factors for Developing Post-Traumatic Stress Disorder Following Childbirth: A Systematic Review. *Acta Obstet Gynecol Scand*. 2012;91(11):1261–1272. doi:10.1111/j.1600-0412.2012.01476.x

41. Beck CT. Birth Trauma and its Sequelae. *J Trauma Dissociation*. 2009;10(2):189–203. doi:10.1080/15299730802624528

42. Beck CT, Casavant S. Synthesis of Mixed Research on Posttraumatic Stress Related to Traumatic Birth. *J Obstet Gynecol Neonatal Nurs*. 2019;48(4):385–397. doi:10.1016/j.jogn. 2019.02.004

43. Etheridge J, Slade P. "Nothing's Actually Happened to Me.": The Experiences of Fathers who Found Childbirth Traumatic. *BMC Pregnancy Childbirth*. 2017;17(1):80. Published 2017 Mar 7. doi:10.1186/s12884-017-1259-y

44. Hollander MH, van Hastenberg E, van Dillen J, van Pampus MG, de Miranda E, Stramrood CAI. Preventing Traumatic Childbirth Experiences: 2192 Women's Perceptions and Views. *Arch Womens Ment Health*. 2017;20(4):515–523. doi:10.1007/s00737-017-0729-6

45. Reed R, Sharman R, Inglis C. Women's Descriptions of Childbirth Trauma Relating to Care Provider Actions and Interactions. *BMC Pregnancy Childbirth*. 2017;17(1):21. Published 2017 Jan 10. doi:10.1186/s12884-016-1197-0

46. Andersson L, Sundström-Poromaa I, Wulff M, Aström M, Bixo M. Implications of Antenatal Depression and Anxiety for Obstetric Outcome. *Obstet Gynecol*. 2004;104(3):467–476. doi:10.1097/01.AOG.0000135277.04565.e9

47. Ayers S, McKenzie-McHarg K, Slade P. Post-Traumatic Stress Disorder after Birth [Editorial]. *Journal of Reproductive and Infant Psychology*. 2015;33(3):215–218. doi.org/10.1080/0264 6838.2015.1030250

48. Boorman RJ, Devilly GJ, Gamble J, Creedy DK, Fenwick J. Childbirth and Criteria for Traumatic Events. *Midwifery*. 2014;30(2):255–261. doi:10.1016/j.midw.2013.03.001

49. Vedam, S., Stoll, K., Taiwo, T.K. *et al*. The Giving Voice to Mothers Study: Inequity and Mistreatment During Pregnancy and Childbirth in the United States. *Reprod Health*. 2019; 16:77. doi.org/10.1186/s12978-019-0729-2

50. van der Pijl MSG, Hollander MH, van der Linden T, et al. Left Powerless: A Qualitative Social Media Content Analysis of the Dutch #breakthesilence Campaign on Negative and Traumatic Experiences of Labour and Birth. *PLoS One*. 2020;15(5):e0233114. doi:10.1371/journal.pone.0233114

51. Webb R, Bond R, Romero-Gonzalez B, Mycroft R, Ayers S. Interventions to Treat Fear of Childbirth in Pregnancy: A Systematic Review and Meta-Analysis. *Psychol Med*. 2021;51(12):1964–1977. doi:10.1017/S0033291721002324

52. Hobfoll SE, Watson P, Bell CC, et al. Five Essential Elements of Immediate and Mid-Term Mass Trauma Intervention: Empirical Evidence. *Psychiatry*. 2007;70(4):283–369. doi:10.1521/psyc.2007.70.4.283

53. Eriksson C, Westman G, Hamberg K. Experiential Factors Associated with Childbirth-Related Fear in Swedish Women and Men: A Population Based Study. *J Psychosom Obstet Gynaecol*. 2005;26(1):63–72. doi:10.1080/01674820400023275

54. Fontein-Kuipers Y, de Groot R, van Staa A. Woman-Centered Care 2.0: Bringing the Concept into Focus. *Eur J Midwifery*. 2018;2:5. doi:10.18332/ejm/91492

55. Karlström A, Nystedt A, Hildingsson I. The Meaning of a Very Positive Birth Experience: Focus Groups Discussions with Women. *BMC Pregnancy Childbirth*. 2015;15:251. doi:10.1186/s12884-015-0683-0

Chapter 8

Birth partners' experiences

Alex Howat

LGBTQ+ BIRTH PARTNERS

Whilst in heterosexual relationships the birth partner is typically male, the biological father of the baby and the romantic partner of the women who has given birth, this may not be true for non-gestational birth partners in LGBTQ+ couples. Lesbian/bisexual women couples may conceive through donated sperm, either through a fertility clinic or known donor. Whilst non-gestational birth partners in these couples do not carry the child during pregnancy, they may be biologically related to the child depending on the method of assisted conception, ie, egg donation. Conversely, cisgender or transgender gay/bisexual men in relationships with cisgender gay/bisexual men may become parents through surrogacy or co-parenting with a single woman, or a cisgender lesbian/bisexual couple, with one of the men donating their sperm. Transgender men and women and non-binary individuals may become a parent as the birth partner of a genetic parent either in a same-gender or different gender relationship, or through being a genetic parent themselves ie, sperm/egg donation. Whilst these are several examples of non-gestational partners in LGBTQ relationships, this list is not exhaustive and may not represent all types of LGBTQ+ birth partners.

To date, most of the limited research on non-gestational LGBTQ+ birth partners has focused on cisgender women who are the non-carrying partner in lesbian or bisexual relationships. No research has explored the experiences of childbirth of non-gestational transgender men and women's, non-binary individuals, or gay/bisexual men. Consequently, this chapter uses findings and examples taken from research with western cisgender lesbian/bisexual parents. However, due to the uniqueness in LGBTQ+ relationships, these are not universal experiences and importantly more research is needed to explore the experiences of these parents.

DOI: 10.4324/9781003305446-9

STRUGGLES WITH PARENTAL IDENTITY AND ROLE DURING BIRTH

Parental identity refers to how someone defines themselves as parent (ie, who am I as a parent? What role do I play?, etc.) and the degree of identification with this role.[1] Parental identity is typically constructed by societal narratives of parenthood. Having a clear parental identity which an individual identifies strongly with may help individuals understand and fulfil the role they are to play during childbirth. For example, although as fathers cisgender heterosexual men expect to be present during the birth and to support their partner,[2] some may also struggle with their parental identity and feel underprepared for childbirth due to conflicting messages from society about what is expected of them as a father.[3, 4] Similarly, some non-gestational LGBTQ+ parents may struggle with their parental identity and their role during childbirth, potentially resulting in a negative experience of childbirth. However, this confusion may be exacerbated for non-gestational LGBTQ+ parents in comparison to cisgender heterosexual fathers for several reasons. First, in contrast to fathers, non-gestational LGBTQ+ parents typically lack well-defined, socially agreed roles and flexible language that capture the complexity of their position when compared with expectations of a heteronormative society.[5-7] In a recent study with non-birthing mothers, one participant reflected:

> *"I guess dads are dads, so dads have their own defined role… I'm her mum but I'm not her **mum**."*[7]

Furthermore, within UK common law as an example, the non-birthing partner in the same-sex couple is neither a mother nor a father but is categorised as a parent, adding to confusion around parental roles.[8] Finally, there is lack of resources or education inclusive of LGBTQ+ parents providing examples of their possible roles and what to do during childbirth. Consequently, non-gestational parents may lack an identity template and expectations for how to behave during and after childbirth, and struggle with pressure to fit within the gendered and restrictive mother/father binary, contributing to role incongruence/confusion, difficulties in embracing their parental identity, feeling unprepared for childbirth, and a sense of isolation.[5, 9-11] This may make the experience of witnessing childbirth additionally stressful by increasing feelings of confusion, helplessness, and panic and consequently decrease their ability to be supportive as a partner and positive birth outcomes. See Box 1 for case example.

Maternity professionals can support non-gestational LGBTQ+ parents who may be struggling with their parental identity and role during childbirth to improve their experiences of birth and help them support their partner by asking appropriate, relevant, and, most importantly, nonintrusive culturally curious questions which offer the opportunity to reflect on their parental identity. By doing this, health care professionals can ensure they are providing culturally sensitive and competent care which involves the careful consideration of the individual social, cultural, and psychological needs of patients and promotes effective cross-cultural communication between patients and health care providers. For example, health care professionals should clarify and use language regarding the role that the non-gestational parent feels most comfortable with. Through doing this, professionals can recognise and validate the non-gestational LGBTQ+ partner's identity in a way that feels safe, which may subsequently have a positive impact on the development of their parental identity by lessening the confusion and anxiety around their role. Furthermore, professionals should also explore non-gestational partner's expectations of their role as a birth partner prior to the birth. Research has demonstrated receiving concrete advice from midwives about how to act during birth felt is positive and is believed to help non-gestational partners support the birthing partner during birth.[12] However, it is highly important that advice and information provided should avoid being gendered and should tailored to LGBTQ+ parents rather than being "catch-all advice," reflecting the nuances of their roles and experiences. Once expectations of roles have been established, professionals should support non-gestational parents to fulfil this role.

BOX 1—PARENTAL IDENTITY AND ROLE DURING BIRTH: SARAH

Sarah (she/her) is the non-gestational parent in a lesbian relationship. Sarah and her wife, Beth, have an 8-month-old daughter, Maeve, together. Sarah is not biologically related to Maeve. Sarah spoke extensively about her difficulties around her identity as the non-birth mother and how this fit into the binary of parental roles. This contributed to confusion of her role during the birth of her daughter and resulted in significant levels of distress for her:

> "Father[s] are there just to run around after the woman and that's kind of their job! And I didn't know what my role was! And the whole like, the man's supposed to run around after the woman! My wife does all the running around! I did, I was the one who packed the hospital bag. I do all of the, I was doing all the Mum's stuff! So I didn't know what I was supposed to do at the hospital and things."[7]

EXCLUSION AND LACK OF SUPPORT

During and after childbirth, the focus of health care professionals is typically on the gestational parent and child, ensuring that both receive appropriate care. Whilst this is understandable, this may mean that non-gestational LGBTQ+ birth partners are likely to experience, at minimum, similar experiences reported by cisgender heterosexual fathers in the paternal literature. For example, many fathers report being left out due to the actions of staff (eg, not receiving adequate information being included in decision making or being ignored) and a lack of support aimed directly at them.[12–14] This contributes to feelings of unimportance and helplessness, which may reduce their supportiveness as a partner and trust in health care professionals, and can intensify distress and anxiety, particularly during traumatic births.[15, 16] Men often qualify this exclusion and lack of support by emphasising that the focus "should" be on the mother and baby, a narrative typically mirrored by services.[13]

Findings within the paternal literature with cisgender heterosexual fathers indicate a significant link to role played in birth and subsequent inclusion/exclusion and lack of support during and after birth. Therefore, it is likely that non-gestational LGBTQ+ parents have similar experiences. Recent research by the author reported experiences of exclusion and feeling on the outside of parenting in contact with maternity services. Some linked this exclusion and lack of support to their role as a non-birthing parent. For example, one participant said:

> *"I think not being the birth parent, I think it gave other people what they felt was the right to exclude me from conversations."*[7]

At times, this exclusion resulted in a perceived lack of control and contributed to uncertainty in role, which negatively impacted on mental health. As with fathers, some non-gestational LGBTQ+ birth partners also justified the lack of inclusion and support being due to the need for gestational parent-centred care, but also spoke about the unsaid expectation within maternity services that non-birthing parent needs were less of a priority, for example, the lack of spaces for partners to sleep on maternity units.

Whilst exclusion during the birth may be a common experience as the non-birthing parent, non-gestational LGBTQ+ parents may be additionally excluded due to their sexual or gender identity. For example, there have been several reports within research and anecdotal evidence of health care professionals questioning or not recognising partner and/or parental status due to pervasive heteronormative assumptions. In Hayman, Wilkes, Halcomb, and Jackson's[17] qualitative study, non-birth mothers reported feeling excluded by maternity services who often failed to recognise non-birth mothers as legitimate parents, preventing them from participating in health-related procedures. This exclusion often led to feelings of anger and sadness and the need to legitimise the non-birth mother's role as a parent. Experiences of non-inclusion of non-gestational LGBTQ+ parents during and after childbirth have been linked to slightly elevated levels of postpartum mental health difficulties,[18] which can have long-term implications on both parents and the baby. Furthermore, whilst exclusion during and after birth and the lack of support being offered for non-gestational birth partners is likely to have been exacerbated during the Covid-19 pandemic, LGBTQ+ birth partners may be more susceptible to being excluded due to stricter visiting protocols and heteronormative assumptions that they are not the partner due to their gender.[19] It is important to recognise some non-gestational LGBTQ+ birth partners may experience high levels of minority stress (ie, experiencing stress based on their sexual orientation). Consequently, some may more hypervigilant (ie, expect and be more aware) to being excluded and discriminated against to protect themselves against these types of experience. However, whilst being hypervigilant serves an important survival function for these parents, there may be times where it results in inadvertently result in misinterpreting some interactions as exclusion and discrimination, increasing parents' stress and anxiety further. See Box 2 for case example.

Services should increase their attempts to include the non-gestational parent during and after the birth regardless of sexuality or gender. However, it may be particularly important to do this for non-gestational LGBTQ+ parents who may be at greater risk of feeling excluded due to additional concerns about their parental role and potential inadvertent consequences of hypervigilance associated with high levels of minority stress. Furthermore, services consider how they can address the negative impact of restrictions relating to pandemics on the inclusion of partners. Health care professionals should be sensitive to the needs of non-gestational LGBTQ+ birth partners, supporting them as a parent-to-be by encouraging them to ask questions and offering guidance and reassurance during the birth. Furthermore, midwives should see them as a valued resource due to their exclusive knowledge of the birthing partner and provide them opportunities to interact with professionals and their partner, for example encouraging them to support with decisions, such as pain relief, and discussing with them about the birthing parent's needs. By supporting non-gestational LGBTQ+ parents and including them in the care of their partner and child, professionals can ensure that childbirth is a mutually shared experience for the couple and that non-gestational birth partners feel recognised, involved, and needed, as well as increasing feelings of being in control while also reducing minority stress.

BOX 2—EXCLUSION DURING BIRTH: BETH

Beth (she/her), a non-gestational birth partner in a cisgender bisexual relationship, reported experiencing high levels of minority stress, including experiences of homophobia and internalised homophobia stemming from her religious background. Beth spoke about how these experiences had increased her sensitivity to perceived exclusion due to her sexuality and the distress she felt as a result. Beth also reflected on the importance of increasing culturally competent care and inclusive amongst maternity services:

> "One of the problems I was having was separating out what was potentially because I was a same-sex partner and what every other parent would have? I think how I was treated was probably the same as all other partners. I think men in a maternity unit tend to be put to one side! Like they're there just to run around after the woman and that's kind of their job! But I think because I was so heightened, I went into that situation feeling like I wasn't supposed to be there! The staff need an understanding that people in same-sex relationships are coming in with all these layers of homophobia and things they have to deal with. So you do have to go the extra mile to try and make them feel more included."[7]

BIRTH AND TRAUMA

Childbirth can be a significantly stressful event for many couples, even if the birth is considered routine, and can have a lasting emotional impact on the non-gestational birth partners. Heterosexual fathers describe childbirth as "a rollercoaster of emotion" due to the speed and unexpectedness of events, with around 8.5% feeling traumatised by experiencing their partners in labour.[15, 20] Non-LGBTQ+ fathers also report feeling worried, fear of the unknown, fear of death, guilt, powerless, overwhelmed helplessness at their inability to support their partner in pain but also a need to suppress their own feelings to focus on their partner.[2, 20, 21] Similar findings are echoed in non-gestational LGBTQ+ parents. Non-birthing mothers in lesbian relationships report feeling powerless to protect or support their partner during birth which resulted in feelings of failure and inadequacy in their role as a supportive partner.[7] For example, one non-birthing mother spoke of her embarrassment and self-criticism when she experienced a panic attack when her partner was given an epidural:

> *"I felt really shit for that happening. I wasn't able to be the supportive partner I wanted to be in that moment and it felt a bit pathetic."*[7]

Feelings of powerlessness and subsequent feelings of failure and guilt are increased if the birth has been traumatic and there is a disparity between expectations and the reality of childbirth. For all birth partners, experiencing childbirth as traumatic is influenced by a lack of, and/or anxiety-provoking, communication by health care professionals.[7] Furthermore, non-gestational LGBTQ+ parents also report feeling that their own needs and feelings are unjustified and suppress them to focus support on the gestational parent. As one non-birthing mother said,

> *"it's not my body that's been ravaged."*[7]

However, there may be instances the trauma of birth may impact differently on the non-gestational partner in LGBTQ+ couples in comparison to heterosexual fathers. In cisgender lesbian, and bisexual relationships, actively deciding that the other partner would carry the pregnancy may exacerbate feelings of inadequacy as a partner and intensify feelings of guilt during childbirth. For example, one lesbian non-birthing mother commented:

> *"I helped as much as I could do, but I did feel a bit guilty that it had been her going through it and not me because it's just being pregnant and giving birth is such a horrible experience."*[7]

Interestingly, same-sex non-gestational parents have reported additional guilt due to physical empathy:

> *"I guess being a woman I could empathise so much with what she'd gone through and how damaged she felt, maybe I found it worse than if I'd been a man."*[7]

During childbirth, non-gestational birth partners are becoming parents and are exposed to everything that occurs during the birth. Whilst good care of the birthing parents is likely to reduce partners' distress, non-gestational partners have different experiences, perspectives, and needs and should receive their own care, especially in more complicated or traumatic births. Receiving clear communication and information is important for non-gestational parents to contextualise experiences and understand what is happening, reducing feelings of powerlessness and helplessness.[21] Non-gestational birth partners focusing on the birthing partners' needs and suppressing their own will frequently mean that they are less likely to ask for support. Therefore, health care professionals need to normalise responses to different birth experiences and acknowledge non-gestational birth partners' needs before the birth (i.e., during antenatal classes), as well as during and after. Within this, birth workers also need to acknowledge the potentially unique dynamics of LGBTQ+ relationships, including decisions about carrying.

BONDING AND BIOLOGICAL CONNECTEDNESS

Concerns about bonding with a new baby are common amongst all non-gestational parents. Whilst these concerns are typically resolved following the birth, for some these difficulties may remain postpartum. Furthermore, there may be additional anxieties about bonding and parental connection amongst non-gestational LGBTQ+ parents arising from concerns about biological connectedness. In McCandlish's qualitative study,[22] lesbian mothers expressed concerns about the closeness of the child's bond with their non-birth mother in comparison to their birth mother.

Some non-gestational parents may struggle with feeling bonded due to not having carried the child, not experiencing the same hormonal processes as birthing parents, or not having a genetic link to their child (see Box 3).[7] Additionally, difficulties with parental connectedness may also be linked to exclusion from the birthing parent-infant-dyad and perceiving preference for the birthing parent as rejection during the breastfeeding period. Whilst cisheterosexual fathers also do not carry the pregnancy, or experience the same hormonal processes, or breastfeed, they are more likely to have a genetic connection to the child than non-gestational LGBTQ+ birth partners. Therefore, anxiety and sensitivity relating to having experiences with and feelings of rejection and disconnection may be increased for non-gestational LGBTQ+ parents during the intrapartum period due to the potential lack of a biological connection and the privilege given to biology in parental roles and bonding, especially in western societies.[18, 23] Interestingly, this lack of bonding may be more difficult to negotiate for non-gestational parents who also have the potential to become gestational parents themselves and made an active choice not to carry.[7, 9]

BOX 3—LINK BETWEEN BOND AND CARRYING: SAM

Sam (she/her), a non-gestational LGBTQ+ birth partner, spoke about the lack of connection they felt to their new-born baby, Thomas, in comparison to their birth partner, Jessica. Sam believes that the experience of carrying Thomas helped develop this bond between birthing parent and baby which Sam did not feel and felt on the outside of. This lack of connection caused additional confusion regarding their parental identity and contributed to the distress they felt after the birth:

> "I didn't give birth to him. So it's not even necessarily about the biology, I think it's about having that experience with him and like him being inside Jessica and stuff. It was almost like they already knew each other. Whereas I was just a bit like oh hello."[7]

Difficulties with bonding may add to confusion regarding parental identity and contribute to feelings of failure or guilt, which feed into their quality of perinatal mental health.[7] Mental health difficulties may be exacerbated by a disparity between expectations and reality of bonding based on messages from society that parents should feel "amazing love" towards their child(ren). For example, one non-birthing mother said:

> "Everyone was saying that you're supposed to feel like this massive rush of love and want to jump in front of a train for your child. But I was there like, you need to stop crying, or I'm going to send you back to the shop."[7]

Moreover, there may be additional stress regarding difficulties bonding due to stigma about being an LGBTQ+ parent and societal expectations of failure increasing the pressure on them to be seen as "successful" in parenthood.[24]

To support non-gestational LGBTQ+ birth partners with their concerns regarding bonding, birth workers should demonstrate an awareness of the anxieties that these parents may be managing internally and actively recognise the parental connection between non-gestational parent and baby during childbirth. Professionals may also help to do this by allowing time and privacy following the birth to be together as a family and engaging non-gestational LGBTQ+ parents in activities to promote feelings of connectedness and bonding, including cutting the umbilical cord, skin-to-skin contact, revisiting activities that were done in utero (ie, singing), or facilitating feeding (ie, co-lactation, bottle-feeding, etc.) Some non-gestational LGBTQ+ parents may be able to and want to breast/chestfeed in addition to the gestational parent. However, there is a lack of guidelines or evidence to guide professionals in supporting non-gestational parents to be involved in feeding their children (ie, prescribing galactagogue, issues with safety profile of medication in relevant population, who prescribes, etc.) Additionally, these discussions frequently do not take priority or, at times, being discouraged by maternity services due to the focus being on supporting the birthing parent to feed and unsubstantiated concerns about supply issues in the gestational parent. For example, when speaking about their wish to be involved in breastfeeding their child, one non-birthing mother said:

> "We didn't find out that the other Mum could take medication breastfeeding until it was too late really! And the medication wouldn't have kicked in in time."[7]

It is important that professionals involved in intrapartum care include non-gestational LGBTQ+ parents in discussions about feeding, exploring their options, and supporting their decisions regarding this and that comprehensive guidelines and evidence base is developed to aid these conversations.

HETEROSEXIST CARE AND EXPERIENCES OF DISCRIMINATION

A distinct experience for non-gestational LGBTQ+ parents may be encountering heterosexist care and discrimination when interacting with maternity services during and after birth. The following two sections will explore these concerns and then recommendations will be provided for how birth workers may address these issues to improve the care they provide for these parents during this time.

Cisheteronormative systems and a lack of social recognition

Despite the increase in LGBTQ+ people creating families, the maternity system is still heterocentric, focusing primarily on heterosexual families.[16, 25] Consequently, there are several cisheteronormative assumptions that plague maternity services, including: that there will be one gestational parent who will be a cisgender woman (and the only person potentially breast/chestfeeding) and one non-gestational partner who will be a cisgender man; that these two are the only parents of the baby; that genetic parents, legal parents, and those raising the baby are the same, so the terms are interchangeable; and that the parents will identity with binary roles of mother/father. Whilst many people conceive within heterosexual relationships, assuming this is true for all people involved in maternity services can be detrimental for LGBTQ+ parents.

Cisheteronormative assumptions are apparent in the attitudes of health care professionals, the care available/provided by services (ie, funded fertility treatment, perinatal mental health support of non-gestational LGBQ+ parents, etc.) and the language used by health care systems in materials and in conversation. Non-gestational LGBTQ+ parents are sometimes met with doubt that they are the partner and/or assumptions that they are the birthing mother (if a woman), biological father or partner of the birth parent (if a man), friend or relative (ie, sibling). For example, Montbaston, a lesbian non-birthing mother, describes a member of hospital staff serving food assuming they had given birth and that their partner was a man meaning she was not able to get food from the trolley for their gestational partner, following introducing herself as a mother and talking about her partner.[26] Furthermore, non-gestational LGBTQ+ parents may be discounted as the other parent due to their gender, with health care professionals speaking exclusively to the birthing parent, or assumptions are made about their involvement as parents, for example that gay/bisexual men will not be involved as a father or that only a genetic father will be involved.[27] Professionals may also misgender non-gestational LBGTQ+ parents due to assumptions based on outward appearance. Conversely, due to differing from cisheteronormative assumptions, some LGBTQ+ couples may be treated as special or a novelty by maternity workers (see Box 4 for case example). Many of the forms, computer records, policies and procedures relating to pregnancy and birth are often stereotyped, only having spaces on forms labelled "mother" and "father." Despite situations where the details of genetic parents are needed (eg, predicting allergies, medical concerns, etc.), using this language fails to recognise that not all parents present at the birth and/or involved with raising the child will identify with the mother/father binary. Finally, many LGBTQ+ parents also report a lack of representation in the available birth resources, with the language and images typically focusing on "second parent" alongside "father," which may not adequately recognise or differentiate their role as a parent.

BOX 4—BEING TREATED AS SPECIAL: ANDREA

Andrea (she/her) is the non-gestational mother in a lesbian relationship. Andrea and her wife, Jennifer, have a two-and-a-half-year-old daughter, Ava, who was carried by Jennifer. Andrea spoke about being perceived as a "novelty" by the ward staff following the birth of their daughter due to being a same-sex couple and whilst she did not view this as a negative experience, she was surprised by how they were treated and the apparent lack of experience with LGBTQ+ families:

> "We were referred to as a special couple. I think they meant that you're a female couple. I was also amazed by how much of a novelty we were and how little some of the staff knew about how two women could have a baby and stuff, that really amazed me."[7]

For non-gestational LGBTQ+ parents, cisheteronormative assumptions in maternity care can result in a lack of social recognition of their role, both as partners and parents. Whilst fathers may also struggle with lack of recognition of their parental role, they are typically recognised as a partner whereas some non-gestational LGBTQ+ parents may face non-recognition in both roles.[7] Experiencing this lack of social recognition in health care systems can contribute to feelings of invisibility, unimportance, invalidation of their sexual, gender, parental and family identity, role confusion, and feelings of discrimination.[17, 28, 29] In turn, this may increase levels of minority stress and contributes to distress.[28, 29] Therefore, social acceptance within societal systems plays a significant role in non-gestational LGBTQ partner's experience. Not all non-gestational LGBTQ+ parents may feel able to challenge professionals about their assumptions due to fear of the reaction they may receive or embarrassment. Those that do may face additional stress due to the burden of (repeated) explanation and potential professional reactions, and increased visibility and potentially vulnerability as LGBTQ+ parents. For example, in a recent study,[7] one non-gestational parent spoke about having to repeatedly remind midwives that she was also a mother which contributed to her distress. In contrast, whilst being seen as special or a novelty isn't necessarily negative and can help non-gestational LGBTQ+ parents feel recognised, for some it may draw attention to differences between themselves and heterosexual parents, increasing feelings of discomfort and vulnerability.

Experiences of hetero-/cisnormative maternity systems during birth which contribute to a lack of recognition of non-gestational LGBTQ+ parents are likely a result of lack of knowledge and cultural competence around working with LGBTQ+ families within these systems. This may arise from the primacy given to biological parenthood in western society and the subsequent lack of a template and terminology for non-gestational LGBTQ+ parents' role.[9, 10, 18] Furthermore, there is a distinct lack of guidelines and policies reflecting the needs of the LGBTQ+ community in maternity services meaning LGBTQ+ parents are underrepresented, and midwives feel ill-equipped and lack confidence in providing care for these parents.[30]

Experiences of homophobic and transphobic discrimination and prejudice

Some non-gestational LGBTQ+ parents may anticipate or experience homophobic and transphobic discrimination and prejudice during or immediately after birth. LGBTQ+ parents experience discrimination through refusal to acknowledge the non-gestational parent entirely or their role as a parent, homophobic and disapproving attitudes by professionals working with these parents, and microaggression in the form of inappropriate and intrusive questions.[7, 31–33] For example, lesbian non-birthing mothers report about being asked intrusive questions about donors, conception and role by professionals which invaded their privacy, invalidated their parental/family identity, and emphasised difference.[7] These discriminatory experiences can lead to nontherapeutic interactions which increase feelings of threat and feed into feelings of internalised homophobia/transphobia, causing non-gestational LGBTQ+ parents to question their right to have children, feelings of inadequacy and contributing to perinatal mental health difficulties.[7, 34] Furthermore, they may also create barriers to the provision of inclusive intrapartum care to LGBTQ+ parents.

Whilst incidents of discrimination should never be tolerated, many of them may result from a lack of sensitivity, knowledge, and training, in addition to clumsy attempts at addressing social difference, rather than being intentionally malicious. For example, one non-birthing mother spoke about their frustration with the lack of cultural competence amongst midwives and how this impacted on their care:

> *"The midwives make comments like oh we didn't know if you were like a friend? Or if you were the other partner and no one wanted to come and ask you cos they thought that you might find it weird!"*[7]

Additionally, some questions may be an attempt by professionals to connect with or learn more about LGBTQ+ parents and their journey. Whilst these questions may be interpreted as curiosity and an opportunity to educate by some non-gestational parents, others may find these more intrusive and threatening as they invalidate their parental/family identity and emphasise difference. Therefore, to ensure that the focus of interactions with LGBTQ+ parents remain on them receiving support and not on parents having to educate their own health care provides, services and individual providers should seek out professional training, many of which is LGBTQ+-led, to increase their awareness and knowledge of relevant issues, and subsequently competence, when working with this community.

In addition to experiences of discrimination, non-gestational LGBTQ+ parents may also need to plan and navigate the possibility of discrimination around how they will be treated that may impact their birth experiences, contributing to distress felt during this time.[29] Research has found that non-gestational LGBTQ+ parents have less positive expectations of birth because of internal fears about having to continually out themselves and being out of place or vulnerable to discrimination by health care systems due to their sexuality and/or family situation.[31, 35, 36] These expectations are frequently dictated by previous discriminatory experiences which contributes to high levels of minority stress and hypervigilance to discrimination (see Box 5 for case example). Living alongside any anxiety about having their parenthood questioned creates doubt and insecurity and potentially negatively impacts parental identity development, suggesting that the anticipation of discrimination and prejudiced events may be just as stressful as the actual events themselves.[10] Consequently, non-gestational LGBTQ+ may be more sensitive to actual or perceived discrimination in interactions with maternity staff, increasing negative experiences of stress and vulnerability.

BOX 5—EXPECTATIONS OF DISCRIMINATION: NATALIE

Natalie (she/her) is a bisexual non-gestational mother who recently had twin daughters, Layla and Ellie, with her wife, Charlotte. For practical reasons, it was decided that Charlotte would be the birth mother. Natalie reported having *"awful"* experiences with health care systems when pursuing assisted conception, during which health care professionals acted like their request to become parents was odd and the couple were put through tests that they did not feel were necessary. This impacted on her expectations for the birth with Natalie feeling highly anxious that these experiences would continue.

Natalie highlighted the importance of training in helping to mitigate some of these experiences:

"I think we'd had those negative experiences with the hospital and GP in the run up to Charlotte getting pregnant, and I was worried those were going to continue with the NHS moving forwards. So that was just a kind of lingering stress that was going on...I think maybe our stress levels wouldn't have been this high in the first place if there was more training for NHS staff about same-sex parents and we hadn't experienced some of the negative experiences that we had experienced."[7]

Recommendations for Providers

The above two sub-sections demonstrate how cisheteronormative assumptions and experiences with and feelings of discrimination and prejudice are distinctive to non-gestational LGBTQ+ parents and can negatively impact their experiences of birth. Health care professionals can address these issues and subsequently improve non-gestational LGBTQ+ parents' experiences in several ways. Most importantly, any discrimination by professionals or services should be acknowledged to be wrong and addressed accordingly. Following on from this, maternity professionals and services need to be mindful of the assumptions they make around conception, pregnancy, and birth, the potential for their actions to be discriminatory (even if this is unintentional), as well as issues relating to minority stress and expectations of discrimination, and how these may impact the experiences of LGBTQ+ birth partners. By developing an awareness of these issues, professionals can be open to alternatives and take action to change how they interact with these families.

Health care professionals should be curious, asking open, considerately worded questions about the families they are working with, such as 'who are the baby's parents?' rather than 'who is the real mother?' However, when asking questions professionals should consider whether these are appropriate or necessary. For example, asking questions about genetic histories or preferences regarding pronouns may be important, whereas questions regarding conception, etc., may not be necessary and some may find these upsetting. Answers should be clearly recorded to avoid questions being repeatedly asked by multiple people and remove the burden of repeated explanation and perpetual outing.[37] Professionals could use genograms, a pictorial display of a person's family relationships, to recognise and document family dynamics and roles without being intrusive. Whilst asking appropriate questions are often received positively by LGBTQ+ families, professionals should not rely on LGBTQ+ parents to educate them on the issues that they face.

Whilst some professionals may feel that it is inclusive and beneficial to treat cisheterosexual and LGTBQ+ non-gestational parents the same,[31] this may be counterproductive as it does not recognise the nuances of non-gestational LGBTQ+ parents' experiences. An individualised approach to care which reflects the unique needs of these parents is likely to be more helpful.[38] Therefore, more training for maternity staff on LGBTQ+ families focusing which recognises diverse family forms and their experiences during and after birth is needed to increase awareness and culturally sensitive/competent care, whilst reducing the likelihood of discrimination and distress caused by the anticipation of these experiences.[39] However, professionals also need to go beyond cultural competence, which can be limited as it may lead to professionals relying on generalisations about specific communities rather than recognising the uniqueness of individuals, and commit to developing cultural humility.[40] In contract to cultural competence, cultural humility is a mindset rather than a goal. It is a life-long process of being aware of social power imbalances, respecting other people's values and continuously reflecting on our own biases (eg, by asking ourselves how these biases might impact on how we treat and understand others), and working to minimise this impact. To practice cultural humility, health care professionals should recognise no culture is superior to another, engage in self-reflection and acknowledge mistakes made, be honest when not sure about something, learn about other cultures with the awareness that they will never reach perfect understanding and be open to what they have not learnt yet, and support colleagues to have open discussions and hold each other accountable. By developing cultural humility, service providers can increase their cultural awareness, ensure that they do not apply a "one-size-fits-all" approach to the care of LGBTQ+ parent and promote equity and inclusion with these families. Importantly, service providers must be willing to discuss the issues faced by these parents and their families in ways that promote safety and understanding, in addition to willingness to get these discussions wrong and recognise when they do so. In doing this, services can reduce some of the stressors within the systems that contribute to negative birth experiences.

Language used by professionals, in addition to language on forms and in resources, needs to be inclusive of all sexual orientations and family structures to increase feelings of being recognised and accepted by health care systems. Improving language starts with recognising that there may be more than two parents, different parents may have different roles, and that role may not be denoted by the parent's gender. Utilising gender-neutral terms (ie, partner or couple) which reflect non-gestational parental roles outside of the binary[41] or avoiding gendered-terms and using names instead may be more inclusive. To acknowledge the agency of partners to identify themselves and demonstrate that birthing and parenting roles can be redefined and reidentified, professionals can ask about and use language preferred by LGBTQ+ parents.[31] Additionally, it may also be useful to create specific information leaflets or groups for LGBTQ+ parents to promote a sense of belonging.

SUMMARY

This chapter has explored birth experiences of non-gestational LGBTQ+ birth partners. Whilst there are some similarities to the experiences of heterosexual fathers, there are also important differences as well as distinctive experiences for non-gestational LGBTQ+ parents. Consequently, it is important that midwives, obstetricians, and other birth workers move away from cisheteronormative assumptions to acknowledge non-gestational LGBTQ+ unique roles and provide culturally competent, inclusive, individualised care that addresses their specific needs. This chapter has highlighted some of the ways in which birth workers may start to do this (see Box 6. Learning Points). By doing this, experiences of childbirth may be more positive for non-gestational parents, which will increase their capacity to support the birthing parent. Importantly, the issues discussed in this chapter may not be representative of the experiences of all non-gestational LGBTQ+ parents. Therefore, it is important for professionals to commit to a process of curiosity and cultural humility to provide meaningful care to these families they work with.

BOX 6—LEARNING POINTS

Experiences of non-gestational LGBTQ+ birth partners are similar but qualitatively distinct to heterosexual fathers. Birth workers can tailor the care they provide to improve their birth experiences by:

- Taking an active stance against discrimination.
- Demonstrating appropriate and nonintrusive cultural curiosity about families by asking only necessary open questions and recording answers in easily accessible ways.
- Engaging in additional training on working with LGBTQ+ families to develop awareness of hetero-/cisnormative assumptions, increase cultural competence and consider alternative ways of working.
- Engaging in a continual process of cultural humility.
- Be willing to have difficult discussions about social difference, get things wrong and acknowledge when this happens.
- Engaging non-gestational LGBTQ+ parents in activities to promote feelings of connectedness and bonding, including involving them in conversations about breast/chestfeeding when appropriate.

- Normalising different birth experiences and acknowledging non-gestational birth partners' needs whilst also acknowledging unique dynamics in LGBTQ+ relationships.
- Providing clear communication and information during the birth.
- Using inclusive language (ie, gender neutral or names) or using language preferred by families in both written and verbal communications which recognises diverse family forms and validates different parental roles.
- Viewing non-gestational partners as a valuable resource and providing them opportunities to interact with professionals and their partner during childbirth.

REFERENCES

1. Piotrowski K. Adaptation of the Utrecht-Management of Identity Commitments Scale (U-MICS) to the Measurement of the Parental Identity Domain. *Scandinavian Journal of Psychology*. 2017;59(2):157–166. doi:10.1111/sjop.12416
2. Premberg Å, Carlsson G, Hellström AL, Berg M. First-Time Fathers' Experiences of Childbirth—A Phenomenological Study. *Midwifery*. 2011;27(6):848–853. doi:10.1016/j.midw.2010.09.002
3. Domoney J, Iles J, Ramchandani, P. Fathers in the Perinatal Period: Taking their Mental Health into Account. In: Leach P. ed. *Transforming Infant Wellbeing: Research, Policy and Practice for the First 1001 Critical Days*. Routledge; 2017:205–214.
4. Dellmann T. "The Best Moment of My Life": A Literature Review of Fathers' Experience of Childbirth. *Australian Midwifery*. 2004;17(3):20–26. doi:10.1016/s1448-8272(04)80014-2
5. Wojnar DM, Katzenmeyer A. Experiences of Preconception, Pregnancy, and New Motherhood for Lesbian Nonbiological Mothers. *Journal of Obstetric, Gynecologic & Neonatal Nursing*. 2014;43(1):50–60. doi:10.1111/1552-6909.12270
6. Brown R, Perlesz A. Not the "Other" Mother: How Language Constructs Lesbian Co-Parenting Relationships. *Journal of GLBT Family Studies*. 2007;3(2–3):267–308. doi:10.1300/j461v03n02_10
7. Howat A, Masterson C, Darwin Z. Non-Birthing Mothers' Experiences of Perinatal Anxiety and Depression: Understanding the Perspectives of the Non-Birthing Mothers in Female Same-Sex Parented Families. *Midwifery*. 2023; 120:103650. doi:10.1016/j.midw.2023.103650.
8. *R (McConnell and YY) v Registrar General for England and Wales*. EWCA Civ 559. 2020. https://www.judiciary.uk/wp-content/uploads/2020/04/McConnell-and-YY-judgment-Final.pdf
9. Paldron MF. *The Other Mother: An Exploration of Non-Biological Lesbian Mothers' Unique Parenting Experience*. [Doctoral Dissertation]. Minneapolis: University of Minnesota; 2014. https://hdl.handle.net/11299/167423.
10. Padavic I, Butterfield J. Mothers, Fathers, and "Mathers." *Gender & Society*. 2011;25(2):176–196. doi:10.1177/0891243211399278

11. Walker, K. What Issues do Lesbian Co-Mothers Face in their Transition to Parenthood? *NCT Perspectives*. 2017;34.

12. Huusko L, Sjöberg S, Ekström A, Hertfelt Wahn E, Thorstensson S. First-Time Fathers' Experience of Support from Midwives in Maternity Clinics: An Interview Study. *Nursing Research and Practice*. 2018;2018:1–7. doi:10.1155/2018/9618036

13. Darwin Z, Galdas P, Hinchliff S, et al. Fathers' Views and Experiences of their Own Mental Health during Pregnancy and the First Postnatal Year: A Qualitative Interview Study of Men Participating in the UK Born and Bred in Yorkshire (BaBY) Cohort. *BMC Pregnancy and Childbirth*. 2017;17(1). doi:10.1186/s12884-017-1229-4

14. Chandler S, Field PA. Becoming a Father. First-Time Fathers' Experience of Labor and Delivery. *Journal of Nurse-Midwifery*. 1997;42(1):17–24. doi:10.1016/s0091-2182(96)00067-5

15. Etheridge J, Slade P. "Nothing's Actually Happened to Me.": The Experiences of Fathers who Found Childbirth Traumatic. *BMC Pregnancy and Childbirth*. 2017;17(1). doi:10.1186/s12884-017-1259-y

16. Cherguit J, Burns J, Pettle S, Tasker F. Lesbian Co-Mothers' Experiences of Maternity Healthcare Services. *Journal of Advanced Nursing*. 2012;69(6):1269–1278. doi:10.1111/j.1365-2648.2012.06115.x

17. Hayman B, Wilkes L, Halcomb E, Jackson D. Marginalised Mothers: Lesbian Women Negotiating Heteronormative Healthcare Services. *Contemporary Nurse*. 2013;44(1):120–127. doi:10.5172/conu.2013.44.1.120

18. McInerney A, Creaner M, Nixon E. The Motherhood Experiences of Non-Birth Mothers in Same-Sex Parent Families. *Psychology of Women Quarterly*. 2021;45(3):279–293. doi:10.1177/03616843211003072

19. Stacey T, Darwin Z, Keely A, Smith A, Farmer D, Heighway K. Experiences of Maternity Care during the COVID-19 Pandemic in the North of England. *British Journal of Midwifery*. 2021;29(9):516–523. doi:10.12968/bjom.2021.29.9.516

20. Vischer LC, Heun X, Steetskamp J, Hasenburg A, Skala C. Birth Experience from the Perspective of the Fathers. *Archives of Gynecology and Obstetrics*. 2020;302(5):1297–1303. doi:10.1007/s00404-020-05714-z

21. Ekström A, Arvidsson K, Falenström M, Thorstensson S. Fathers' Feelings and Experiences during Pregnancy and Childbirth: A Qualitative Study. *Journal of Nursing & Care*. 2013; 02(02). doi:10.4172/2167-1168.1000136

22. McCandlish B. Against all Odds: Lesbian Mother Family Dynamics. In: Bozett FW, Bozett FW. eds. *Gay and Lesbian Parents*. Greenwood Publishing Group. 1987:23–38.

23. Goldberg, AE, Smith JZ. The Social Context of Lesbian Mothers' Anxiety during Early Parenthood. *Parenting: Science and Practice*. 2008;8(3):213–239.

24. Bos HMW, van Balen F, van den Boom DC, Sandfort ThGM. Minority Stress, Experience of Parenthood and Child Adjustment in Lesbian Families. *Journal of Reproductive and Infant Psychology*. 2004;22(4):291–304. doi:10.1080/02646830412331298350

25. McManus AJ, Hunter LP, Renn H. Lesbian Experiences and Needs during Childbirth: Guidance for Health Care Providers. *Journal of Obstetric, Gynecologic & Neonatal Nursing*. 2006;35(1):13–23. doi:10.1111/j.1552-6909.2006.00008.x

26. Montbaston J de. *My Daughter's Birth*. Published March 30, 2017. Accessed July 3, 2022. https://readingmedievalbooks.wordpress.com/2017/03/30/my-daughters-birth/

27. Malmquist A, Nelson KZ. Efforts to Maintain a "Just Great" Story: Lesbian Parents' Talk about Encounters with Professionals in Fertility Clinics and Maternal and Child Healthcare Services. *Feminism & Psychology*. 2013;24(1):56–73. doi:10.1177/0959353513487532

28. Goldberg AE, Perry-Jenkins M. The Division of Labor and Perceptions of Parental Roles: Lesbian Couples Across the Transition to Parenthood. *Journal of Social and Personal Relationships*. 2007;24(2):297–318. doi:10.1177/0265407507075415

29. Abelsohn KA, Epstein R, Ross LE. Celebrating the "Other" Parent: Mental Health and Wellness of Expecting Lesbian, Bisexual, and Queer Non-Birth Parents. *Journal of Gay & Lesbian Mental Health*. 2013;17(4):387–405. doi:10.1080/19359705.2013.771808

30. Fish J. Conceptualising Social Exclusion and Lesbian, Gay, Bisexual and Transgender People: The Implications for Promoting Equity in Nursing Policy and Practice. *J Res Nurs*. 2010;15 (4):303–312. doi.org/10.1177/1744987110364691

31. Goldberg L, Harbin A, Campbell S. Queering the Birthing Space: Phenomenological Interpretations of the Relationships Between Lesbian Couples and Perinatal Nurses in the Context of Birthing Care. *Sexualities*. 2011;14(2):173–192. doi:10.1177/1363460711399028

32. Erlandsson K, Linder H, Häggström-Nordin E. Experiences of Gay Women during their Partner's Pregnancy and Childbirth. *British Journal of Midwifery*. 2010;18(2):99–103. doi:10. 12968/bjom.2010.18.2.46407

33. McKelvey MM. The Other Mother: A Narrative Analysis of the Postpartum Experiences of Nonbirth Lesbian Mothers. *Advances in Nursing Science*. 2014;37(2):101–116. doi:10.1097/ ans.0000000000000022

34. Touroni E, Coyle A. Decision-Making in Planned Lesbian Parenting: An Interpretative Phenomenological Analysis. *Journal of Community & Applied Social Psychology*. 2002; 12(3):194–209. doi:10.1002/casp.672

35. Kazyak E, Finken E. Law and Same-Sex Couples' Experiences of Childbirth. In: Liu H, Reczek C, Wilkinson L. eds. *Marriage and Health: The Well-Being of Same-Sex Couples*. Rutgers University Press; 2020:176–187.

36. Kerppola J, Halme N, Perälä ML, Maija-Pietilä A. Empowering LGBTQ Parents: How to Improve Maternity Services and Child Healthcare Settings for this Community – "She Told us that We are Good as a Family." *Nordic Journal of Nursing Research*. 2019;40(1):41–51. doi:10.1177/2057158519865844

37. Rickards T, Wuest J. The Process of Losing and Regaining Credibility When Coming-Out at Midlife. *Health Care for Women International*. 2006;27(6):530–547. doi:10.1080/073993 30600770254

38. Lee E. Lesbian Users of Maternity Services: Appropriate Care. *British Journal of Midwifery*. 2004;12(6):353–358. doi:10.12968/bjom.2004.12.6.13132

39. Wilton T, Kaufmann T. Lesbian Mothers' Experiences of Maternity Care in the UK. *Midwifery*. 2001;17(3):203–211. doi:10.1054/midw.2001.0261

40. Tervalon M, Murray-García J. Cultural Humility Versus Cultural Competence: A Critical Distinction in Defining Physician Training Outcomes in Multicultural Education. *Journal of Health Care for the Poor and Underserved*. 1998;9(2):117–125. doi:10.1353/hpu.2010.0233

41. Röndahl G, Bruhner E, Lindhe J. Heteronormative Communication with Lesbian Families in Antenatal Care, Childbirth and Postnatal Care. *Journal of Advanced Nursing*. 2009;65(11): 2337–2344. doi:10.1111/j.1365-2648.2009.05092.x

Chapter 9

Infant feeding

Nina A Juntereal and Diane L Spatz

INTRODUCTION

The United Nations Children's Fund and World Health Organization describe feeding of human milk as one of the most effective interventions to promote child wellbeing and survival.[1] Professional organizations across the globe continue to recommend that infants receive human milk only during the first six months of life.[2-6] The Association of Women's Health, Obstetric and Neonatal Nurses (AWHONN), Academy of Breastfeeding Medicine (ABM), American College of Obstetricians and Gynecologists (ACOG), American Academy of Family Physician (AAFP), International Lactation Consultant Association (ILCA), and La Leche League International (LLLI) have updated their position statements on infant feeding in recognition of LGBTQ+ families who breast/chestfeed or lactate.[2, 7-11] All health care professionals providing lactation care to members of the LGBTQ+ community should align their clinical practice to these position statements and advocate for other professional organizations to develop their own statements to ensure that respect and care is given to all individuals building families.

LACTATION-RELATED LANGUAGE

Lactation-related language has historically been discussed from a gendered maternal domain.[12] The evolutionary perspective has designated that humans who were assigned female at birth and identify their gender as woman have a physiological function for childbearing and that the hormones involved in pregnancy would promote human milk production.[13] This evolutionary perspective assumes that humans assigned female at birth therefore identify their gender as women and has resulted in the frequent use of gendered lactation-related language in both clinical practice and published literature.[12] To avoid assumptions

DOI: 10.4324/9781003305446-10

and misrepresenting identities, health care professionals must ask patients their preferred bodily and lactation related terminology and then use this language when talking to that patient. Some examples of inclusive language include "mammary tissue" or "chest" as opposed to "breast," "human milk" as opposed to "breast milk," and "chestfeeding," "lactating," "human milk feeding," or "infant feeding" as opposed to "breastfeeding."[8] For families with more than one person providing human milk to their infant, the term "co-lactation" or "milk sharing" may be preferred and used.[14]

INFANT FEEDING OPTIONS FOR LGBTQ+ FAMILIES

The evidence surrounding the value and benefits of human milk feeding to infants, parents, and society is well-documented.[3, 15–17] Beyond physiologic and economic benefits, human milk feeding offers the opportunity to build additional emotional capacity and bonds between parents and infants.[18] The science of human milk and anticipatory guidance on the options available related to lactation need to be communicated by health care professionals to LGBTQ+ individuals during antenatal clinical encounters such as antenatal check-ups or antenatal education programs. Health care professionals should communicate that LGBTQ+ individuals who are building families have options regarding infant feeding.

Health care professionals should also avoid assuming that all parents desire to breast/chestfeed or lactate.[19] Like any other family, human milk as the primary source of nutrition may not be a desired goal for LGBTQ+ parents, when building their family. All parents should discuss their expectations and goals related to lactation to facilitate a positive relationship with infant feeding. The process of lactation occurs during pregnancy when hormonal levels change and the mammary tissue undergoes development. This lactation process may not happen as expected with parents undergoing gender-affirming treatments or practices.[14] The decision to choose gender-affirming treatments or practices such as hormones, chest binders, top surgery, or breast augmentation may affect the ability to lactate and make breast/chestfeeding challenging or uncomfortable.[14, 20] Parents who forego or pause gender-affirming treatments or practices in order to develop their milk supply may have feelings of gender dysphoria.[14, 20] Parents who decide to carry and birth their infant but choose not to pursue lactation for any reason should seek clinical support to reduce their milk supply safely and swiftly as feasible. Health care professionals must balance between providing appropriate information and resources while avoiding assumptions or judgments on parents' infant feeding decisions.[19, 21]

All parents interested in human milk feeding are likely to need an in-depth consultation with a lactation consultant, and various other health care professionals who may provide health and medical advice to parents choosing to provide their own human milk to their babies to make an informed decision on their infant feeding plan.[14] To support and develop a long-term milk supply for infant feeding requires early and proactive counseling during the antepartum period.[22] Either partner who is able to undergo pregnancy and lactate may decide to conceive, give birth and feed their infant. Most commonly, the gestational parent will be the primary lactating parent. However, the non-gestational parent can also produce and/or provide human milk.[23, 24] Case descriptions of infant feeding options for LGBTQ+ families including same-gender male parents, same-gender female parents, and trans parents involving trans men and/or trans women partners are described below.

SAME-GENDER MALE PARENTS

Infant feeding options for same-gender male parents (eg, gay, bisexual, and other queer identified cis men) may depend on the pathway they choose to build their family such as through surrogacy or adoption. Cisgender men who use hormonal therapy involving suppression of testosterone and promotion of prolactin may produce milk but the amount of milk produced will not lead to an adequate milk supply for infant feeding.[7] Other methods for parents to gain access to human milk include contracting with their surrogate or through donor human milk.[25] Parents may choose to bottle feed their newborn formula. An Australian cross-sectional survey conducted in 2012 found that 22% of children of same-gender male couples were fed human milk at some point under the age of five.[26] Surrogates who express their milk may share this milk with same-gender male parents to bottle feed their infants.[27] Same-gender male parents may also consider using a supplemental nursing system (SNS) to feed surrogate milk, donor milk, or formula to their infant.[28]

Same-gender male couples may choose to obtain donor human milk to feed their infant. Donor human milk is indicated as the first alternative nutrition source for any infant if the gestational parent's own milk is unavailable.[29] However, same-gender male couples may face challenges in accessing donor human milk from non-profit milk banks because non-profit milk banks prioritize donor human milk to families of infants in the neonatal intensive care unit.[30] Donor human milk may be obtained from for profit milk banks in countries where legislation permits the sale of human milk but the associated price tag may be too expensive for couples.[29, 31] Further information on the use of donor human milk for infant feeding is discussed in the *Donor Human Milk and Informal Milk Sharing* section.

TRANS MEN

The infant feeding options for trans men include chestfeeding, donor human milk, or formula feeding. Health care professionals should recognize that not all trans men who give birth want to chestfeed their infant due to concerns around gender dysphoria or mental health amongst other reasons.[20, 32] For trans men who have given birth, as for any other birthing person, the decision to provide human milk is personal. The ability of trans men to lactate depends on the presence of mammary tissue and use of any gender-affirming treatments.[14, 33, 34] The type, strength, and timing of gender-affirming treatments such as chest binding, chest masculinization surgery, or testosterone therapy may affect the development of mammary tissue and the related hormones for lactation.[14, 35] Trans men who plan to provide human milk may consider delaying gender-affirming treatments until after birth and postpartum to ensure they produce enough milk.[20, 34, 35] Health care professionals should offer open discussions to trans men about their plans for infant feeding and whether they use (or have used) gender-affirming treatments.

Chest binding is a gender-affirming and non-invasive method that compresses mammary tissue using constrictive materials to create the physical appearance of a flat chest.[20, 35] Hormonal levels are likely unaffected, but the use of chest binders may contribute to atrophy of mammary tissue and potential scarring over time.[14] Chest binding for short time intervals and/or with light pressure will minimize these risks.[20] During early postpartum, the use of chest binders may elevate the risk of mastitis, an infection of mammary tissue, and blocked milk ducts.[20, 28, 36] Trans men parents who wish to lactate but use chest binders may be less likely to develop their milk supply.[14, 28, 36] Some parents may be able to safely practice chest binding after their milk supply is established during postpartum.[20] Trans men who plan to bind their chests while lactating should connect with health care professionals to monitor their chest health.

Trans men may pursue chest masculinization surgery or top surgery to change the shape and appearance of the chest to address dysphoria and affirm one's gender.[20] A number of considerations must be taken into account for trans men who intend to become pregnant and/or lactate. The surgery may involve removal or repositioning of the nipple and areola which may damage or sever milk ducts, thus increasing the risk of engorgement, ie, excess milk in mammary tissue, during postpartum.[20, 35] Preservation of the nipple and/or areola will result in less damage to milk ducts during the lactating period.[20, 35] A review of breast reduction studies demonstrates a more positive correlation of human lactation if the subareolar parenchyma, the lactating tissue under the areola, remains intact.[37] Those who have already had top surgery should be aware that mammary tissue may or may not develop during pregnancy.[20] Human milk production after top surgery is feasible but may require supplementation with donor human milk or formula.[20, 34] Of the chestfeeding positions, health care professionals recommend that parents who underwent top surgery choose the crossover hold and rugby hold.[34, 35] The reclined position is not recommended because this position stretches the mammary tissue and may cause difficulties with infant latching.[34, 35] Trans men with infant latching challenges due to a flatter chest may consider a nipple shield as an option.[36] A supplemental nursing system (SNS) is another low-cost and accessible option for trans men who would like to provide supplemental milk (expressed milk, donor milk, or formula) simultaneously with their own milk while chestfeeding.[28]

The use of testosterone therapy as part of gender affirming care may interrupt lactation-related physiology including mammary tissue development and/or the hormonal profile for milk production such as prolactin, insulin, or hydrocortisone.[33, 35] Some individuals naturally produce higher levels of testosterone than others including those diagnosed with polycystic ovarian syndrome, adrenal pathology, or pituitary pathology.[38, 39] However, evidence on testosterone use and lactation among trans men is limited. A qualitative study on transmasculine experiences found that testosterone use was a positive decision for one participant while chestfeeding his child into toddlerhood.[20] Only one case study exists that reported the safety of testosterone during lactation in which this hormone was secreted in insignificant amounts through human milk without any adverse effects on the infant.[3] Due to the paucity of evidence, more research is needed to determine the safety and efficacy of testosterone use on trans men who choose to lactate.

INDUCED LACTATION

Currently, no standard clinical guidelines exist for induced lactation for any population of parents. The most relevant induced lactation protocols available include the Mount Sinai/Zil Goldstein case study and the Newman-Goldfarb protocol.[40–42] Induced lactation requires the use of galactagogues which are pharmacological substances to increase prolactin levels for milk production.[24] Domperidone is an anti-emetic medication used off-label as a galactagogue and is available over the counter in many countries across Europe and in Canada.[43] In the United States, domperidone is unavailable because the Food and Drug Administration is concerned about the association of high dosing of domperidone intravenously and cardiac arrhythmias and cardiac arrest.[44] However, in other contexts, it is important to note that this medication when used for lactation is only given orally at a maximum dosage of 20 mg three times per day (ie, 60 mg daily maximum dose) compared to a maximum of 120 mg/daily oral dose for adults requiring domperidone therapy for nausea or vomiting.[45, 46] Individuals with pre-existing arrhythmias, history of cardiac disease, or those using medications that can prolong the QTc interval should not take domperidone in any instances.[45, 47]

Two reviews were published on the safety and efficacy of domperidone as a galactagogue.[48, 49] Both studies noted the limitations in the sample sizes of the included studies and found domperidone to be effective in increasing milk production with no adverse effects observed among infants exposed to domperidone through transfer of milk during breastfeeding.[48, 49] A randomized controlled trial was conducted on 46 mothers of preterm infants comparing domperidone to placebo treatment and found that domperidone did not modify human milk's nutrient composition or risks to mothers or infants as no adverse events were observed.[50] This trial showed that milk volume increased by 267% in the domperidone group compared to 18.5% in the placebo group by day 14 postpartum ($p = 0.005$).[50]

Any parent planning to induce lactation should seek support from health care professionals, especially lactation consultants who can provide additional information and resources such as supplemental nursing systems, flanges, or nipple shields during the process.[14, 24, 28] A cross-sectional study surveying health care professionals working in trans health found induced lactation services were primarily available in the United States or Canada.[51] It is also worth noting that although, induced lactation allows a parent to produce mature milk.[41, 52] Colostrum, the first form of milk rich in antibodies and immunoglobulins, has not yet been reported in previous cases of parents who have achieved milk production through lactation induction.[14, 40, 53]

SAME-GENDER FEMALE PARENTS

Partnered sexual minority women (eg, lesbian, bisexual, and other queer identified cis women) may choose the gestational parent to solely lactate, the non-gestational parent to solely lactate, or both parents to contribute human milk, sometimes termed co-lactation or to feed their baby infant formula.[54] Any cis women who undergo breast augmentation or reduction can breastfeed their infants without complications.[55] A study using data from the 2006 to 2017 National Survey of Family Growth female pregnancy questionnaire compared breastfeeding outcomes between sexual minority women and heterosexual women.[56] The results showed no difference in breastfeeding outcomes between bisexual women and their heterosexual counterparts.[56] However, this study reported that infants born to women who identify as lesbians were less likely to receive human milk compared to infants born to women who identify as heterosexual, even after adjustment of several demographic and pregnancy-related factors.[56] The researchers described demographics including racial and class inequities as contributing to lesbian parents' breastfeeding experiences but are unable to completely explain the relationship and suggested the need for future research on the barriers that lesbian parents encounter while breastfeeding.[56] It is important to note that this research used a dataset that spanned a time frame of 5 to 16 years ago and breastfeeding initiation rates have increased since this time period. A more recent mixed methods study on the breastfeeding experiences of same-gender mothers found that same-gender mothers are motivated and committed to breastfeeding, with many providing milk for a year or more.[57]

Non-gestational parents can contribute to feeding their infant through induced lactation.[23, 24] This process is defined as stimulation of human milk outside of the physiology of pregnancy.[24] The most widely used protocol, appears to be the Newman-Goldfarb protocol for induced lactation. This involves time and effort of the non-gestational partner during antepartum through a combination of galactagogues, non-pharmacological stimulation of the mammary tissue, and hormonal supplementation.[24, 58] Juntereal and Spatz conducted a mixed-methods study on the breastfeeding experiences of same-gender mothers.[57] Birth mothers were enrolled in the study because they identified as the primary lactating parent.[57] Out of 68 survey respondents, the researchers found that only 21% (n=14) of participants received information on induced lactation from health care professionals and that only 13% (n=9) of participants reported that their partner, the non-gestational parent, practiced induced lactation with education and information on induced lactation obtained from non-clinical outside sources.[57] The *Induced Lactation* section provides further description on the process.

Both parents can contribute to their newborn's feeding experience in other ways. Skin-to-skin contact following birth or during postpartum can be practiced by both parents and contributes to initiation of breastfeeding.[28, 57] For gestational parents, skin-to-skin contact physiologically stimulates secretion of oxytocin, the hormone needed for milk ejection.[59] Parents who are expressing after birth can share responsibilities in bottle feeding their infant. Both parents can contribute to cleaning and care of these feeding items.[57] Infants of LGBTQ+ parents may find comfort in non-nutritive sucking from both parents as well.[28, 58]

TRANS WOMEN

Development of breast tissue by gender-affirming breast augmentation is a common aspect of the transition of trans women which provides important implications for lactation.[60, 61] However, research on gender-affirming breast augmentation and lactation is limited and trans women without this procedure are also able to lactate.[60] A review conducted in 2018 found that approximately 60% of trans women augmented their breasts.[61] Available data suggests that most trans women ages 18 and older are not likely to achieve full breast maturity and may have physically smaller breasts on average compared to cisgender women.[60] Breast implants are the most common method for breast augmentation.[62] Health care professionals should acknowledge that breast augmentation may actually hide the true size and volume of mammary tissue available.[14] Trans women who received breast augmentation may experience pressure atrophy of any remaining mammary tissue.[14] Health care professionals should counsel all parents about feeding or expressing their milk appropriately during postpartum to avoid engorgement, mastitis, or low milk supply.[28] Supplementation may be required, which can be fulfilled by gaining access to milk through human milk banks, informal milk sharing, formula feeding, or by co-lactation with the baby's gestational parent.[28, 60]

Additional hormonal therapy involving estrogen and progesterone, as specified in induced lactation protocols, is needed for trans women to be able to secrete milk, however they may be unlikely to establish a full milk supply.[40, 53] Reisman & Goldstein (2018) described a case report of a trans woman on a gender-affirming hormone regimen of estrogen, progesterone, spironolactone for 6 years without breast augmentation who experienced induced lactation.[40] The patient was able to produce 8 ounces of milk per day 2 weeks before the infant's due date and also serve as the sole source of nutrition for her infant for 6 weeks postpartum.[40] The researchers did not report the specific total amount of milk the patient could produce postpartum.[40] Wamboldt and colleagues (2021) reported another case of a trans woman who achieved milk production within 1 month of initiation of an induced lactation protocol.[53] The woman was able to produce 3 to 5 ounces of milk per day via hand expression which supported the immunological health of her child, despite not meeting her goals for full nutrition and development.[53] Induced lactation, the process of mimicking lactogenesis, for trans women is similar to those followed by non-gestational same-gender mothers. This regimen involves progressive dosing of the hormones estrogen and progesterone followed by a withdrawal period.[60] The hormonal regimen is combined with a galactagogue, a medication that promotes secretion of prolactin for milk production, and non-pharmacological stimulation of the mammary tissue using strategies such as a breast pump or hand expression.[60]

The primary difference for induced lactation between cisgender women and trans women is the use of androgen-blocking medication such as spirononlactone.[60, 63] This medication inhibits the effects of androgens including testosterone for trans women who have not received gender-affirming treatments such as an orchiectomy, the removal of one or both of the testicles, or have conditions that elevate testosterone such as polycystic ovary syndrome, adrenal pathology, or pituitary pathology.[38, 39, 60, 63] The Drugs and Lactation Database (2022) specifies spironolactone use during lactation as acceptable.[64] According to *Hale's Medications and Mothers' Milk 2019*, spironolactone is categorized as "probably compatible" with breastfeeding because the evidence of adverse effects following spironolactone use is remote.[45] Hale's manual also reported that spironolactone is metabolized into the metabolite canrenone which is known to be secreted in human milk and is likely too low and clinically insignificant.[45]

TWO OR MORE CO-LACTATING PARENTS

Health care professionals need to counsel families with two or more co-lactating parents that lactation physiology requires frequent maintenance involving breast/chest emptying with minimal to no prolonged pauses to ensure an adequate long-term milk supply.[14] Families may consider co-lactation if one or more parents decide to induce lactation or because one parent has experience feeding a previous child or may still be lactating at the time their partner gives birth. Families with more than two parents may refer to co-lactation as milk sharing. Families who share in the experience and bonding of co-lactation with their infant must take into consideration other parental duties and available resources and develop a co-lactation plan to minimize feeling fatigued or overwhelmed and optimize human milk feeding.

Parents should discuss expectations and goals related to milk feeding because co-lactation may not always reduce the gestational parent's workload.[14] Rotating responsibilities such as skin-to-skin contact, feeding schedules, and the maintenance of multiple milk supplies by expressing or feeding require thorough discussion and decision-making. Because colostrum production begins as early as the second trimester of pregnancy, families should consider expressing colostrum prior to the pregnancy ending and prioritizing colostrum feeding for the first few days after birth by the gestational parent when possible.[14, 65] The Academy of Breastfeeding Medicine developed a sample co-lactation plan that families can tailor and share with their health care team prior to birth.[14]

Families who begin planning during antepartum for the non-gestational parent to induce lactation and share in co-lactating should prepare to test the non-gestational parent's milk for transmissible infections.[14] Hospital laboratories recommend this practice during prenatal care to guide lactation management.[41] Birth hospitals located in areas with populations at high risk for various transmissible diseases, may also require non-gestational parents who want to provide their milk to undergo laboratory tests for infections including HIV, syphilis, tuberculosis, and hepatitis B and C prior to offering their milk to their infants.[66] Other tests that may be performed include cytomegalovirus or human T-lymphotropic virus types I and II.[66] These services are available in some neonatal intensive care units in the United States and highly endemic regions such as southern Japan, west and central Africa, the Caribbean, and parts of South America.[14, 66] Some parents may consider such tests discriminating or stigmatising.[35, 63] Health care professionals should emphasize to parents who plan to lactate that these screening tests are routine for gestational parents.[14] Gestational parents who give birth at home or outside of hospital settings and want the non-gestational parent to provide milk may consider these screening tests as potential safety measures.[14]

DONOR HUMAN MILK AND INFORMAL MILK SHARING

Pasteurised donor human milk is recognised as a safe and viable nutrition source for infants of mothers with insufficient milk supply.[67, 68] The safety recognition of pasteurised donor human milk is based upon acceptable measures for screening, collecting, storing, and pasteurising human milk followed by distribution to accredited human milk banks.[69] However, many countries limit the availability and affordability of pasteurised donor human milk at both non-profit and for-profit milk banks to preterm, low-birth weight, or critically-ill infants in the neonatal intensive care unit.[30] Access to pasteurised donor human milk in countries which allow the sale of human milk can be too expensive for some families as price ranges from $3.50 to $6 per ounce.[70] Health insurance may cover a portion of the expense as part of the inpatient hospital stay in the United States or Canada.[31] Without health insurance coverage, the cost of pasteurised donor human milk may reach more than $1000 per week.[31] Any LGBTQ+ family planning to only feed a human milk diet to their infant and who cannot or choose not to provide the full supply from a parent(s) may face challenges in sourcing pasteurised donor human milk.

Non-pasteurised donor human milk, also known as informal milk sharing or wet-nursing is a prevalent alternative for LGBTQ+ families seeking to gain access to human milk.[71] Because of the inability to assess safety, the American Academy of Pediatrics and Food and Drug Administration does not endorse the practice of informal milk sharing.[67, 69] The Academy of Breastfeeding Medicine published a position statement acknowledging the risks and benefits of informal milk sharing and provides guidelines on screening of donor milk and home pasteurisation to minimise risk and maximise safety.[72] Health care professionals should appropriately counsel families about the risk of viral or bacterial contaminants in non-pasteurized donor human milk and potential exposure of other contaminants including allergens, medications or drugs when practicing informal milk sharing.[69]

The largest networks for informal milk sharing include Human Milk 4 Human Babies (https://www.hm4hb.net/) and Eats on Feets (http://eatsonfeets.org/) and have an estimated membership of more than 42,000 people across 52 countries.[70] Both websites connect individuals interested in informal milk sharing on social media and provide guidance and resources on safety and expectations for informal milk sharing.[31, 70] These networks do not interact with the physical exchange of milk and strictly promote commerce-free human milk sharing.[31, 70] The American Academy of Pediatrics and Academy of Breastfeeding Medicine recommend against internet-based human milk sharing.[14] The American Academy of Nursing and World Health Organization acknowledge informal milk sharing and wet nursing as an option for families wanting to reach their personal lactation goals.[73, 74]

CONCLUSION

All LGBTQ+ parents who want to breast/chestfeed or lactate deserve equitable evidence-based lactation care, interventions, and support. Health care professionals should ensure service users who are building families have access to appropriate resources to reach their feeding goals. Anticipatory guidance involving discussion of the risks and benefits of the various feeding options should be offered as early as antepartum so that families are able to make informed feeding decisions for their infant. Systemic investments must be made such as continued education for health care professionals, revised policies on donor milk and informal milk sharing, and further research on induced lactation and co-lactation to improve infant feeding for LGBTQ+ families.

MAIN LEARNING POINTS

- All families should have the opportunity to make informed feeding choices and learn about the science of human milk and its benefits for a child.
- Health care professionals should provide inclusive, evidence-based lactation support, care, and services.

- If mammary tissue is present, the person has the ability to lactate/produce milk without being pregnant.
- Any parent or support person can be involved in the care of the child and the lactation journey based on the desires of each household.
- The United States policies and recommendations surrounding the use of certain medications (Domperidone) and informal milk sharing differ from other countries and global recommendations.

KEY PRACTICE RECOMMENDATIONS

- Health care professionals should be aware of the differing lactation needs of LGBTQ+ families.
- Open, honest, inclusive, and evidence-based lactation conversations and care are important and valued by families.
- Even if a parent can not provide milk to their child, there are many ways for the parent to be involved in care and infant feeding (eg, skin-to-skin contact).
- Inducing lactation requires advanced planning and preparation, as well as dedication and commitment by the parent who is undergoing the process.
- While the FDA warns against informal milk sharing, the WHO supports wet-nursing as an option, therefore parents should be offered evidence-based information about the risks and benefits of all infant feeding choices.

SUGGESTIONS FOR FURTHER READING

- Academy of Breastfeeding Medicine Clinical Protocol #33: Lactation Care for Lesbian, Gay, Bisexual, Transgender, Queer, Questioning, Plus Patients (https://www.urmc.rochester.edu/MediaLibraries/URMCMedia/breastfeeding/documents/lactation-care-protocol.pdf)
- *Where's the Mother?: Stories from a Transgender Dad* by Trevor MacDonald
- *Breastfeeding Without Birthing* by Alyssa Schnell (https://www.alyssaschnellibclc.com/book)
- University of Rochester: LGBTQI+, Lactating, Breastfeeding, and Chestfeeding (https://www.urmc.rochester.edu/breastfeeding/services/lgbtqi-and-breastfeeding.aspx)
- Institute for the Advancement of Breastfeeding & Lactation Education (https://lacted.org/shop/crs-lgbtq-lactation/)
- Breastfeeding and parenting from a transgender perspective (http://www.milkjunkies.net/)

REFERENCES

1. United Nations Children's Fund & World Health Organization. Global Breastfeeding Scorecard 2021: Protecting Breastfeeding through Bold National Actions during the COVID-19 Pandemic and Beyond. World Health Organization. Published October 2021. Accessed May 24, 2022. https://apps.who.int/iris/bitstream/handle/10665/348546/WHO-HEP-NFS-21.45-eng.pdf?sequence=1&isAllowed=y

2. American Academy of Family Physicians. Breastfeeding, Family Physicians Supporting (position paper). American Academy of Family Physicians. Published January 1, 2015. Updated April 2021. Accessed May 24, 2022. https://www.aafp.org/about/policies/all/breastfeeding-position-paper.html

3. American Academy of Pediatrics Section on Breastfeeding. Breastfeeding and the use of human milk. *Pediatrics*. 2012;129(3):e827–e841. doi:10.1542/peds.2011-3552

4. Chantry CJ, Eglash A, Labbok M. ABM Position on Breastfeeding-Revised 2015. *Breastfeed Med*. 2015;10(9):407–411. doi:10.1089/bfm.2015.29012.cha

5. American College of Obstetricians and Gynecologists' Committee on Obstetric Practice; Breastfeeding Expert Work Group. Committee Opinion No. 658: Optimizing Support for Breastfeeding as Part of Obstetric Practice. *Obstet Gynecol*. 2016;127(2):e86–e92. doi:10.1097/AOG.0000000000001318

6. World Health Organization. Statement: Exclusive Breastfeeding for Six Months Best for Babies Everywhere. World Health Organization. Published January 15, 2011. Accessed May 24, 2022. https://www.who.int/mediacentre/news/statements/2011/breastfeeding_20110115/en/

7. Spatz DL. Provision of Human Milk in the Context of Gender Diversity: AWHONN Practice Brief Number 15. *Nurs Womens Health*. 2021;25(5):e12–e14. doi:10.1016/j.nwh.2021.07.002

8. Bartick M, Stehel EK, Calhoun SL, et al. Academy of Breastfeeding Medicine Position Statement and Guideline: Infant Feeding and Lactation-Related Language and Gender. *Breastfeed Med*. 2021;16(8):587–590. doi:10.1089/bfm.2021.29188.abm

9. American College of Obstetricians and Gynecologists' Committee on Gynecologic Practice; American College of Obstetricians and Gynecologists' Committee on Health Care for Underserved Women. Health Care for Transgender and Gender Diverse Individuals: ACOG Committee Opinion, Number 823. *Obstet Gynecol*. 2021;137(3):e75–e88. doi:10.1097/AOG.0000000000004294

10. International Lactation Consultant Association. Introducing the New ILCA Style Guidelines for Written Professional Resources. Lactation Matters. Published January 3, 2017. Accessed May 24, 2022. https://lactationmatters.org/2017/01/03/introducing-the-new-ilca-style-guidelines-for-written-professional-resources/

11. La Leche League International. Transgender and Non-Binary Parents. Llli.org. Published 2016. Accessed May 24, 2022. https://www.llli.org/breastfeeding-info/transgender-non-binary-parents/

12. Dinour LM. Speaking Out on "Breastfeeding" Terminology: Recommendations for Gender-Inclusive Language in Research and Reporting. *Breastfeed Med*. 2019;14(8):523–532. doi:10.1089/bfm.2019.0110

13. Brines J, Billeaud C. Breast-Feeding from an Evolutionary Perspective. *Healthcare*. 2021 Oct 28;9(11):1458. doi:10.3390/healthcare9111458

14. Ferri RL, Rosen-Carole CB, Jackson J, Carreno-Rijo E, Greenberg KB; Academy of Breastfeeding Medicine. ABM Clinical Protocol #33: Lactation Care for Lesbian, Gay, Bisexual, Transgender, Queer, Questioning, Plus Patients. *Breastfeed Med*. 2020;15(5):284–293. doi:10.1089/bfm.2020.29152.rlf

15. Chowdhury R, Sinha B, Sankar MJ, et al. Breastfeeding and Maternal Health Outcomes: A Systematic Review and Meta-Analysis. *Acta Paediatr*. 2015;104(467):96–113. doi:10.1111/apa.13102

16. Ip S, Chung M, Raman G, et al. Breastfeeding and Maternal and Infant Health Outcomes in Developed Countries. *Evid Rep Technol Assess (Full Rep)*. 2007;(153):1–186.

17. Walters DD, Phan LTH, Mathisen R. The Cost of Not Breastfeeding: Global Results from a New Tool. *Health Policy Plan*. 2019;34(6):407–417. doi:10.1093/heapol/czz050

18. Krol KM, Grossmann T. Psychological Effects of Breastfeeding on Children and Mothers. Psychologische Effekte des Stillens auf Kinder und Mütter. *Bundesgesundheitsblatt Gesundheitsforschung Gesundheitsschutz*. 2018;61(8):977–985. doi:10.1007/s00103-018-2769-0

19. Chetwynd EM, Facelli V. Lactation Support for LGBTQIA+ Families. *J Hum Lact*. 2019; 35(2):244–247. Doi:10.1177/0890334419831269

20. MacDonald T, Noel-Weiss J, West D, et al. Transmasculine Individuals' Experiences with Lactation, Chestfeeding, and Gender Identity: A Qualitative Study. *BMC Pregnancy Childbirth*. 2016;16:106. Published May 16, 2016. doi:10.1186/s12884-016-0907-y

21. Wolfe-Roubatis E, Spatz DL. Transgender Men and Lactation: What Nurses Need to Know. *MCN Am J Matern Child Nurs*. 2015;40(1):32–38. doi:10.1097/NMC.0000000000000097

22. Spatz DL. Getting it right: The Critical Window to Effectively Establish Lactation. *Infant*. 2020;16(2):58–60.

23. Biervliet FP, Maguiness SD, Hay DM, Killick SR, Atkin SL. Induction of Lactation in the Intended Mother of a Surrogate Pregnancy: Case report. *Hum Reprod*. 2001;16(3):581–583. doi:10.1093/humrep/16.3.581

24. Wittig SL, Spatz DL. Induced Lactation: Gaining a Better Understanding. *MCN Am J Matern Child Nurs*. 2008;33(2):76–83. doi:10.1097/01.NMC.0000313413.92291.0f

25. Logan R Jr. Gay Fatherhood in the NICU: Supporting the "Gayby" Boom. *Adv Neonatal Care*. 2020;20(4):286–293. doi:10.1097/ANC.0000000000000712

26. Crouch SR, Waters E, McNair R, Power J, Davis E. Parent-Reported Measures of Child Health and Wellbeing in Same-Sex Parent Families: A Cross-Sectional Survey. *BMC Public Health*. 2014 Dec;14(1):1–2. doi: 10.1186/1471-2458-14-635

27. Carone N, Baiocco R, Lingiardi V. Italian Gay Fathers' Experiences of Transnational Surrogacy and their Relationship with the Surrogate Pre- and Post-Birth. *Reprod Biomed Online*. 2017;34(2):181–190. doi:10.1016/j.rbmo.2016.10.010

28. Griggs KM, Waddill CB, Bice A, Ward N. Care During Pregnancy, Childbirth, Postpartum, and Human Milk Feeding for Individuals Who Identify as LGBTQ. *MCN Am J Matern Child Nurs*. 2021;46(1):43–53. doi:10.1097/NMC.0000000000000675

29. Bai Y, Kuscin J. The Current State of Donor Human Milk Use and Practice. *Journal of Midwifery & Women's Health*. 2021 Jul;66(4):478–485. doi:10.1111/jmwh.13244

30. Paynter MJ, Goldberg L. A Critical Review of Human Milk Sharing Using an Intersectional Feminist Framework: Implications for Practice. *Midwifery*. 2018;66:141–147. doi:10.1016/j.midw.2018.08.014

31. Martino K, Spatz D. Informal Milk Sharing: What Nurses Need to Know. *MCN Am J Matern Child Nurs*. 2014;39(6):369–374. doi:10.1097/NMC.0000000000000077

32. Charter R, Ussher JM, Perz J, Robinson K. The Transgender Parent: Experiences and Constructions of Pregnancy and Parenthood for Transgender Men in Australia. *International Journal of Transgenderism*. 2018 Jan 2;19(1):64–77. doi:10.1080/15532739.2017.1399496

33. Oberhelman-Eaton S, Chang A, Gonzalez C, Braith A, Singh RJ, Lteif A. Initiation of Gender-Affirming Testosterone Therapy in a Lactating Transgender Man. *J Hum Lact*. 2022;38(2):339–343. doi:10.1177/08903344211037646

34. MacLean LR. Preconception, Pregnancy, Birthing, and Lactation Needs of Transgender Men. *Nurs Womens Health*. 2021;25(2):129–138. doi:10.1016/j.nwh.2021.01.006

35. García-Acosta JM, San Juan-Valdivia RM, Fernández-Martínez AD, Lorenzo-Rocha ND, Castro-Peraza ME. Trans* Pregnancy and Lactation: A Literature Review from a Nursing Perspective. *Int J Environ Res Public Health*. 2019;17(1):44. Published December 19, 2019. doi:10.3390/ijerph17010044

36. MacDonald TK. Lactation Care for Transgender and Non-Binary Patients: Empowering Clients and Avoiding Aversives. *J Hum Lact*. 2019;35(2):223–226. doi:10.1177/0890334419830989

37. Kraut RY, Brown E, Korownyk C, et al. The Impact of Breast Reduction Surgery on Breastfeeding: Systematic Review of Observational Studies. *PLoS One*. 2017;12(10):e0186591. Published October 19, 2017. doi:10.1371/journal.pone.0186591

38. Liu M, Murthi S, Poretsky L. Polycystic Ovary Syndrome and Gender Identity. *Yale J Biol Med*. 2020 Sep 30;93(4):529–537.

39. Maheshwari A, Nippoldt T, Davidge-Pitts C. An Approach to Nonsuppressed Testosterone in Transgender Women Receiving Gender-Affirming Feminizing Hormonal Therapy. *J Endocr Soc*. 2021 Apr 16;5(9):bvab068. doi:10.1210/jendso/bvab068

40. Reisman T, Goldstein Z. Case Report: Induced Lactation in a Transgender Woman. *Transgend Health*. 2018;3(1):24–26. Published January 1, 2018. doi:10.1089/trgh.2017.0044

41. Goldfarb L, Newman J. The Protocols for Induced Lactation a Guide for Maximizing Breastmilk Production. Asklenore.info. Published March 24, 2002. Accessed June 8, 2022. https://www.asklenore.info/breastfeeding/induced_lactation/protocols4print.shtml

42. Newman J. Inducing lactation. International Breastfeeding Centre. Published August 10, 2017. Accessed June 9, 2022. http://ibconline.ca/induction/

43. Newman J, Pitman T. Revised ed. *Dr. Jack Newman's Guide to Breastfeeding*. Pinter and Martin; 2014.

44. United States Food and Drug Administration. FDA Talk Paper: FDA Warns Against Women Using Unapproved Drug, Domperidone, to Increase Milk Production. FDA.gov. Published June 7, 2004. Updated April 18, 2016. Accessed June 8, 2022. https://www.fda.gov/drugs/information-drug-class/fda-talk-paper-fda-warns-against-women-using-unapproved-drug-domperidone-increase-milk-production

45. Hale TW. Eighteenth ed. *Hale's Medications and Mothers' Milk*. Springer Publishing Company; 2019.

46. Ortiz A, Cooper CJ, Alvarez A, Gomez Y, Sarosiek I, McCallum RW. Cardiovascular Safety Profile and Clinical Experience with High-Dose Domperidone Therapy for Nausea and Vomiting. *Am J Med Sci*. 2015;349(5):421–424. doi:10.1097/MAJ.0000000000000439

47. Osborne RJ, Slevin ML, Hunter RW, Hamer J. Cardiac Arrhythmias during Cytotoxic Chemotherapy: Role of Domperidone. *Hum Toxicol*. 1985;4(6):617–626. doi:10.1177/096032718500400608

48. Paul C, Zénut M, Dorut A, et al. Use of Domperidone as a Galactagogue Drug: A Systematic Review of the Benefit-Risk Ratio. *J Hum Lact*. 2015;31(1):57–63. doi:10.1177/0890334414561265

49. Zuppa AA, Sindico P, Orchi C, Carducci C, Cardiello V, Romagnoli C. Safety and Efficacy of Galactogogues: Substances that Induce, Maintain and Increase Breast Milk Production. *J Pharm Pharm Sci*. 2010;13(2):162–174. doi:10.18433/j3ds3r

50. Campbell-Yeo ML, Allen AC, Joseph KS, et al. Effect of Domperidone on the Composition of Preterm Human Breast Milk. *Pediatrics*. 2010;125(1):e107–e114. doi:10.1542/peds.2008-3441

51. Trautner E, McCool-Myers M, Joyner AB. Knowledge and Practice of Induction of Lactation in Trans Women among Professionals Working in Trans Health. *Int Breastfeed J*. 2020;15(1):63. Published July 16, 2020. doi:10.1186/s13006-020-00308-6

52. Perrin MT, Wilson E, Chetwynd E, Fogleman A. A Pilot Study on the Protein Composition of Induced Nonpuerperal Human Milk. *J Hum Lact*. 2015;31(1):166–171. doi:10.1177/0890334414552827

53. Wamboldt R, Shuster S, Sidhu BS. Lactation Induction in a Transgender Woman Wanting to Breastfeed: Case Report. *J Clin Endocrinol Metab*. 2021;106(5):e2047–e2052. doi:10.1210/clinem/dgaa976

54. Zizzo G. Lesbian Families and the Negotiation of Maternal Identity through the Unconventional Use of Breast Milk. *Gay Lesbian Iss Psychol Rev*. 2009;5(2):96–109.

55. Jewell ML, Edwards MC, Murphy DK, Schumacher A. Lactation Outcomes in More Than 3500 Women Following Primary Augmentation: 5-Year Data From the Breast Implant Follow-Up Study. *Aesthet Surg J*. 2019;39(8):875–883. doi:10.1093/asj/sjy221

56. Jenkins V, Everett BG, Steadman M, Mollborn S. Breastfeeding Initiation and Continuation Among Sexual Minority Women. *Matern Child Health J*. 2021;25(11):1757–1765. doi:10.1007/s10995-021-03218-z

57. Juntereal NA, Spatz DL. Breastfeeding Experiences of Same-Sex Mothers. *Birth*. 2020;47(1):21–28. doi:10.1111/birt.12470

58. Juntereal NA, Spatz DL. Same-Sex Mothers and Lactation. *MCN Am J Matern Child Nurs*. 2019;44(3):164–169. doi:10.1097/NMC.0000000000000519

59. Moberg KU, Prime DK. Oxytocin Effects in Mothers and Infants during Breastfeeding. *Infant*. 2013;9(6):201–206.

60. Reisman T, Goldstein Z, Safer JD. A Review of Breast Development in Cisgender Women and Implications for Transgender Women. *Endocr Pract*. 2019;25(12):1338–1345. doi:10.4158/EP-2019-0183

61. Sonnenblick EB, Shah AD, Goldstein Z, Reisman T. Breast Imaging of Transgender Individuals: A Review. *Curr Radiol Rep*. 2018;6(1):1. doi:10.1007/s40134-018-0260-1

62. Bekeny JC, Zolper EG, Fan KL, Del Corral G. Breast Augmentation for Transfeminine Patients: Methods, Complications, and Outcomes. *Gland Surg*. 2020;9(3):788–796. doi:10.21037/gs.2020.03.18

63. Paynter MJ. Medication and Facilitation of Transgender Women's Lactation. *J Hum Lact*. 2019;35(2):239–243. doi:10.1177/0890334419829729

64. Drugs and Lactation Database (LactMed) [Internet]. Bethesda (MD): National Library of Medicine (US); 2006–. Spironolactone. [Updated January 18, 2022]. Available from: https://www.ncbi.nlm.nih.gov/books/NBK501101/

65. Juntereal NA, Spatz DL. Integrative Review of Antenatal Milk Expression and Mother-Infant Outcomes During the First 2 Weeks After Birth. *J Obstet Gynecol Neonatal Nurs*. 2021;50(6):659–668. doi:10.1016/j.jogn.2021.07.003

66. Prendergast AJ, Goga AE, Waitt C, et al. Transmission of CMV, HTLV-1, and HIV through Breastmilk. *Lancet Child Adolesc Health*. 2019;3(4):264–273. doi:10.1016/S2352-4642(19)30024-0

67. Committee on nutrition; Section on breastfeeding; Committee on fetus and newborn. Donor Human Milk for the High-Risk Infant: Preparation, Safety, and Usage Options in the United States. *Pediatrics*. 2017;139(1):e20163440. doi:10.1542/peds.2016-3440

68. Tyeballly Fang M, Chatzixiros E, Grummer-Strawn L, et al. Developing Global Guidance on Human Milk Banking. *Bull World Health Organ*. 2021;99(12):892–900. doi:10.2471/BLT.21.286943

69. United States Food and Drug Administration. Use of Donor Human Milk. FDA.gov. Published March 22, 2018. Accessed June 9, 2022. https://www.fda.gov/science-research/pediatrics/use-donor-human-milk

70. McNally D, Spatz DL. Mothers Who Engage in Long-Term Informal Milk Sharing. *MCN Am J Matern Child Nurs*. 2020;45(6):338–343. doi:10.1097/NMC.0000000000000660

71. Palmquist AE, Doehler K. Human Milk Sharing Practices in the U.S. *Matern Child Nutr*. 2016;12(2):278–290. doi:10.1111/mcn.12221

72. Sriraman NK, Evans AE, Lawrence R, Noble L; Academy of Breastfeeding Medicine's Board of Directors. Academy of Breastfeeding Medicine's 2017 Position Statement on Informal Breast Milk Sharing for the Term Healthy Infant. *Breastfeed Med*. 2018;13(1):2–4. doi:10.1089bfm.2017.29064.nks

73. American Academy of Nursing on Policy. Position Statement Regarding use of Informally Shared Human Milk. *Nurs Outlook*. 2016;64(1):98–102. doi:10.1016/j.outlook.2015.12.004

74. World Health Organization. Frequently Asked Questions: Breastfeeding and COVID-19 for Health Care Workers. World Health Organization. Published May 12, 2020. Accessed June 29, 2022. https://www.who.int/mediacentre/news/statements/2011/breastfeeding_20110115/en/

Chapter 10

Processing birth experiences

Mari Greenfield, El Molloy, Sofia Klittmark, and Anna Malmquist

INTRODUCTION

The birth of a child is assumed to be a happy event for the whole family in almost every culture. New baby cards congratulating the parents are ubiquitous. Research shows that for many cis women, childbirth is a positive event.[1-4] Figures for experiencing giving birth as a negative or traumatic event vary by study and by country, but a systematic review found that globally between 6.8% and 44% of women had a negative experience of childbirth.[2] For some, childbirth is not just a negative experience, it is experienced as a traumatic event. The consequences of experiencing birth as a traumatic event include difficulties in breastfeeding[5, 6] and probably chestfeeding (although no research has investigated this), enduring mental health problems,[7, 8] compromised maternal infant relationships,[9] poorer quality intimate relationships[10] and can mean people change their plans about having more children.[11-13]

The enduring mental health problems that can be linked to a traumatic birth include postnatal depression,[14] post-traumatic stress disorder (PTSD),[15] and psychotic-like experiences (PLEs).[16] A meta-analysis found that 3.1% of women (non-binary people and trans men were not included in the research) develop PTSD following birth.[17] However, in groups who had more risk factors, this rose to 15.7%.[17]

Research shows that factors that make experiencing birth as a traumatic event more likely amongst cis women fall into two main categories—previous life experiences, and experiences that occur during birth (no comparable research has been carried out with non-binary people or trans men).[18] Having experienced sexual abuse, physical abuse, domestic violence, or previous traumatic events make it more likely that birth will be a traumatic event.[19] Having an existing mental health diagnosis, including fear of childbirth, also increases the risk of a traumatic

DOI: 10.4324/9781003305446-11

birth.[20, 21] Factors related to the birth that increase this risk include threat of harm or actual harm to the mother or baby, unplanned medical interventions, and care which is perceived as uncaring, disrespectful, or unsupportive.[21] LGBTQ+ people are more likely than cisheterosexual women to have these previous life experiences.[22, 23] Studies have also found that many LGBTQ+ people experience poor intrapartum care.[13, 24] In Chapter 7 we also examined potential risk factors that are not experienced by cisheterosexual women such as gender dysphoria and tokophobia in nulliparous people who have been present when their partner gave birth, which might place LGBTQ+ people at greater risk of a traumatic birth.

PROMOTING POSITIVE BIRTH EXPERIENCES

Good care has repeatedly been identified as the most protective factor in promoting positive births and preventing a traumatic birth. Even where an expectant parent is predisposed, in relation to their life history, to experience birth as a traumatic event, and then goes on to experience adverse events during labour and birth, good care can protect their emotional wellbeing, and ensure the birth is not experienced as traumatic.[15, 25] Good care in this context is well-defined in the literature—it is care which is individualised, ensures the birthing person makes the decisions, and trauma-informed.[26] Experiencing continuity of carer from the antenatal period through labour and/or birth and into the postnatal period is proven to have a significant effect on whether the care given is perceived as good.[27] The continuity allows for a trusting relationship to be built and makes it more likely that the health care professional is aware of the parent's birth choices.

Given that we have a significant body of evidence about the risk factors that make negative or traumatic birth experiences more likely, and the factors that make a positive birth experience more likely, these high rates of birth trauma are avoidable. Providing care that promotes a positive birth experience and reduces the likelihood of birth trauma should be a priority for all intrapartum services, and wherever possible, midwives, obstetricians, and other health care professionals caring for people giving birth should provide care that protects against birth trauma. Sometimes, the objective events of the birth make this a significant challenge. More often, the challenges to promoting positive birth experiences and preventing birth trauma come from constraints imposed by the health services themselves. These include:

- Understaffing
- Staffing organised in ways that do not prioritise known protective factors, such as continuity of carer

- Guidelines for care which do not allow all birthing people access to all birth choices (such as age, BMI, or other restrictions on access to some birth services or birth choices)
- Organisational cultures which coerce pregnant people into agreeing to give birth in the way that a health care professional thinks they ought to
- Organisational cultures which do not value factors that promote positive birth experiences[28]

The current rates of birth trauma reflect the choices made by health services.

When faced with these challenges, it is unsurprising that so many people experience birth as a negative or traumatic event. If we have failed to prevent a traumatic birth, appropriately identifying and supporting those who are experiencing the negative sequalae should be our next priority. In the remainder of this chapter, we will explore what we know about the identification and treatment of birth trauma and secondary fear of childbirth, and why both might be different for LGBTQ+ parents.

IDENTIFYING BIRTH TRAUMA AND SECONDARY FEAR OF CHILDBIRTH IN LGBTQ+ PEOPLE

Cisheterosexist assumptions about family formation results in binary divisions in perinatal mental health provision, whereby services are largely aimed at cis women, who are assumed to be or have been pregnant. Services for processing fear of childbirth (FOC) during pregnancy will therefore require that the person who is treated is themselves pregnant, and postnatal maternal mental health services will usually only be available to someone who has given birth. Services for non-gestational parents are usually less well developed and resourced, but where they do exist are based on the assumption that the non-gestational parent is a cis man and the father of the baby, and who is assumed not to have given birth.

In LGBTQ+ families, divisions which equate gender and gestational/non-gestational status may not be so simple, and the cisheterosexist assumptions which underpin the services available may prevent the identification of LGBTQ+ people who need help to process a traumatic birth or secondary FOC.

Women, non-binary people, and trans men who have watched their partners experience a traumatic birth may themselves need support in dealing with the immediate psychological consequences to themselves, but if they have not given birth, they are unlikely to be considered a maternity services' patient, and are then unlikely to be eligible to access services labelled "maternal mental health."

They may be able to access services for partners, but as those services are primarily aimed at cis fathers, support which encompasses the challenges a partner might face about decisions around their own future conception choices or which reflect on their own previous experiences of having given birth are unlikely to be provided. Such services may also lack appropriate literature and women and non-binary people may not see themselves reflected in the images or terminology used within service information. This may potentially further invalidate their parental role at a time when they are already emotionally vulnerable.

If these people later become pregnant, the consequences of their partner's traumatic birth, including a secondary fear of childbirth, may not be recognised by health care professionals. Reproductive histories are usually taken as part of an initial booking appointment in order to provide appropriate care, but these histories do not generally include the conception attempts or pregnancies of a partner. Medical terms such as "primiparous" may make LGBTQ+ people's experiences of the birth of their non-gestational children invisible, and the lack of questions about the family's reproductive history on forms routinely used by health care professionals may mean that no opportunity is created to discuss the potential impact of previous birth experiences.

For trans men and non-binary people, whether they are the gestational or non-gestational parent, the services provided may be inappropriate. If a trans man is a non-gestational parent, accessing support aimed at fathers may come with the same challenges as it does for women whose partners have had a traumatic birth. If they are the gestational parent, accessing services for women who have given birth may also feel invalidating of their gender, again at a time when they are already vulnerable. For non-binary people, accessing services which present gender both as binary and as linked to a binary model of reproduction has the potential to cause further harm, rather than support the processing of the birth experience.

CASE STUDY—LAILA AND AMARA

Laila and her wife Amara have a six-year-old, who Laila gave birth to. Laila was cared for poorly postnatally in hospital.

Amara is currently pregnant with their second child, and is fearful about giving birth. Laila is very worried about the care that Amara will receive. As the birth draws closer, Laila is experiencing flashbacks to the time she spent in hospital after giving birth.

The couple have planned a homebirth, so that Laila can look after Amara postnatally. Laila has developed significant anxiety about the possibility that Amara might need to transfer into hospital after the birth. Laila wants to attend all Amara's antenatal appointments and talk about reasons for postnatal transfer and how to reduce this possibility with the midwives. This is creating strain between the couple, as Amara doesn't want to focus on the things that might go wrong. The appointments are short, and the midwives are finding it difficult to deliver the care they need to and have these conversations during the appointment. The midwives also cannot give Laila the reassurance that she needs. Whilst they recognise her anxiety, she is not their patient, and they are concerned about the impact her anxiety is having on Amara. One midwife suggests to Laila that she should stop attending the appointments, and trust the midwives to look after Amara.

The local hospital offers Birth Choices meetings, where women who have previously had a traumatic birth and are pregnant again can talk with a senior midwife about the choices available for this birth. As Laila is primiparous and Amara is not pregnant, they do not fit the criteria for Birth Choices, and so their midwife does not think to suggest this.

Amara continues to feel fearful about the birth, and watching the deteriorating relationship between her wife and the midwives makes it difficult for her to trust the midwives or to feel supported by her wife. Even though she wants a second child, and going through IVF represented a significant financial and emotional investment, she sometimes wishes she had never got pregnant.

Key learning points

- Terms such as "mother," "maternal," "father," "paternal," "nulliparous," and "primiparous" may make parts of LGBTQ+ people's reproductive experiences invisible
- Identifying LGBTQ+ people who require help in processing birth experiences is hampered by binary care models which equate gender with gestational/non-gestational parenthood
- Making treatment accessible only through such binary care models risks causing harm to LGBTQ+ new and expectant parents

PROCESSING BIRTH TRAUMA

A body of evidence about the effectiveness of different interventions in treating birth trauma does exist. This evidence base has, however, been based on either cisheterosexual populations, or on populations where gender and sexual orientation were not known or were assumed. As no literature exists about the efficacy of interventions amongst an LGBTQ+ population exists, we will discuss the evidence from cisheterosexual populations and then consider why and how interventions might need to be different for LGBTQ+ people.

Immediate interventions

When a potentially traumatic birth has occurred, it may be possible with trauma sensitive early interventions to deliver immediate help after the birth that helps to alleviate or protect the parents from acute posttraumatic stress symptoms.[29] The principles of psychological first aid (PFA) are widely used in general crisis support aiming at stabilizing after an overwhelming experience, and facilitate the natural recovery after a stressful experience.[30] The PFA alone seem not to prevent from a development of PTSD, and should therefore be followed by an invitation to more traditional interventions for persons with abundant symptoms of acute stress.[31] Trauma sensitive care is based on awareness that both patients and HCP may have experienced previous trauma, and aims to prevent retraumatising as well as enhancing posttraumatic recovery.[32]

It is worth noting that none of the previous studies are conducted in an LBTQ context, which underlines the need for trauma sensitive LBTQ competence amongst HCPs.

If a parent wishes to chestfeed or breastfeed, ensuring they have qualified, consistent support to do so may help prevent further trauma. Some research has also found that a midwife-led counselling intervention delivered within the first 72 hours can assist those whose births were potentially traumatic—however identifying who would benefit from this intervention is a challenge.

Longer-term interventions

A range of interventions and therapies exist that are used to help people process negative or traumatic birth experiences. We will look at the evidence base for four popular interventions:

- Eye-Movement Desensitization and Reprocessing (EMDR)
- Cognitive behavioural therapy (CBT) especially Prolonged Exposure and Therapeutic writing

- Rewind technique
- Birth Reflections meetings

To be classed as successful, an intervention should help to reduce the severity of some of the distressing consequences of a traumatic birth, but it should be noted that these interventions will not remove all the consequences or resolve mental health problems. It is also important to note that some therapies, including those listed above, may cause further trauma if delivered at the wrong time or by a poorly trained practitioner.

There is not a significant evidence base for the use of these interventions following a birth, although there are many anecdotal reports that some treatments have helped some parents, and a few peer-reviewed research papers. The lack of a larger evidence base stems from two facts. First, most studies which evaluate the interventions above are carried out with people who have PTSD. Not everyone who experiences a negative or traumatic birth will go on to develop PTSD, and those who do not are missed out of the evaluations. Second, in general studies analysing the effectiveness of interventions for PTSD, postpartum parents are rarely included, meaning that even for those parents who do develop PTSD, the evidence base is smaller.

Eye-Movement Desensitization and Reprocessing (EMDR)

EMDR is a structured therapy that integrates techniques from cognitive behavioural, psychodynamic, and body-oriented therapy. It takes place over a limited number of sessions, typically 6–12, although some people require as few as 3 sessions. Unlike most trauma-focused treatments, EMDR does not seek to decrease fear, change how people think, or reduce avoidant behaviours. Instead, EMDR therapy works on changing how traumatic memories have been stored. EMDR therapy is based on the Adaptive Information Processing (AIP) model, which hypothesises that memories of traumatic events are not processed in the same way as other memories.[33] Memories are normally processed in a way that allows the person to learn useful lessons from the event and are then filed away. This might include thinking, talking, or dreaming about the event for a short while, but then no longer doing so. When a traumatic event happens, the mind is not able to process the memory in this way. Instead,

> "the information acquired at the time of the event, including images, sound, affect and physical sensations, is retained neurologically in its disturbing state."[33]

External events and internal thoughts can trigger these original memories, causing the person to instantly re-experience the original memory in as vivid a way as they did at the time. This might be experienced as flashbacks, intrusive thoughts, or nightmares.

To help re-process traumatic memories, patients are encouraged to focus briefly on the traumatic memory while simultaneously experiencing bilateral stimulation (typically eye movements, but can involve hearing, touch, or other bilateral stimulation). Bilateral stimulation has been shown to have an effect on memory retrieval and storage, although the mechanism by which this works is not fully understood.[33] Perhaps the most persuasive hypothesis is that bilateral stimulation approximates the movements of the eyes—or of the attention when auditory or touch stimulants are used—during the rapid eye movement stage of sleep. REM sleep is crucial for the consolidation and movement of recent memories into long-term storage.[34] It is thought that replicating these movements whilst briefly recalling the traumatic event may therefore support the patient's neuropsychological systems to re-process the traumatic memory appropriately as something which happened in the past, rather than continuing to re-experience it as a current event.[33]

Research shows that EMDR can help reduce PTSD symptoms in those with a diagnosis. For those who have experienced a traumatic event but who do not have PTSD it can result in a reduction in the vividness and overwhelming emotions associated with memories of traumatic events. Research shows positive clinical outcomes for EMDR use in people with a variety of diagnoses including anxiety, depression, obsessive compulsive disorder, and other distressing life experiences.[33, 35] EMDR is recommended in a number of international guidelines as one of the very few treatments of choice for people who have experienced a traumatic event.[36–38] Perhaps most importantly in this context, research has proven EMDR to be effective in treating cis women who have post-traumatic stress after childbirth.[39, 40]

Trauma-focused cognitive behavioural therapy

Trauma-focused cognitive behavioural therapy (TF-CBT) is a form of structured therapy which takes place across a pre-set number of sessions (typically 8–25). The programme may be dictated by patient need or organisational restrictions, but will include several key components, typically: psychoeducation, relaxation training, imaginal or real-life exposure to the trauma, cognitive restructuring, homework exercises, and discussions around social support.[41] Unlike EMDR, TF-CBT aims to help patients change their thoughts, beliefs, and behaviours.

In common with EMDR, key features of the therapy include exposure to the traumatic memory—for those who have experienced a traumatic birth this would usually be through recalling the birth—and simultaneous cognitive processing of the meaning or interpretations of the trauma.[42] Similarly to EMDR, it is thought that TF-CBT effects changes in the symptoms experienced by patients through the re-processing of the traumatic memories.

Meta-analyses of interventions for a general population of people with PTSD have shown that TF-CBT is highly effective at reducing symptoms, with a similar impact to EMDR.[43] It is also effective in reducing the symptoms of anxiety and depression. Alongside EMDR, TF-CBT is advised as a first-choice intervention for people with diagnoses of PTSD.[36–38] It has also been proven to be effective in reducing PTSD symptoms in cis women who have experienced a traumatic birth.[44] Based on this, UK guidance recommends that EMDR and TF-CBT are the only suitable treatments for those who experience PTSD after a traumatic birth.[45]

A word of caution is needed here, as the distinction between TF-CBT and general cognitive behavioural therapy (CBT) is both essential and not always well understood. Using general psychological therapies rather than trauma-informed versions is inappropriate. Several meta-analyses have demonstrated that using CBT as an intervention for PTSD is, at best, significantly less effective than using TF-CBT.[43, 46] Even when a specialist trauma-focused therapy such as TF-CBT is used, if it is not adapted for use with parents after a traumatic birth, it can be ineffective, or cause harm.

Rewind technique

Therapies based on the Rewind technique have become popular recently for treating those who have experienced a traumatic birth.[47] Several companies are training a variety of birth workers in the technique. There is a limited evidence base of peer-reviewed articles proving any success, with most of the evidence based on case studies of one or two patients. In some countries the use of the Rewind techniques has been promoted by health services—for example, in the UK, the Royal College of Midwives have accredited the technique despite the lack of evidence of its effectiveness.[48]

The general availability of Rewind technique training in many countries to those without knowledge of or training in psychological support has been flagged as a concern,[47] as this lack of appropriate education and understanding of the practitioner may cause further psychological harm. A further concern is the lack of a standardised curriculum or substantive quality control amongst the various companies offering training.

Specialist listening and psychological debriefing

Psychological debriefing is contraindicated for people with PTSD, as it has consistently been shown to increase symptoms rather than reduce them. In national health care guidance, some forms of psychological debriefing are advised against not just for those people who meet the criteria for PTSD, but also for those who have had a traumatic birth:

> "Do not offer single-session high-intensity psychological interventions with an explicit focus on 're-living' the trauma to women who have a traumatic birth."[45]

In many countries, a specialist form of listening and psychological debriefing after a negative or traumatic birth is offered. It is referred to by different names in different countries, but common terms include Birth Reflections meetings, Birth Afterthoughts, and midwife-led debriefing. These sessions usually consist of a single postnatal meeting between the parent(s) and a medical person who was not involved directly in the perinatal care, frequently a senior midwife. In the session the labour, birth, and antenatal or postnatal care if relevant will be discussed, using the antenatal and intrapartum health care notes and the parents' recollections as a basis.

Unlike EMDR or TF-CBT, Birth Reflections–style sessions have no agreed content or structure, and are driven by the patient and the HCP. A review of the research about these sessions unsurprisingly found a large amount of variance in which parents were offered a meeting, who carried out the meetings, how they were structured, what the goal of the meeting was for the professional(s) involved, and what was discussed.[49] They concluded that debriefings of this type were sometimes useful, when targeted at cis women who both described their birth as traumatic, and met some of the criteria for PTSD. However, the effectiveness of the intervention was dependent on the purpose ascribed to the meeting by the HCP involved, and their skillset. If the meeting was intended to prevent a complaint or litigation, for example, it was unlikely to help resolve trauma, and may cause further harm. Primary research which has found that specialist midwife-led debriefing has a positive effect on PTSD symptoms report that it has no effect on depressive symptoms.[50] Taking this together with the challenges posed by variability, these sessions should not be used as an alternative to EMDR or TF-CBT, but may be a helpful addition if such therapies cannot be provided imminently.

Availability of, and access to, interventions

In order to treat an illness, it must first be diagnosed and assessed. For this to happen the person in need of support, and/or their family members first need to recognise their illness and seek support. Research around perinatal mental health for cisgender parents suggests that approximately half of all parents struggling with mental health issues in the perinatal period do not seek support for this.[51] Other research has indicated that despite an increase in awareness of PNMH illness some parents find it hard to access services and seek support. This may be because of a fear of judgement around their parenting and the safety of their infant, or because they assume, or are told when seeking support, that all new parents find the postnatal period challenging, and therefore assume their emotional struggles are down to inherent weaknesses.[52]

Parents today are often more likely, in the Global North and other Westernised societies, to seek support and information through online means. UK focused parent facing information[53] discusses EMDR and CBT trauma focused therapy with references to NICE guidelines for care for PTSD.[54] But even this can only be offered as a limited resource in those areas which have capacity and capability to offer it.[55] In Australia, although birth trauma is mentioned on some parent facing sites, the focus of much the information is still around PND, and PTSD is a "see your GP" signpost.[56] Information available through the Australian Birth Trauma Association signposts again to GP and talks about an "array of psychological therapies and/or medication."[57] The current version of the City Birth Trauma Scale is in use in research in the UK, and has been validated in various languages for use in diverse populations including Hebrew, Croatian, French, Chinese, Turkish, Slovenian, Spanish, and Swedish[58-60] as well as being assessed for construct validity in Australasian populations,[61] but is not routinely used in postnatal checks. The Centre for Perinatal Excellence (COPE) provides resources for health care professionals including a variety of downloadable information sheets (COPE, 2022) which are derived from the National Perinatal Mental Health Guidelines. Again, these sheets specifically relate to anxiety, depression, schizophrenia, postpartum psychosis, borderline personality disorders, bipolar disorder, and assessing woman and infant interactions and safety in the perinatal period but no mention is made of PTSD. Within the Australian National Clinical Guidelines[62] the consensus guidelines are to suggest counselling for women with PTSD (highlighted as low-quality evidence from National Institute for Health and Care Excellence) in order to reduce symptoms of depression, and no other information about treatment for CB-PTSD.

All of these sources use predominantly gendered terminology and may further disenfranchise and invalidate LGBTQ+ parents. As highlighted previously, access to services is dependent on fulfilling threshold referral criteria, and where services are badged as "maternal" they assume this means cis hetero birthing woman. Furthermore, there is still a huge amount of trans- and homophobia which is made explicit both across social media and in media in general which incorrectly conflates LGBTQ+ with sexual predation, and therefore may also act as a barrier to support seeking for PMNH.

SECONDARY FEAR OF CHILDBIRTH TREATMENT

Secondary FOC is defined as a FOC that has its origin in a previous traumatic birth experience. This often has components of posttraumatic stress (sometimes even fulfilling the criteria of PTSD), generally influencing the individual's expectation of the forthcoming birth. It is common that the person only becomes aware of the fear during a prospective pregnancy, resulting in the need for treatment often arising when planning the forthcoming birth. The point of departure of the treatment is to creating understanding of the traumatic experience. Sometimes a review of the medical record together with an obstetrician or senior midwife can bring an understanding which supports the birthing person, couple, or family. A treatment plan would then need to be formulated, which highlights the need for LBTQ competence in antenatal care. In couples where both people have a childbearing capacity, it is important to remember that the non-gestational partner may also be a prospective gestational parent, meaning that both partners should be recognised and included in the treatment.

The standard differentiation between primary and secondary FOC is that primary FOC is experienced before the first childbirth, while secondary FOC is caused by birth trauma. This may not however always be applicable for LGBTQ+ people. A person may be pregnant for the first time, but carry FOC that began, or was intensified when witnessing their partner giving birth previously. This specific experience constitutes a FOC that has similarities with both primary and secondary FOC.

Secondary FOC may influence decisions about whether to become pregnant again. In couples with two potential gestational parents, secondary FOC may influence the choice about who conceives in the future. It is important to stress that these decisions can take many directions. Either partner may or may not be afraid to give birth (again) themselves. In addition, either partner may or may not be afraid for their partner if they want to be pregnant and give birth. In any scenario, support can be needed before both feel safe and comfortable in approaching a new pregnancy.

DO LGBTQ+ PARENTS HAVE DIFFERENT NEEDS WHEN PROCESSING BIRTH EXPERIENCES?

Research suggests that experiencing homophobia or transphobia during birth can contribute to a negative or traumatic birth experience.[13] No research has, as of yet, established whether experiencing homophobia or transphobia during birth can cause birth trauma when no other factors are present. Given the centrality of respectful, individualised care to the perception of the birth experience however, it seems likely that these experiences would affect whether giving birth was a positive, negative, or traumatic experience. If a parent required help in processing a birth experience in which transphobia, homophobia, or misgendering formed a part of the traumatic experience, it is unlikely that practitioners would be sufficiently trained in LGBTQ+ issues to provide appropriate support. This might particularly be the case in therapies such as TF-CBT where the practitioner takes an active role in helping the patient to change their thoughts and beliefs.

Misgendering may not only affect the birth experience, but may impact the provision of interventions to support people in processing those experiences. It is an issue which may affect trans and non-binary people directly either if they have not chosen to disclose their gender to an HCP, or if after disclosure the HCP continues to use incorrect pronouns or gendered terms without apology. Misgendering also affects same-gender couples when HCPs make heterosexist assumptions, such as using "he" to refer to a pregnant woman's partner when they have no met the partner or been informed of their gender. Another commonly experienced form of misgendering occurs when a HCP assumes that a same-gender partner is a friend or relative, because they have made the heterosexist assumption that the person's partner will be different-gender. Again, this can happen when the person has not disclosed their sexual orientation to the HCP, or following disclosure if the HCP uses incorrect pronouns or gendered terms when referring to the person's partner. Misgendering can therefore happen for three reasons; because the HCP does not have the correct information, by mistake, or deliberately to indicate disapproval of gender and sexual minority people. Where services to help parents process birth experiences are provided on a gendered basis, or with gendered names (such as paternal mental health services), or with underlying heterosexist assumptions, further misgendering may be experienced by parents every time they access the service. This can turn an intervention in birth trauma processing into a further trauma, potentially without the HCP being aware of this.

LGBTQ+ parents may be affected by birth experiences in ways which cisheterosexual parents are not. Non-gestational parents who have the ability to be gestational parents may experience secondary tokophobia even if they are nulliparous. There is currently a very small evidence base about interventions for those in this situation, and it does not form a core part of the birth trauma training for therapists that we have examined. Similarly, if a trans man or non-binary person also experiences gender dysphoria, this may be exacerbated by pregnancy and birth.[63] Gender dysphoria is not currently recognised as a perinatal mental health concern, and again does not form a core part of the birth trauma training for therapists that we have examined.

HOW COULD WE DESIGN SERVICES FOR TREATING LGBTQ+ FEAR OF CHILDBIRTH AND BIRTH TRAUMA?

Services to help LGBTQ+ people process birth experiences therefore need to be organised in a way which does not assume heterosexuality or equate gender with parental role. They need to ask for information about gender, pronouns, sexual orientation, and partners, suggestions for which are made in the good practice box below. Introducing data collection cannot be the first step though—services must first create an environment in which it is safe for LGBTQ+ people to provide that information. Once information is collected, it must be used. Most importantly, HCPs and therapists must also be equipped to support LGBTQ+ people's birth experiences.

BOX 2—GOOD PRACTICE SUGGESTIONS

1. Ask about gender, sexual orientation, and family make-up
2. Ensure all forms throughout all services can contain accurate information
3. Use inclusive terminology in all policies and service information
4. Use diverse imagery in service information
5. Ensure diverse examples are used in any training
6. Ensure training includes non-clinical staff, for example reception staff

---

REFERENCES

1. Menhart L, Prosen M. Women's Satisfaction with the Childbirth Experience: A Descriptive Research. *Obz Zdr Nege*. 2017;51(4):298–311. doi:10.14528/snr.2017.51.4.189
2. Hosseini Tabaghdehi M, Kolahdozan S, Keramat A, Shahhossein Z, Moosazadeh M, Motaghi Z. Prevalence and Factors Affecting the Negative Childbirth Experiences: A Systematic Review. *J Matern Fetal Neonatal Med*. 2020;33(22):3849–3856. doi:10.1080/14767058.2019.1583740

3. Fumagalli S, Colciago E, Antolini L, Riva A, Nespoli A, Locatelli A. Variables Related to Maternal Satisfaction with Intrapartum Care in Northern Italy. *Women Birth*. 2021;34(2): 154–161. doi:10.1016/j.wombi.2020.01.012

4. Martins ACM, Giugliani ERJ, Nunes LN, et al. Factors Associated with a Positive Childbirth Experience in Brazilian Women: A Cross-Sectional Study. *Women Birth*. 2021;34(4):e337–e345. doi:10.1016/j.wombi.2020.06.003

5. Beck CT, Watson S. Impact of Birth Trauma on Breast-Feeding: A Tale of Two Pathways. *Nurs Res*. 2008;57(4):228–236. doi:10.1097/01.NNR.0000313494.87282.90

6. Cook N, Ayers S, Horsch A. Maternal Posttraumatic Stress Disorder during the Perinatal Period and Child Outcomes: A Systematic Review. *J Affect Disord*. 2018;225:18–31. doi:10. 1016/j.jad.2017.07.045

7. Beck CT. Post-Traumatic Stress Disorder Due to Childbirth: The Aftermath. *Nurs Res*. 2004;53(4):216–224. doi:10.1097/00006199-200407000-00004

8. Forssén ASK. Lifelong Significance of Disempowering Experiences in Prenatal and Maternity Care: Interviews with Elderly Swedish Women. *Qual Health Res*. 2012;22(11): 1535–1546. doi:10.1177/1049732312449212

9. Nicholls K, Ayers S. Childbirth-Related Post-Traumatic Stress Disorder in Couples: A Qualitative Study. *Br J Health Psychol*. 2007;12(4):491–509. doi:10.1348/135910706X120627

10. Ayers S, Eagle A, Waring H. The Effects of Childbirth-Related Post-Traumatic Stress Disorder on Women and their Relationships: A Qualitative Study. *Psychol Health Med*. 2006;11(4):389–398. doi:10.1080/13548500600708409

11. Fenech G, Thomson G. 'Tormented by Ghosts from their Past': A Meta-Synthesis to Explore the Psychosocial Implications of a Traumatic Birth on Maternal Well-Being. *Midwifery*. 2014;30(2):185–193. doi:10.1016/j.midw.2013.12.004

12. Malmquist A, Nieminen K. Negotiating Who Gives Birth and the Influence of Fear of Childbirth: Lesbians, Bisexual Women and Transgender People in Parenting Relationships. *Women Birth*. 2021;34(3):e271–e278. doi:10.1016/j.wombi.2020.04.005

13. Klittmark S, Malmquist A, Karlsson G, Ulfsdotter A, Grundström H, Nieminen K. When Complications Arise during Birth: LBTQ People's Experiences of Care. *Midwifery*. 2023; 121:103649. doi:10.1016/j.midw.2023.103649

14. Bell AF, Andersson E. The Birth Experience and Women's Postnatal Depression: A Systematic Review. *Midwifery*. 2016;39:112–123. doi:10.1016/j.midw.2016.04.014

15. Kendall-Tackett K. Birth Trauma: The Causes and Consequences of Childbirth-Related Trauma and PTSD. In: Barnes DL, ed. *Women's Reproductive Mental Health Across the Lifespan*. Springer International Publishing; 2014:177–191. doi:10.1007/978-3-319-05 116-1_10

16. Holt L, Sellwood W, Slade P. Birth Experiences, Trauma Responses and Self-Concept in Postpartum Psychotic-Like Experiences. *Schizophr Res*. 2018;197:531–538. doi:10.1016/ j.schres.2017.12.015

17. Grekin R, O'Hara MW. Prevalence and Risk Factors of Postpartum Posttraumatic Stress Disorder: A Meta-Analysis. *Clin Psychol Rev*. 2014;34(5):389–401. doi:10.1016/j.cpr.2014. 05.003

18. Greenfield M, Jomeen J, Glover L. What is Traumatic Birth? A Concept Analysis and Literature Review. *Br J Midwifery*. 2016;24(4):254–267. doi:10.12968/bjom.2016.24.4.254

19. LoGiudice JA. A Systematic Literature Review of the Childbearing Cycle as Experienced by Survivors of Sexual Abuse. *Nurs Womens Health*. 2016;20(6):582–594. doi:10.1016/j.nwh.2016.10.008

20. Ayers S, Bond R, Bertullies S, Wijma K. The Aetiology of Post-Traumatic Stress Following Childbirth: A Meta-Analysis and Theoretical Framework. *Psychol Med*. 2016;46(6):1121–1134. doi:10.1017/S0033291715002706

21. Simpson M, Catling C. Understanding Psychological Traumatic Birth Experiences: A Literature Review. *Women Birth*. 2016;29(3):203–207. doi:10.1016/j.wombi.2015.10.009

22. Hafeez H, Zeshan M, Tahir MA, Jahan N, Naveed S. Health Care Disparities Among Lesbian, Gay, Bisexual, and Transgender Youth: A Literature Review. *Cureus*. Published online April 20, 2017. doi:10.7759/cureus.1184

23. Alencar Albuquerque G, De Lima Garcia C, Da Silva Quirino G, et al. Access to Health Services by Lesbian, Gay, Bisexual, and Transgender Persons: Systematic Literature Review. *BMC Int Health Hum Rights*. 2016;16(1):2. doi:10.1186/s12914-015-0072-9

24. LGBT Foundation. *Improving Trans and Non-Binary Experiences of Maternity Services (ITEMS) Report*.; 2022:63. Accessed December 6, 2023. https://dxfy8lrzbpywr.cloudfront.net/Files/97ecdaea-833d-4ea5-a891-c59f0ea429fb/ITEMS%2520report%2520final.pdf

25. Sword W, Heaman MI, Brooks S, et al. Women's and Care Providers' Perspectives of Quality Prenatal Care: A Qualitative Descriptive Study. *BMC Pregnancy Childbirth*. 2012;12(1):29. doi:10.1186/1471-2393-12-29

26. Sperlich M, Seng JS, Li Y, Taylor J, Bradbury-Jones C. Integrating Trauma-Informed Care into Maternity Care Practice: Conceptual and Practical Issues. *J Midwifery Womens Health*. 2017;62(6):661–672. doi:10.1111/jmwh.12674

27. Sandall J, Hatem M, Devane D, Soltani H, Gates S. Discussions of Findings from a Cochrane Review of Midwife-Led Versus Other Models of Care for Childbearing Women: Continuity, Normality and Safety. *Midwifery*. 2009;25(1):8–13. doi:10.1016/j.midw.2008.12.002

28. Patterson J, Hollins Martin CJ, Karatzias T. Disempowered Midwives and Traumatised Women: Exploring the Parallel Processes of Care Provider Interaction that Contribute to Women Developing Post Traumatic Stress Disorder (PTSD) Post Childbirth. *Midwifery*. 2019;76:21–35. doi:10.1016/j.midw.2019.05.010

29. Horsch A, Vial Y, Favrod C, et al. Reducing Intrusive Traumatic Memories after Emergency Caesarean Section: A Proof-of-Principle Randomized Controlled Study. *Behav Res Ther*. 2017;94:36–47. doi:10.1016/j.brat.2017.03.018

30. Everly GS, Lating JM. Psychological First Aid (PFA) and Disasters. *Int Rev Psychiatry*. 2021;33(8):718–727. doi:10.1080/09540261.2021.2016661

31. Figueroa RA, Cortés PF, Marín H, Vergés A, Gillibrand R, Repetto P. The ABCDE Psychological First Aid Intervention Decreases early PTSD Symptoms but Does not Prevent it: Results of a Randomized-Controlled Trial. *Eur J Psychotraumatology*. 2022;13(1):2031829. doi:10.1080/20008198.2022.2031829

32. Sachdeva J, Nagle Yang S, Gopalan P, et al. Trauma Informed Care in the Obstetric Setting and Role of the Perinatal Psychiatrist: A Comprehensive Review of the Literature. *J Acad Consult-Liaison Psychiatry*. 2022;63(5):485–496. doi:10.1016/j.jaclp.2022.04.005

33. Shapiro F. *Eye Movement Desensitization and Reprocessing (EDMR) Therapy: Basic Principles, Protocols, and Procedures*. Third edition. The Guilford Press; 2018.

34. Boyce R, Williams S, Adamantidis A. REM Sleep and Memory. *Curr Opin Neurobiol.* 2017;44:167–177. doi:10.1016/j.conb.2017.05.001

35. Maxfield L. A Clinician's Guide to the Efficacy of EMDR Therapy. *J EMDR Pract Res.* 2019;13(4):239–246. doi:10.1891/1933-3196.13.4.239

36. APA. *Practice Guidelines for the Treatment of Patients with Acute Stress Disorder and Posttraumatic Stress Disorder.* Published online 2004.

37. INSERM. *Psychotherapy: An Evaluation of Three Approaches.* Published online 2004.

38. NICE. *Post Traumatic Stress Disorder (PTSD): The Management of Adults and Children in Primary and Secondary Care.* Published online 2005.

39. Sandström M, Wiberg B, Wikman M, Willman AK, Högberg U. A Pilot Study of Eye Movement Desensitisation and Reprocessing Treatment (EMDR) for Post-Traumatic Stress after Childbirth. *Midwifery.* 2008;24(1):62–73. doi:10.1016/j.midw.2006.07.008

40. Stramrood CAI, van der Velde J, Doornbos B, Marieke Paarlberg K, Weijmar Schultz WCM, van Pampus MG. The Patient Observer: Eye-Movement Desensitization and Reprocessing for the Treatment of Posttraumatic Stress Following Childbirth. *Birth.* 2012;39(1):70–76. doi:10.1111/j.1523-536X.2011.00517.x

41. Lowe C, Murray C. Adult Service-Users' Experiences of Trauma-Focused Cognitive Behavioural Therapy. *J Contemp Psychother.* 2014;44(4):223–231. doi:10.1007/s10879-014-9272-1

42. Forbes D, Creamer M, Phelps A, et al. Australian Guidelines for the Treatment of Adults with Acute Stress Disorder and Post-Traumatic Stress Disorder. *Aust N Z J Psychiatry.* 2007;41(8):637–648. doi:10.1080/00048670701449161

43. Bisson JI, Ehlers A, Matthews R, Pilling S, Richards D, Turner S. Psychological Treatments for Chronic Post-Traumatic Stress Disorder: Systematic Review and Meta-Analysis. *Br J Psychiatry.* 2007;190(2):97–104. doi:10.1192/bjp.bp.106.021402

44. Nieminen K, Berg I, Frankenstein K, et al. Internet-Provided Cognitive Behaviour Therapy of Posttraumatic Stress Symptoms Following Childbirth—A Randomized Controlled Trial. *Cogn Behav Ther.* 2016;45(4):287–306. doi:10.1080/16506073.2016.1169626

45. NICE. *Antenatal and Postnatal Mental Health: Clinical Management and Service Guidance, Clinical Guideline [CG192].* Published online 2014. Accessed March 10, 2023. https://www.nice.org.uk/guidance/cg192/chapter/Recommendations#treating-specific-mental-health-problems-in-pregnancy-and-the-postnatal-period

46. Ehring T, Welboren R, Morina N, Wicherts JM, Freitag J, Emmelkamp PMG. Meta-Analysis of Psychological Treatments for Posttraumatic Stress Disorder in Adult Survivors of Childhood Abuse. *Clin Psychol Rev.* 2014;34(8):645–657. doi:10.1016/j.cpr.2014.10.004

47. Delicate A, Ayers S, McMullen S. Health Care Practitioners' Views of the Support Women, Partners, and the Couple Relationship Require for Birth Trauma: Current Practice and Potential Improvements. *Prim Health Care Res Dev.* 2020;21:e40. doi:10.1017/S1463423620000407

48. Mullan J. Birth Trauma Resolution. *MIDIRS Midwifery Dig.* 2017;27(3):345–348. Accessed March 10, 2023. https://www.birthtraumaresolution.com/wp-content/uploads/2020/01/Midirs-Birth-Trauma-published-Paper.pdf

49. Sheen K, Slade P. The Efficacy of 'Debriefing' after Childbirth: Is there a Case for Targeted Intervention? *J Reprod Infant Psychol.* 2015;33(3):308–320. doi:10.1080/02646838.2015.1009881

50. Meades R, Pond C, Ayers S, Warren F. Postnatal Debriefing: Have we Thrown the Baby out with the Bath Water? *Behav Res Ther*. 2011;49(5):367–372. doi:10.1016/j.brat.2011.03.002

51. NCT. *The Hidden Half – Bringing Postnatal Mental Illness out of Hiding*. Accessed December 6, 2023. https://www.nct.org.uk/sites/default/files/2019-04/NCT%20The%20Hidden%20Half_0.pdf

52. Molloy E, Biggerstaff DL, Sidebotham P. A Phenomenological Exploration of Parenting after Birth Trauma: Mothers Perceptions of the First year. *Women Birth*. 2021;34(3):278–287. doi:10.1016/j.wombi.2020.03.004

53. NCT. *Traumatic Birth and Post-Traumatic Stress Disorder*. Published November 2018. Accessed December 6, 2023. https://www.nct.org.uk/labour-birth/you-after-birth/traumatic-birth-and-post-traumatic-stress-disorder#:~:text=Psychological%20therapies,of%20these%20methods%20work%20well.

54. NICE. *Post-Traumatic Stress Disorder Nice Guideline [NG116]*; 2018. Accessed December 6, 2023. https://www.nice.org.uk/guidance/ng116

55. Williamson E, Pipeva A, Brodrick A, Saradjian A, Slade P. The Birth Trauma Psychological Therapy Service: An Audit of Outcomes. *Midwifery*. 2021;102:103099. doi:10.1016/j.midw.2021.103099

56. Pregnancy, Birth and Baby. Birth Trauma (Emotional). Published May 2021. Accessed December 6, 2023. https://www.pregnancybirthbaby.org.au/birth-trauma-emotional#treated

57. Australasian Birth Trauma Association. Potspartum Trauma Disorders (e.g. PTSD). Published 2020. Accessed December 6, 2023. https://www.birthtrauma.org.au/postpartum-trauma-disorders-e-g-ptsd/

58. Caparros-Gonzalez RA, Romero-Gonzalez B, Peralta-Ramirez MI, Ayers S, Galán-Paredes A, Caracuel-Romero A. Assessment of Posttraumatic Stress Disorder among Women after Childbirth Using the City Birth Trauma Scale in Spain. *Psychol Trauma Theory Res Pract Policy*. 2021;13(5):545–554. doi:10.1037/tra0001007

59. Bayrı Bingöl F, Bal MD, Dişsiz M, Sormageç MT, Yildiz PD. Validity and Reliability of the Turkish Version of the City Birth Trauma Scale (CityBiTS). *J Obstet Gynaecol*. 2021;41(7):1023–1031. doi:10.1080/01443615.2020.1821354

60. Handelzalts JE, Hairston IS, Matatyahu A. Construct Validity and Psychometric Properties of the Hebrew Version of the City Birth Trauma Scale. *Front Psychol*. 2018;9:1726. doi:10.3389/fpsyg.2018.01726

61. Dobson H, Malpas C, Kulkarni J. Measuring Posttraumatic Stress Disorder Following Childbirth. *Australas Psychiatry*. 2022;30(4):476–480. doi:10.1177/10398562221077900

62. Austin MP, Highet N, Expert Working Group. *Mental Health Care in the Perinatal Period: Australian Clinical Practice Guideline*; 2017.

63. Greenfield M, Darwin Z. Trans and Non-Binary Pregnancy, Traumatic Birth, and Perinatal Mental Health: A Scoping Review. *Int J Transgender Health*. 2021;22(1–2):203–216. doi:10.1080/26895269.2020.1841057

Chapter 11

Postnatal mental health

Zoe Darwin and Lucy Warwick-Guasp

INTRODUCTION

Mental health in the perinatal period includes mental health difficulties, psychological distress and psychological wellbeing in the time spanning conception, birth, and the first postnatal year.[1] Research with cisheterosexual mothers and fathers show that perinatal mental health difficulties are common.[2, 3] Any parent or person pursuing parenthood can themselves be affected, regardless of gender and whether the person is themselves pregnant. This reflects that, whilst some mental health conditions (eg, postpartum psychosis) have strong biological components, we must not underestimate the critical role of psychosocial factors. The perinatal period is a time of transition, accompanied by not only biological changes, but also psychological and social changes. For example, changes in roles, identity, and relationships, often accompanied by changes to material circumstances such as finances, employment, and housing.

The consequences of perinatal mental health difficulties can be long-lasting, for parents, for their babies and other children in the family. These impacts can endure across generations. For example, children of parents who experience perinatal mental health difficulties face increased chance of adverse socioemotional outcomes and their own perinatal mental health difficulties. However, these impacts are not inevitable. Early identification of need and prompt treatment is vital.[2] Children's relationships with other caregivers can also be protective (ie, they can buffer the possible effects), indicating the value of supporting any parents and the family as a whole.[4]

In this chapter, we begin by summarising perinatal mental health conditions, what is known about their prevalence in LGBTQ+ populations and the case for monitoring gender and sexuality in perinatal services. Consistent with the shift in research, policy and practice away from an emphasis on postnatal depression, we

DOI: 10.4324/9781003305446-12

summarise the wide range of conditions that can impact during pregnancy, birth and postpartum, including new onset conditions (eg, postpartum psychosis, childbirth-related post-traumatic stress disorder) and pre-existing conditions that may continue, recur or worsen.[5] This shift carries implications for services, both in terms of identifying need, for example the key role played by midwifery/maternity services, as well as prevention, through understanding and tackling the ways that services and practitioners may directly and indirectly contribute to traumatic experiences.

We next consider the evidence concerning vulnerability and protective factors in LGBTQ+ populations, ie, those factors that may affect the likelihood of someone being affected by perinatal mental health difficulties. We encourage reflection on the comparisons being made and challenge perspectives on maternal and paternal mental health [see Reflective Box 1]. We then outline barriers to seeking and accepting help, both through informal support mechanisms and through statutory services, followed by considerations for in-patient mental health services and services that assess and support parent-infant relationships. After summarising knowledge gaps in LGBTQ+ perinatal mental health, we present the chapter's key learning points. Boxes are used to present reflective questions to help readers in developing their own awareness in this field and consider what they may be able to do differently in their own practice. As authors, we note that the content is informed by our own experiences with perinatal services as LGBTQ+ parents, including direct personal experience of being cared for by perinatal mental health services.

REFLECTIVE BOX 1—MATERNAL MENTAL HEALTH AND PATERNAL MENTAL HEALTH?

Work in academic, clinical, and policy spaces continue to focus on maternal mental health, while using cisheteronormative language and an emphasis on women and mothers as gestational parents and commonly the focus of services. Whilst there is growing awareness of paternal mental health, this is used to refer to fathers and men, consistently positioned as non-gestational parents. We argue the need to challenge these false dichotomies and conflation of gender and role (ie, mother = female, father = male), which limit our learning, understanding and provision of care.[6] For example, in examining the experiences of a non-gestational mother's experiences, is it appropriate to compare with the existing cisheterosexual maternal literature, cisheterosexual paternal health literature, or both? In considering a birthing trans man's experiences, what (if anything) does the broader paternal health literature offer about feeling excluded or invisible as fathers?

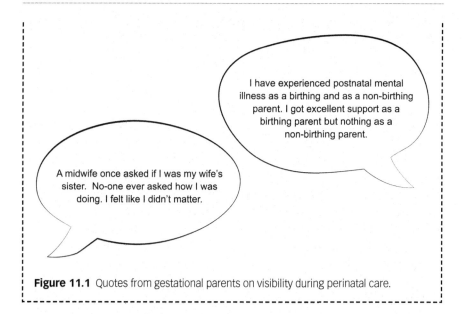

Figure 11.1 Quotes from gestational parents on visibility during perinatal care.

PERINATAL MENTAL HEALTH DIFFICULTIES AND THEIR PREVALENCE

There is now established evidence on rates of perinatal mental health conditions in cisheterosexual mothers and, to a lesser extent (limited to a subset of conditions), cisheterosexual fathers. Whilst it is reasonable to assume that LGBTQ+ people may experience any of these conditions, rates are unknown in sexual and gender minority groups and could indeed be higher. Where evidence is available, this remains confined to individual studies with LGBTQ+ people and we currently lack estimates that are generated by statistically combining results from multiple studies (referred to as meta-analysis). We therefore first summarise here what is known from evidence with cisgender people in heterosexual relationships, recognising that some of these people may not identify as heterosexual and that identity may be fluid.

Overall, around one in five birthing women experience mental health difficulties in the perinatal period.[7] The focus of research and practice has been on perinatal depression and perinatal anxiety. These are the most common difficulties, both for birthing mothers and for cisgender fathers. Statistical evidence that has been combined across studies finds approximately 5–10% of fathers experience depression and 5–15% experience anxiety.[3, 8] Most research has focused on fathers who are resident and currently in a relationship with their baby's mother, whereas rates are likely higher in other fathers. Although evidence is limited, it suggests that rates increase dramatically for fathers whose partners are themselves experiencing mental health difficulties, with estimates of affecting around half of those fathers.[9]

Research with cisgender parents in heterosexual relationships has also identified that any parents may experience childbirth-related post-traumatic stress; for example, around 3% of birthing women experience post-traumatic stress disorder (PTSD) following childbirth and there is evidence of non-birthing fathers also developing PTSD through observing traumatic birth.[10, 11] Post-traumatic stress can follow any birth, regardless of the level or type of interventions involved or the outcomes; ultimately, trauma is "in the eye of the beholder."[12] Closely related to traumatic birth is severe fear of childbirth, also known as tokophobia. This can affect people who have never birthed (known as primary tokophobia) or can follow a previous traumatic birth (known as secondary tokophobia); worldwide prevalence of tokophobia in pregnant women has been estimated at 14% however this reduced to less than 1% when focusing on those where it is accompanied by avoidance behaviours.[13]

Another condition that has received growing attention, both concerning cisgender mothers and fathers is parental obsessive compulsive disorder (OCD). In birthing women, prevalence is identified as greater in the perinatal period (recently estimated at around 8% in pregnancy and 17% postpartum) and more likely to concern intrusive thoughts concerning harm to the child.[14] Prevalence is not established in non-birthing fathers but has been estimated at approximately 2–4%.[3]

Whilst there is evidence of cisgender fathers experiencing psychosis in the perinatal period, this is focused on fathers with existing histories of severe mental illness. Although any parent may experience a psychotic episode in this period, current thinking about postpartum psychosis—a psychiatric emergency that is linked to the rapid hormonal changes accompanying birth—is that this condition is unique to birthing parents.

Within LGBTQ+ research relating to the perinatal period, most researched has been the experiences of lesbian and bisexual cisgender women who are gestational parents, followed by lesbian cisgender women as non-gestational parents, and then research with trans and non-binary gestational parents. Little exists concerning trans and non-binary non-gestational parents, although a recent exception is notable.[15] This body of evidence varies in the extent to which perinatal mental health is a focus however research on wider perinatal experiences, including relating to experiences of services and transition to parenthood, nonetheless offers insight into potential vulnerability and protective factors. Where specific conditions have been examined, a great deal of research has focused on depression, anxiety, traumatic birth, and fear of birth. Most research with trans and non-binary birthing people relating to psychological health has focused on gender dysphoria.

In the minimal literature that has attempted to make quantitative comparisons, findings have thus far been inconsistent. For example, a Canadian study[16] where women accessing maternity services (as gestational parents) were asked to complete a measure of depression symptoms (the Edinburgh Postnatal Depression Scale, EPDS) found that amongst women whose sexual histories included partners of more than one gender, scores were higher for those who were currently partnered with men than those currently partnered with women or not partnered. The authors suggested that this observed difference may be linked to invisibility in maternity services in sexual minority women who are currently partnered by men; however, study design precluded exploration of other possible reasons (eg, other factors associated with perinatal distress including partner support, intendedness of pregnancy). In apparent contrast, another study reported higher depression scores (using the EPDS) in sexual minority birthing and non-birthing mothers than expected based on population scores[17] and a recent survey study conducted in the UK during the early period of the COVID-19 pandemic[18] found higher rates of postnatal anxiety (measured using a postpartum-specific anxiety tool) in LGBQ+ gestational mothers, compared with cisheterosexual gestational mothers in the same sample.

Together, these studies highlight that learning is limited by treating LGBTQ+ people as a homogenous group and point to the need for further visibility in research, policy, and practice.[6] This includes determining the involvement of LGBTQ+ parents within research that involves wider samples of (predominantly cisheterosexual) parents and understanding who is accessing services in the perinatal period.[19]

CASE STUDY—AUTHOR'S OWN EXPERIENCES AS A GESTATIONAL MOTHER IN A SAME-SEX RELATIONSHIP

"When my wife and I decided we'd like to start a family we went to our GP to discuss our options. Our GP was unaware of anything and said perhaps 'somewhere like Canada' would offer such services. We left feeling even less informed than when we went in! We scoured policy documents and liaised with our Trust to eventually figure out that we would have to pay for 6 rounds of IUI (intrauterine insemination) before being referred for fertility treatment. We knew at this point we would have to save and fund all treatment ourselves and used a highly-recommended LGBTQ+ inclusive clinic in Denmark. After two rounds of IUI we were very excited to announce that we were pregnant.

From then on, every antenatal appointment was with a different midwife requiring us to 'come out' every time, tell our story and put ourselves in a position of potential acceptance or discrimination. Disconcertingly, we were once asked if our pregnancy was planned. We went on a tour of the local hospital's Birth Centre where all imagery and references were of 'mums and dads'.

I experienced, and my wife was witness to, a long and traumatic birth. After 36 hours of labour, where we had been moved from the Birth Centre to the maternity ward, we were prepared for surgery and our daughter was eventually delivered via forceps.

After this experience I went on to develop postnatal depression and anxiety. We struggled for a long time trying to find and access various forms of formal and informal support. And any information there was, was targeted at 'mums and dads'. There was no mention of LGBTQ+ parent families anywhere to at least signal that we would be welcomed and included. Any advice or support for my wife who was trying to navigate all of this was targeted at 'dads'. It was very isolating. After 7 months of asking for help from many GPs I was admitted to our local Mother and Baby Unit. Mixed in with the relief of finally getting help, there was fear in once again not knowing what to expect, but the care here was excellent and we both felt very supported."

(Lucy Warwick-Guasp)

Inequalities and the need for monitoring

Increasingly, countries in the Global North have routine mental health assessment within universal services (ie, primary care, maternity, child health) as part of their national clinical guidance and local guidelines. However, this alone does not ensure that needs will be identified or met. Even with awareness of perinatal mental health, both in the general population and within perinatal services, inequalities continue around access. This is relevant across the full pathway of accessing care, including disclosure, identification, and management, including referral, uptake, and ongoing access (sometimes referred to as engagement). Our ability to determine levels of inequalities depends on the available data. For example, despite being no less likely to experience perinatal mental health difficulties, it has been found that women from minoritised ethnic backgrounds are less likely to be asked about their mental health in maternity services.[20] Relevant here is that we lack gender and sexuality monitoring in perinatal services and this limits our ability to understand inequalities in prevalence and access to services. Considerations are presented in Reflective Box 2.

REFLECTIVE BOX 2—INTRODUCING ROUTINE MONITORING: QUESTIONS FOR DEVELOPING YOUR SERVICE

What could be monitored? You may consider monitoring gender and sexuality of the "index patient" (eg, birthing person). Would it also be relevant to monitor gender of any co-parents or partners?

What would be your concerns about introducing monitoring? Are these concerns for the service, for parents, for you as a practitioner? Do your concerns differ depending on what you are monitoring? Why may this be?

Even if your local sociolegal context means that disclosing gender and/or sexuality feel safe, may this vary within the communities that are cared for by your service?

How could you explore these concerns within your service? How could you involve users in these conversations?

Whilst acknowledging that considerations will necessarily vary within different sociocultural and legal context in different settings, may monitoring be a possibility within your workplace? If not, what would need to change in order for this to be possible? How could you include monitoring within your existing systems and forms?

What training would be needed for staff?

How could you capture any impact that may follow from introducing monitoring?

Remember: anyone who is subject to monitoring needs to feel safe to share this information and be made aware of where the information is going and the purpose of monitoring.

VULNERABILITY FACTORS

Anyone can experience mental health difficulties in the perinatal period however certain factors can increase vulnerability, ie, increase the chances. For example, perinatal depression and anxiety are more likely for people with histories of previous mental health difficulties, with limited or no partner support, or experiencing conflict in their relationship with an intimate partner.[3, 21] Additional vulnerability factors both for childbirth-related post-traumatic stress and for tokophobia (severe fear of childbirth) include history of trauma, including childhood sexual violence/abuse, obstetric complications, and poor care.[22] Whilst these are taken from research with wider populations (predominantly assumed to be cisheterosexual), it seems likely that these vulnerability factors are relevant regardless of gender or sexuality, ie, factors may be common across parents. Moreover, some of these vulnerability factors may be disproportionately higher in LGBTQ+ people who are pregnant or pursuing parenthood given what is known about LGBTQ+ people in the general population. For example, rates of mental health conditions are disproportionately higher in LGBTQ+ people and there is evidence suggesting these disparities extend to suicidality and to severe mental illness,[23, 24] and can be understood in a minority stress framework, ie, with recognition of stressors connected to intersecting minoritised identities.[25] Rates of trauma in childhood, including sexual abuse are higher[26] and research also finds increased rates of family estrangement or breakdown in relationships, sometimes linked to experiencing discrimination where gender and sexual diversity is considered unacceptable within people's own birth families.[27]

Turning to those aspects that may be amplified or distinct, research on traumatic birth and on tokophobia offer sites for learning (for further information about traumatic birth and tokophobia see Chapter 7). For example, research by Malmquist and colleagues with lesbians, trans men and non-binary people who had the ability to become pregnant cited presence at their partner's traumatic birth as contributing to their own tokophobia, thus experiencing birth as traumatic may create additional challenges for non-gestational parents who themselves have "childbearing capacity."[28]

Other vulnerability factors that may be amplified for LGBTQ+ parents, particularly those in non-gestational roles, concern role insecurity and feelings of invalidation as a parent and as a partner (eg,[29, 30]), which for some individuals connects with a felt lack of role models.[31] Whilst these aspects echoes findings in cisgender paternal mental health research concerning feelings of exclusion, there may be further complexity for several reasons. As discussed in Chapter 6 of this book, these may include an absence of biological connectedness and social recognition of their role as a part,[29] including a potential absence of legal recognition as parent[32] and also relate to conscious decision-making about who will carry a pregnancy. For example, a UK study[31] exploring lived experiences of perinatal anxiety and depression in co-mothers identified role resentment, both for gestational and non-gestational parents. Howat[31] proposed that whilst non-gestational mothers' feelings of exclusion, rejection and jealousy were similar to those of cisheterosexual fathers' (eg, reported in[33]), they may be heightened, potentially linked to a desire and potential to have themselves carried.[31] Similarly, as a partner of someone who has experienced a traumatic birth, there may be further complexity through not only feeling powerless to protect during the event, but also feeling implicated in the partner going through this, which may be heightened in families where there has been a conscious decision about who will be the gestational parent.[31]

Interactions with services in the perinatal period and pre-conception

Key to any exploration of vulnerability factors in LGBTQ+ people is the role played by services. Research with LGBTQ+ people repeatedly demonstrates the negative impact caused by perinatal services being inherently cisheteronormative,[34] for example language used in administrative processes (eg, health records) and interactions with staff, which may not correctly recognise peoples' genders or relationships, either with their partner or their baby. There are instances where assumptions or failures to take appropriate action have been dangerous, for example resulting in delayed access to care.[35] There is evidence of microaggressions and structural discrimination[36, 37] across assisted conception services, maternity services (antenatal care, intrapartum, and postpartum) and child health services. For example, despite anti-discriminatory policies being in place, access to assisted conception remains unfair,[38–40] and carries psychosocial stress including the impact of financial burden and unnecessary medicalisation. There are also multiple documented examples of LGBTQ+ people experiencing discriminatory attitudes in interactions with practitioners in perinatal services.[37, 41]

These aspects relating to stigma and discrimination act as stressors, whereby LGBTQ+ people pursuing parenthood are subjected to minority stress—discussed further in Chapter 13—with increased vulnerability for mental health difficulties. Critically, this relates not only to *experienced* difficult experiences with services but *anticipated* poor care from midwives and other practitioners due to homophobia or transphobia. This has been found in relation to tokophobia in lesbian women, trans men, and non-binary people.[28] Similarly, the salience of both experienced and anticipated poor care was evident in reviewing literature on traumatic birth in trans and non-binary people.[35] This links with findings in the wider perinatal mental health literature citing the ways in which anticipated poor care can be felt in marginalised communities, for example those from minoritised ethnic backgrounds,[42] and highlights the need to be aware of potential fears that parents may be affected by, with implications for their relationships with services and practitioners.

REFLECTIVE BOX 3—INTERACTIONS WITH SERVICES MATTER

In this chapter, we have highlighted the potential impact of poor experiences of care and also anticipated poor experiences. Conversely, experiencing good care can be protective; for example, even in the event of physical complications during birth, good care may prevent birth from being experienced as psychologically traumatic. Applying learning about anticipated experiences, providing inclusive care may offer benefits that extend beyond the individual family, building trust in services throughout the wider LGBTQ+ community.

Consider how learning presented in the NHS good practice guide on trauma-informed care in maternity services and mental health services in the perinatal period[43] may apply here, regardless of whether someone has a history of traumatic experiences. For example, can you consider prioritising continuity of carer when working with LGBTQ+ people? How can you reduce the need for people to repeatedly share their information?

PROTECTIVE FACTORS

It is common in mental health research to focus on vulnerability factors (often described as risk factors) but protective factors equally warrant consideration. There is some emerging evidence from qualitative research with cisgender sexual minority birthing and non-birthing parents in the context of perinatal depression. One suggested protective factor is relationship satisfaction related to increased likelihood of a more equitable division of roles in the transition to parenthood in co-mother families[32, 41] and increased likelihood of feeling more in agreement with each other concerning parenting compared with cisheterosexual parents.[44] Preparation for parenthood may be another protective factor given that unplanned pregnancy is an established vulnerability factor for perinatal depression and many LGBTQ+ people have used assisted conception, requiring in-depth planning.[45] However, this may be highly variable within LGBTQ+ populations, varying with identity and with age; for example, transmasculine people are more likely than their cisgender peers to have an adolescent or unplanned pregnancy.[46] More recently, a study with non-gestational co-mothers identified examples where previous experiences of mental health difficulties were identified as protective, through applying established coping strategies, and examples of drawing on social networks that had a shared social identity concerning sexuality.[31] Although research on protective factors is limited, including concerning populations and types of mental health difficulty, it remains important to consider these possibilities when caring for people in the perinatal period. This is consistent with a wider call for strengths-based approaches to promoting health with LGBTQ+ people,[47] noting the need to consider resilience and social support and that, within the LGBTQ+ population, different groups may be more marginalised than others.

REFLECTIVE BOX 4—NURTURING POSSIBLE PROTECTIVE FACTORS

Consider what could be done to help parents become aware of possible protective factors they may have. For example, could this include facilitating reflection on social support that is available within their family or friends, or wider social networks where there is a shared social identity (for example, LGBTQ+ groups)? How may previous experiences with mental health have equipped parents with coping strategies in navigating the transition to parenthood? May the lack of expectations around what LGBTQ+ parental roles "look like" offer opportunities (or "freedom") to think about their own preferences without feeling limited by others' expectations? Discuss with families how their relationship could enable them to share parenting roles.

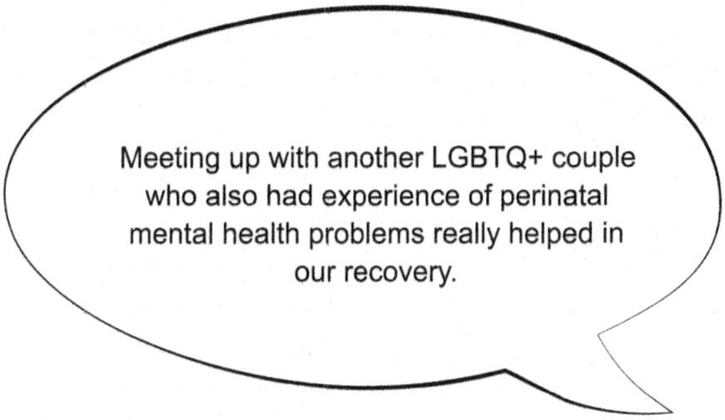

Meeting up with another LGBTQ+ couple who also had experience of perinatal mental health problems really helped in our recovery.

Figure 11.2 Quote about intra-community support as a protective factor.

GENDER DYSPHORIA

LGBTQ+ people are often treated as a homogenous (ie, single) group in research and in clinical practice recommendations despite comprising multiple groups.[48] Gender dysphoria warrants specific consideration in addressing the needs of non-binary people and trans men and is one area that illustrates the ways in which experiences and needs may vary considerably within LGBTQ+ individuals.

It is important to be aware that not all trans people in the general population experience gender dysphoria; similarly, in the context of the perinatal period, experiences can be diverse. Gender dysphoria has largely not been framed through a perinatal mental health lens however we argue its relevance here. First, it has relevance within a broad approach to mental health and wellbeing, and second, omitting gender dysphoria from discussion of perinatal mental health may risk that parents' needs are missed or dismissed. For example, it has been argued that tools routinely used to assess perinatal depression do not assess gender dysphoria, and that both gender dysphoria and suicidal ideation should be monitored in trans men in perinatal services.[49]

Without neglecting individualised experiences and the need for care to be personalised, it is helpful to be aware of certain areas that have been found to present challenges relating to hormonal changes (including discontinuation of testosterone therapy and hormonal changes directly arising through being pregnant), changes to the chest, visibility and recognition as a pregnant person, birthing, and lactation. In our scoping review,[35] we framed dysphoria broadly to encompass both "intrinsic physical dysphoria" (ie, embodied physical experiences) and "extrinsic social dysphoria" (ie, relating to anticipated or experienced reactions or treatment by others).

Faced with bodily changes, some people experienced disconnection from their body[50, 51] however others described improvements in gender dysphoria[52] or a new relationship with their body.[53] Similarly, whereas some found the possibility of vaginal birth traumatic, including relating to distress at the prospect of having their genitals exposed,[49, 50] some who experienced a vaginal birth found it to be personally meaningful and experienced a lack of inhibition during labour and birth that differed to their usual concerns.[50] This illustrates that assumptions should not be made about preferred birth choices and, as Chapter 6 discusses, practitioners should make people aware of different birthing options. People may negotiate their visibility[37] which carries implications for monitoring (see Reflective Box 2) and for seeking and accepting help relating to mental health and wellbeing during the perinatal period. There may also be lack of availability of suitable mental health assessment tools.

BARRIERS TO SEEKING AND ACCEPTING HELP

Any parent may face barriers to seeking and accepting help concerning their perinatal mental health. These barriers relate to the influence of their own beliefs and perceptions, the influence of health care services (including administrative systems and practitioners) and the influence of others (eg, those relating to partners, other family members or community, etc.).[54] Examples within these include own or professionals' limited knowledge and awareness of perinatal mental health, limited ability to recognise symptoms, stigma and shame relating to mental health, fear of consequences (eg, social care involvement, particular types of mental health treatment) anticipated or experienced reactions of others, and aspects relating to the organisation of services (eg, limited time within appointments, extent to which mental health appears to be the focus, lack of continuity with practitioners, disconnected care pathways or unclear policies, limited access due to transport costs or lack of childcare provision, provision of language support).[54, 55] Research with cisgender fathers also indicates stigma relating to men's mental health, questioning the legitimacy of own mental health needs and entitlement to health professionals' support (as a non-gestational parent) and concerns of compromising the support offered to their partner.[1]

Whilst any of these may be relevant for LGBTQ+ parents, there may also exist additional specific barriers. Within health services, this may include reduced visibility for LGBTQ+ parents, including non-gestational parents who may not be recognised by practitioners or services as co-parents. Anticipated or experienced discrimination relating to sexuality or gender is likely to create additional barriers. For example, people may hold concerns that they face additional scrutiny as parents and that their parenting may be judged more harshly.[56] These aspects may potentially combine with internalised homophobia or transphobia, for example questioning own right to have children and feelings of inadequacy.[57] People may fear that they are hypervisible as an LGBTQ+ parents and that disclosing their mental health difficulties may wrongly confirm other people's negative judgments about LGBTQ+ parents more broadly.[31] In parallel, they may view their LGBTQ+ community as less accessible as parents and this may vary with different family formations.[58]

Barriers to disclosure also exist where there may be limited support available. For example, female and non-binary non-gestational parents may feel excluded by support that is targeted at fathers.[31] It similarly seems questionable that birthing fathers would feel validation or belonging in such provision. Whilst there are moves towards introducing mental health assessment of non-gestational parents in settings that routinely assess gestational parents,[59] these have often been framed as the need for gendered approaches, again conflating gender and role and risking further marginalisation of LGBTQ+ parents. In light of these barriers, it is important that practitioners and systems normalise perinatal mental health difficulties for all parents and consider non-judgemental assessment for any parents.

REFLECTIVE BOX 5—IN-PATIENT STAYS

Possible barriers concerning seeking or accepting help may have further considerations when making decisions about accessing in-patient mental health services or residential services. These may differ for general adult mental health settings and settings that are specialised to the perinatal period or early parenting.

People may have concerns about possible discrimination—from practitioners but also from other families. They may hold concerns about needing to explain their family make-up. For trans and non-binary birthing parents, there may be concerns for physical and emotional safety about staying in a gendered environment or even on wards. Others may be concerned that non-male non-gestational parents will not be welcomed at groups for "fathers" or "partners."

Ensure that any materials for in-patient stays are inclusive of LGBTQ+ parents.

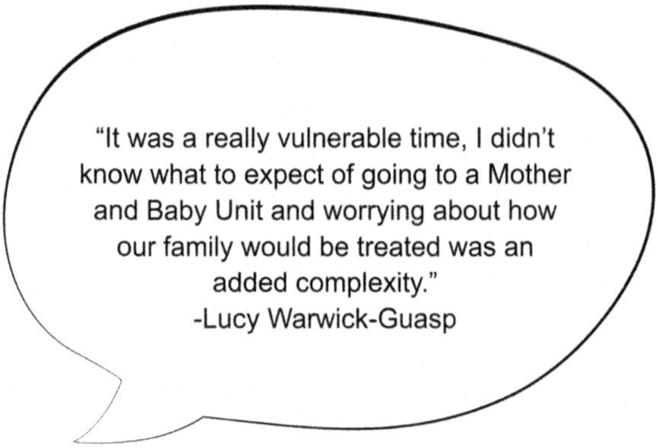

"It was a really vulnerable time, I didn't know what to expect of going to a Mother and Baby Unit and worrying about how our family would be treated was an added complexity."
-Lucy Warwick-Guasp

Figure 11.3 Quote from author about experience as an LGBTQ+ parent.

LIMITATIONS OF EXISTING LITERATURE AND AREAS FOR FUTURE LEARNING

We recognise that research with seldom-heard and seldom-asked communities can have inherent challenges. For example, large sample sizes can be difficult to achieve and this can preclude statistical testing. There can also exist challenges about recruitment methods and sampling bias; for example, it can be more feasible to recruit through LGBTQ+ focused organisations and/or social media because relatively smaller numbers can mean that recruiting through mainstream health services would require numerous study sites or recruitment for a long time period. However, the rates of mental health difficulties and the nature of experiences amongst those accessing LGBTQ+ focused organisations may be different to those who do not access such organisations, including those for whom having a public LGBTQ+ identity would present considerable negative repercussions, potentially including discrimination in their community, place of work, or compromising their physical safety or freedom. This has implications not only for estimates of prevalence but also for aspects explored elsewhere in this chapter. For example, support needs and barriers to accessing services may be qualitatively different in people who are active users of social media compared with those who are not. Further challenges can exist about ethical aspects such as potentially over-burdening people with research, for example in inviting birthing fathers to take part in multiple research projects.

A further limitation in this research is the lack of intersectionality, eg, participants predominantly being from white backgrounds with high levels of formal education, and from the Global North. This is relevant in light of findings such as the recent research in England on Improving Trans and Non-binary People's Experiences of Maternity Services,[37] which found that experiences of racism and transphobia interact. In addition, literature often treats individuals with diverse sexual identities and genders as one group, rather than individual communities.[51] This, combined with the use of varied terminologies, has implications for what is known about pregnancy outcomes more widely[48] and the same can be argued for perinatal mental health outcomes, as well as experiences and needs. For example, reviewing literature on trans men and non-binary parents' experiences identified that pregnant non-binary people were frequently excluded by eligibility criteria used in research, or assumed to have the same needs and experiences as trans men.[35] There is an urgent need for consultation and research with trans and non-binary communities. This includes with non-gestational parents who are themselves trans or non-binary, or whose partners are.

A further limitation reflects trends in the development of the wider (cisheterosexual) perinatal mental health literature whereby we have seen an initial exploration on postnatal depression, followed by perinatal depression and anxiety, then traumatic birth and fear of birth, with other conditions not yet explored (eg, parental obsessive compulsive disorder and eating disorders). In addition, the existing focus has concerned self-report measures of symptoms of distress in community samples. Research, audit, and service evaluation is needed with parents who have been referred to or accessed formal support for their mental health needs, including support relating to parent-infant relationships. Routine monitoring is a key part of this, to explore inequalities and consider how to make access to services fair for anyone who may want to or need to use them.

In addressing these areas of future learning, we urge that practitioners and researchers hold in mind that people may hold different roles in different pregnancies or conception attempts, that language concerning parity may be physically but not psychologically appropriate, and that the perinatal period may be experienced as beginning earlier, including in planning conception.[19]

SUMMARY LEARNING POINTS

- Anyone can experience mental health difficulties during the perinatal period, spanning conception and the first year following birth; difficulties may also arise pre-conception. Research with presumed cisheterosexual participants consistently shows that these difficulties are common, meaning it is likely relevant to LGBTQ+ people as well.
- Be aware that non-gestational parents and co-parents can also experience perinatal mental health concerns independently of the gestational parent.
- In the absence of established rates in LGBTQ+ people, it is reasonable to assume that rates may be comparable with cisheterosexual parents, or indeed higher given the vulnerability factors that may be amplified or distinct for LGBTQ+ people, including those relating to interactions with services and to social and legal recognition as parents. This is a sizeable group warranting support and existing approaches within services may not be suitably tailored to meet these needs.
- LGBTQ+ parents may be affected both by anticipated and experienced poor experiences with services. Through services being anti-discriminatory and inclusive, there are opportunities to reduce vulnerability, identify needs and respond appropriately.
- Services and practitioners need to become aware of their own assumptions and stay curious to what a family may look like. Language matters, including in spoken and written communication with individuals, families, and more widely in the service as a whole; for example, attending to inclusivity and diversity within paperwork and imagery used.
- Ensure that inpatient facilities are inclusive of all families in order to limit anticipated discrimination from staff, other service users and visitors by LGBTQ+ parents.

- Remain open to the possibility of psychological distress and mental health difficulties manifesting in different ways. This may include behavioural signs as well as visible emotions. Give consideration to all caregivers.
- LGBTQ+ parents are not a homogenous group. There may be diverse experiences and needs within the LGBTQ+ community. In addition, identity may be fluid and people may hold different roles in different pregnancies. Research findings are taken mostly from the Global North and in settings where LGBTQ+ people have greater rights; these may not necessarily be transferable elsewhere.
- Monitoring sexual identity and gender within services facilitates understanding of need, including inequalities in prevalence, access to services, and outcomes.
- Consultation with parents is important, including attention to intersectionality, in designing, implementing, and evaluating services.

REFERENCES

1. Darwin Z, Galdas P, Hinchliff S, et al. Fathers' Views and Experiences of their Own Mental Health during Pregnancy and the First Postnatal Year: A Qualitative Interview Study of Men Participating in the UK Born and Bred in Yorkshire (BaBY) Cohort. *BMC Pregnancy & Childbirth*. 2017;17(1):1–15. doi:10.1186/s12884-017-1229-4
2. Howard LM, Piot P, Stein A. No Health Without Perinatal Mental Health. *The Lancet*. 2014;384(9956):1723–1724. doi:10.1016/S0140-6736(14)62040-7
3. Leach LS, Poyser C, Cooklin AR, Giallo R. Prevalence and Course of Anxiety Disorders (and Symptom levels) in Men across the Perinatal Period: A Systematic Review. *Journal of Affective Disorders*. 2016;190:675–686. doi:10.1016/j.jad.2015.09.063
4. Darwin Z, Domoney J, Iles J, Bristow F, McLeish J, Sethna V. *Involving and Supporting Partners and Other Family Members in Specialist Perinatal Mental Health Services: Good Practice Guide*. London: NHS England and NHS Improvement; 2021. Available at: https://www.england.nhs.uk/mental-health/perinatal/perinatal-mental-health-resources/
5. O'Hara MW, Wisner KL. Perinatal Mental Illness: Definition, Description and Aetiology. *Best Practice Research Clinical Obstetrics & Gynaecology*. 2014;28(1):3–12. doi:10.1016/j.bpobgyn.2013.09.002
6. Darwin Z, Greenfield M. Mothers and Others: The Invisibility of LGBTQ People in Reproductive and Infant Psychology. *Journal of Reproductive & Infant Psychology*. 2019;37(4):341–343. doi:10.1080/02646838.2019.1649919
7. Pilav S, De Backer K, Easter A, et al. A Qualitative Study of Minority Ethnic Women's Experiences of Access to and Engagement with Perinatal Mental Health Care. *BMC Pregnancy and Childbirth*. 2022;22(421). doi:10.1186/s12884-022-04698-9
8. Cameron EE, Sedov ID, Tomfohr-Madsen LM. Prevalence of Paternal Depression in Pregnancy and the Postpartum: An Updated Meta-Analysis. *Journal of Affective Disorders*. 2016;206:189–203. doi:10.1016/j.jad.2016.07.044

9. Lovestone S, Kumar R. Postnatal Psychiatric Illness: The Impact on Partners. *The British Journal of Psychiatry*. 1993;163(2):210–216. doi:10.1192/bjp.163.2.210

10. Daniels E, Arden-Close E, Mayers A. Be Quiet and Man Up: A Qualitative Questionnaire Study into Fathers who Witnessed their Partner's Birth Trauma. *BMC Pregnancy & Childbirth*. 2020;20(236). doi:10.1186/s12884-020-02902-2

11. Inglis C, Sharman R, Reed R. Paternal Mental Health Following Perceived Traumatic Childbirth. *Midwifery*. 2016;41:125–131. doi:10.1016/j.midw.2016.08.008

12. Beck CT. Birth Trauma: In the Eye of the Beholder. *Nursing Research*. 2004;53(1):28–35. doi:10.1097/00006199-200401000-00005

13. Jomeen J, Martin C, Jones C, et al. Tokophobia and Fear of Birth: A Workshop Consensus Statement on Current Issues and Recommendations for Future Research. *Journal of Reproductive & Infant Psychology*. 2021;39(1):2–15. doi:10.1080/02646838.2020.1843908

14. Hudepohl N, MacLean JV, Osborne LM. Perinatal Obsessive-Compulsive Disorder: Epidemiology, Phenomenology, Etiology, and Treatment. *Current Psychiatry Reports*. 2022:1–9. doi:10.1007/s11920-022-01333-4

15. Bower-Brown S. Beyond Mum and Dad: Gendered Assumptions about Parenting and the Experiences of Trans and/or Non-Binary Parents in the UK. *LGBTQ+ Family: An Interdisciplinary Journal*. 2022;18(3):223–240. doi:10.1080/27703371.2022.2083040

16. Flanders CE, Gibson MF, Goldberg AE, Ross LE. Postpartum Depression among Visible and Invisible Sexual Minority Women: A Pilot Study. *Archives of Women's Mental Health*. 2016;19(2):299–305. doi:10.1007/s00737-015-0566-4

17. Ross LE, Steele L, Goldfinger C, Strike C. Perinatal Depressive Symptomatology among Lesbian and Bisexual Women. *Archives of Women's Mental Health*. 2007;10(2):53–59. doi:10.1007/s00737-007-0168-x

18. Greenfield M, Payne-Gifford S, McKenzie G. Between a Rock and a Hard Place: Considering "Freebirth" during Covid-19. *Frontiers in Global Women's Health*. 2021:5. doi:10.3389/fgwh.2021.603744

19. Darwin Z, Greenfield M. Gestational and Non-Gestational Parents: Challenging Assumptions. *Journal of Reproductive & Infant Psychology*. 2022;40(1):1–2. doi:10.1080/02646838.2021.2020977

20. Prady SL, Endacott C, Dickerson J, Bywater TJ, Blower SL. Inequalities in the Identification and Management of Common Mental Disorders in the Perinatal Period: An Equity Focused Re-Analysis of a Systematic Review. *PloS One*. 2021;16(3):e0248631. doi:10.1371/journal.pone.0248631

21. Lancaster CA, Gold KJ, Flynn HA, Yoo H, Marcus SM, Davis MM. Risk Factors for Depressive Symptoms during Pregnancy: A Systematic Review. *American Journal of Obstetrics & Gynecology*. 2010;202(1):5–14. doi:10.1016/j.ajog.2009.09.007

22. Andersen LB, Melvaer LB, Videbech P, Lamont RF, Joergensen JS. Risk Factors for Developing Post-Traumatic Stress Disorder Following Childbirth: A Systematic Review. *Acta Obstetricia et Gynecologica Scandinavica*. 2012;91(11):1261–1272. doi:doi.org/10.1111/j.1600-0412.2012.01476.x

23. Kidd SA, Howison M, Pilling M, Ross LE, McKenzie K. Severe Mental Illness in LGBT Populations: A Scoping Review. *Psychiatric Services*. 2016;67(7):779–783. doi:10.1176/appi.ps.201500209

24. McNeil J, Ellis SJ, Eccles FJ. Suicide in Trans Populations: A Systematic Review of Prevalence and Correlates. *Psychology of Sexual Orientation and Gender Diversity*. 2017;4(3):341–353. doi:10.1037/sgd0000235

25. Mongelli F, Perrone D, Balducci J, et al. Minority Stress and Mental Health among LGBT Populations: An Update on the Evidence. *Minerva Psychiatry*. 2019;60(1):27–50. doi:10.23736/S0391-1772.18.01995-7

26. Schneeberger AR, Dietl MF, Muenzenmaier KH, Huber CG, Lang UE. Stressful Childhood Experiences and Health Outcomes in Sexual Minority Populations: A Systematic Review. *Social Psychiatry and Psychiatric Epidemiology*. 2014;49(9):1427–1445. doi:10.1007/s00127-014-0854-8

27. Ross LE, Steele L, Sapiro B. Perceptions of Predisposing and Protective Factors for Perinatal Depression in Same-Sex Parents. *Journal of Midwifery & Women's Health*. 2005;50(6):e65–e70. doi:10.1016/j.jmwh.2005.08.002

28. Malmquist A, Jonsson L, Wikström J, Nieminen K. Minority Stress Adds an Additional Layer to Fear of Childbirth in Lesbian and Bisexual Women, and Transgender People. *Midwifery*. 2019;79:102551. doi:10.1016/j.midw.2019.102551

29. Abelsohn KA, Epstein R, Ross LE. Celebrating the "Other" Parent: Mental Health and Wellness of Expecting Lesbian, Bisexual, and Queer Non-Birth Parents. *Journal of Gay & Lesbian Mental Health*. 2013;17(4):387–405. doi:10.1080/19359705.2013.771808

30. Hayman B, Wilkes L, Halcomb E, Jackson D. Marginalised Mothers: Lesbian Women Negotiating Heteronormative Healthcare Services. *Contemporary Nurse*. 2013;44(1):120–127. doi:10.5172/conu.2013.44.1.120

31. Howat A. *Exploring Non-Birth Mothers' Experiences of Perinatal Anxiety and Depression: Understanding the Perspectives of the Non-Carrying Parent in Same-Sex Parented Families*. Leeds: School of Medicine, University of Leeds; 2021. Available at: https://etheses.whiterose.ac.uk/29750/

32. Goldberg AE, Perry-Jenkins M. The Division of Labor and Perceptions of Parental Roles: Lesbian Couples across the Transition to Parenthood. *Journal of Social and Personal Relationships*. 2007;24(2):297–318. doi:10.1177/0265407507075415

33. Goodman J. Becoming an Involved Father of an Infant. *Journal of Obstetric, Gynecologic, & Neonatal Nursing*. 2005;34(2):190–200. doi:10.1177/0884217505274581

34. Kirubarajan A, Barker LC, Leung S, et al. LGBTQ2S+ Childbearing Individuals and Perinatal Mental Health: A Systematic Review. *BJOG: An International Journal of Obstetrics & Gynaecology*. 2022. doi:10.1111/1471-0528.17103

35. Greenfield M, Darwin Z. Trans and Non-Binary Pregnancy, Traumatic Birth, and Perinatal Mental Health: A Scoping Review. *International Journal of Transgender Health*. 2021;22(1-2):203–216. doi:10.1080/26895269.2020.1841057

36. Falck F, Frisén L, Dhejne C, Armuand G. Undergoing Pregnancy and Childbirth as Trans Masculine in Sweden: Experiencing and Dealing with Structural Discrimination, Gender Norms and Microaggressions in Antenatal Care, Delivery and Gender Clinics. *International Journal of Transgender Health*. 2020;22(1-2):42–53. doi:10.1080/26895269.2020.1845905

37. LGBT Foundation. *Trans and Non-Binary Experiences of Maternity Services: Survey Findings, Report and Recommendations*. 2022. Available at: https://lgbt.foundation/news/revealed-improving-trans-and-non-binary-experiences-of-maternity-services-items-report/475

38. Carvalho PGCd, Cabral CdS, Ferguson L, Gruskin S, Diniz CSG. 'We are not Infertile': Challenges and Limitations Faced by Women in Same-Sex Relationships when Seeking Conception Services in São Paulo, Brazil. *Culture, Health & Sexuality*. 2019;21(11):1257–1272. doi:10.1080/13691058.2018.1556343

39. Charter R, Ussher JM, Perz J, Robinson K. The Transgender Parent: Experiences and Constructions of Pregnancy and Parenthood for Transgender Men in Australia. *International Journal of Transgenderism*. 2018;19(1):64–77. doi:10.1080/15532739.2017.1399496

40. Dempsey D, Power J, Kelly F. A Perfect Storm of Intervention? Lesbian and Cisgender Queer Women Conceiving through Australian Fertility Clinics. *Critical Public Health*. 2022;32(2):206–216. doi:10.1080/09581596.2020.1810636

41. Maccio EM, Pangburn JA. Self-Reported Depressive Symptoms in Lesbian Birth Mothers and Comothers. *Journal of Family Social Work*. 2012;15(2):99–110. doi:10.1080/10522158.2012.662860

42. Darwin Z, Blower S, Nekitsing C, Masefield S, Willan K, Dickerson J. Understanding and Tackling Inequalities in Identifying and Managing Perinatal Mental Health Difficulties through Application of a Socio-Technical Framework. *Frontiers in Global Women's Health*. 2022;3:1028192. doi:10.3389/fgwh.2022.1028192

43. Law C, Wolfenden L, Sperlich M, Taylor S. *A Good Practice Guide to Support Implementation of Trauma-Informed Care in the Perinatal Period*. London: NHS England and NHS Improvement; 2021. Available at: https://www.england.nhs.uk/mental-health/perinatal/perinatal-mental-health-resources/

44. Bos HM, Van Balen F, Van Den Boom DC. Experience of Parenthood, Couple Relationship, Social Support, and Child-Rearing Goals in Planned Lesbian Mother Families. *Journal of Child Psychology and Psychiatry*. 2004;45(4):755–764. doi:10.1111/j.1469-7610.2004.00269.x

45. Ross LE. Perinatal Mental Health in Lesbian Mothers: A Review of Potential Risk and Protective Factors. *Women & Health*. 2005;41(3):113–128. doi:10.1300/J013v41n03_07

46. Charlton BM, Reynolds CA, Tabaac AR, et al. Unintended and Teen Pregnancy Experiences of Trans Masculine People Living in the United States. *International Journal of Transgender Health*. 2020;22(1–2):65–76. doi:10.1080/26895269.2020.1824692

47. Gahagan J, Colpitts E. Understanding and Measuring LGBTQ Pathways to Health: A Scoping Review of Strengths-Based Health Promotion Approaches in LGBTQ Health Research. *Journal of Homosexuality*. 2017;64(1):95–121. doi:10.1080/00918369.2016.1172893

48. Croll J, Sanapo L, Bourjeily G. LGBTQ+ Individuals and Pregnancy Outcomes: A Commentary. *BJOG: An International Journal of Obstetrics & Gynaecology*. 2022. doi:10.1111/1471-0528.17131

49. Brandt JS, Patel AJ, Marshall I, Bachmann GA. Transgender Men, Pregnancy, and the "New" Advanced Paternal Age: A Review of the Literature. *Maturitas*. 2019;128:17–21. doi:10.1016/j.maturitas.2019.07.004

50. Ellis SA, Wojnar DM, Pettinato M. Conception, Pregnancy, and Birth Experiences of Male and Gender Variant Gestational Parents: It's How We Could Have a Family. *Journal of Midwifery & Women's Health*. 2015;60(1):62–69. doi:10.1111/jmwh.12213

51. Obedin-Maliver J, Makadon HJ. Transgender Men and Pregnancy. *Obstetric Medicine*. 2016;9(1):4–8. doi:10.1177/1753495X15612658

52. Hoffkling A, Obedin-Maliver J, Sevelius J. From Erasure to Opportunity: A Qualitative Study of the Experiences of Transgender Men around Pregnancy and Recommendations for Providers. *BMC Pregnancy and Childbirth*. 2017;17(332):1–14. doi:10.1186/s12884-017-1491-5

53. Light AD, Obedin-Maliver J, Sevelius JM, Kerns JL. Transgender Men who Experienced Pregnancy after Female-to-Male Gender Transitioning. *Obstetrics & Gynecology*. 2014;124(6):1120–1127. doi:10.1097/AOG.0000000000000540

54. Newman TC, Hirst J, Darwin Z. What Enables or Prevents Women with Depressive Symptoms Seeking Help in the Postnatal Period? *British Journal of Midwifery*. 2019;27(4):219–227. doi:10.12968/bjom.2019.27.4.219

55. Sambrook Smith M, Lawrence V, Sadler E, Easter A. Barriers to Accessing Mental Health Services for Women with Perinatal Mental Illness: Systematic Review and Meta-Synthesis of Qualitative Studies in the UK. *BMJ Open*. 2019;9(1):e024803. doi:10.1136/bmjopen-2018-024803

56. Alang SM, Fomotar M. Postpartum Depression in an Online Community of Lesbian Mothers: Implications for Clinical Practice. *Journal of Gay & Lesbian Mental Health*. 2015;19(1):21–39. doi:10.1080/19359705.2014.910853

57. Touroni E, Coyle A. Decision-Making in Planned Lesbian Parenting: An Interpretative Phenomenological Analysis. *Journal of Community & Applied Social Psychology*. 2002;12(3):194–209. doi:10.1002/casp.672

58. Manley MH, Goldberg AE, Ross LEJ. Invisibility and Involvement: LGBTQ Community Connections among Plurisexual Women during Pregnancy and Postpartum. *Psychology of Sexual Orientation and Gender Diversity*. 2018;5(2):169–181. doi:10.1037/sgd0000285

59. Darwin Z, Domoney J, Iles J, Bristow F, Siew J, Sethna V. Assessing the Mental Health of Fathers, Other Co-Parents, and Partners in the Perinatal Period: Mixed Methods Evidence Synthesis. *Frontiers in Psychiatry*. 2021;11:585479. doi:10.3389/fpsyt.2020.585479

Chapter 12

Infant health surveillance services

Sarah Arnold

WHAT IS HEALTH VISITING FOR?

Most countries in the Global North have an infant or child health surveillance service available to families from the birth of their baby for the first few years of their life. The role of these services is to act as a triage system for other health or social care services, offering universal support for all families, and referral into specialist services. Child health surveillance services are usually staffed by qualified nurses or midwives who have additional training in child development, and whose remit for universal family support includes issues around infant weight gain and growth, feeding, sleep, development, vaccinations, and parental mental health. Referral to specialist services might occur in cases where a potential health or developmental need in the infant is identified, or where there is a potential safeguarding issue. In addition, referrals for parents and carers to specialist services might occur where a postnatal mental or physical health need is identified.

Within the UK, this service is referred to as Health Visiting. Specialist Community Public Health Nurses, commonly referred to as Health Visitors, are qualified professionals who are already registered with the Nursing and Midwifery Council, who undertake a further year of specialist training. The UK Institute of Health Visiting identifies four overlapping roles for Health Visitors:

1. Physical health—Health Visitors can monitor and promote the physical health, primarily of the infant(s), but also of their carers. Health promotion work can include providing supporting breastfeeding, providing sexual health information, and information about healthy lifestyles. In some locations Health Visitors can make referrals to Food Banks for families who are facing poverty and hunger.

DOI: 10.4324/9781003305446-13

2.   Mental health—Health Visitors have specialist knowledge about postnatal mental health and bonding. They will have knowledge about local postnatal mental health services and can make referrals to these where a referral is required.
3.   Child development—Health Visitors have specialist knowledge about child development and offer support with common developmental issues such as sleep, weaning, speech and behaviours. Support includes offering parents information about these issues, reassurance, support with low level difficulties, or referrals to specialist services as appropriate.
4.   Social needs and safeguarding—Health Visitors build relationships with families and local community groups and support services. Health Visitors frequently also provide groups for new parents. They can use the knowledge they have about local provision to assist families in creating a social support network of other new parents and accessing appropriate services, including parent and infant groups, playgroups, chest/breastfeeding support, disability support groups, mental health services, and domestic violence and substance misuse services. Their connection to the family means they may be aware of infants who are at risk of neglect or abuse, and can make the appropriate referrals for further investigation in these cases.

WHAT ARE THE ISSUES FOR LGBTQ+ PARENTS?

Cisheterosexism and mono-normativity are built into the structure of perinatal services, including Health Visiting. As we have seen in Chapters 2 and 6, these assumptions begin at the first encounter with perinatal services, either in preconception care, or with midwifery "booking in forms" for those who have conceived without medical involvement. Perinatal services assumptions that a family means two people in a monogamous sexual relationship affect the recording of medical and social information (see Chapter 6), medical terminology (eg, primiparous), informal language used (mum and baby groups), the rights of expectant parents (visiting hours for fathers, see Chapter 8), and the design of services (maternal and paternal mental health services, see Chapter 11). As Health Visiting services are available towards the end of the perinatal journey, both the experiences of parents and the information available to Health Visitors in their first encounters with parents are shaped by the previous cisheterosexist mono-normative services.

Whilst many LGBTQ+ parents will have positive encounters with Health Visiting services, these factors can affect whether some LGBTQ+ parents are able to access the services that Health Visitors provide, and how useful those services are, including: information provision, universal wellbeing services, specialist services, and ultimately the relationship between the parent(s) and the Health Visitor.

Information

Whilst great effort has been put into creating some general resources that apply to parents in a couple relationship, regardless of gender or sexual orientation,[1] images of LGBTQ+ families rarely appear on leaflets unless they are specific to LGBTQ+ families, and families that include more than two partners are not ever mentioned. If specialist, rather than universal information is required, it is rarely suitable for LGBTQ+ families. For example, most sexual health information provided by Health Visiting services and by the NHS assumes that contraception will be necessary "You can get pregnant as little as 3 weeks after the birth of a baby, even if you're breastfeeding and your periods haven't started again."[2, 3] NHS information about resuming sex after birth includes statements such as "Men may worry about hurting their partner,"[2] which of course they may, but so may women and non-binary non-gestational new parents. There are no resources available which refer to lesbian sexual health and practices (for example, the use of hands, fingers, or sex toys, as opposed to assuming sex is always about a penis in a vagina, or how suitable the use of harnesses or straps may be following caesarean birth).

Looking at the information about lactation, we can see that there is an assumption that the person who gives birth will be a woman, and that if breastfeeding happens, she will be the only person to breastfeed the baby. Currently, there is one page within the NHS website that offers advice about chestfeeding for trans men and non-binary people,[4] and a further paragraph on a separate page about testosterone and chestfeeding.[5] There is however no information about co-breastfeeding, or induced lactation. In fact, most leaflets about breastfeeding specifically exclude the possibility that a non-gestational parent might be breastfeeding, suggesting (ironically in a leaflet entitled "Breastfeeding for everyone") that

"Fathers/partners can do skin-to-skin, cuddle, carry and bath their baby."[6]

So far, there is no research investigating Health Visitors' knowledge about issues such as lesbian sexual health, breastfeeding by non-gestational mothers and chestfeeding. Given the dearth of information available for parents, it is likely that Health Visitors also face a dearth of information about LGBTQ+ families. This prevents them from being able to offer appropriate universal services to all LGBTQ+ families.

Universal services—check-ups and group settings

Alongside information, Health Visitors offer universal wellbeing check-ups for well infants. This includes weighing babies when they are young, visual and physical checks of their body, and developmental checks as they get a little older. Such check-ups are often delivered in a less proscriptive and private setting than doctor's appointments might be, and may be provided in health centres, community centres, or children's centres.[7] A common model in the UK involves several Health Visitors working in a large room, each with one family, with an attached waiting room, and access to private rooms for discussion between the parent(s) and Health Visitor if needed. These services may be run on a booked appointment, or a drop-in basis. This way of organising wellbeing checks for well infants has several benefits. First, as many of these check-ups are only a few minutes long, it is a more efficient use of time than the Health Visitors making visits to families' homes. It also means Health Visitors can quickly access a second opinion from colleagues who might have specialist knowledge if a potential issue is noticed. As babies can be unpredictable in terms of feeding and sleeping needs, the drop-in clinic can reduce the pressure on parents that a set appointment might cause. Finally, social connections and friendships between new parents who live in the area are likely to arise spontaneously in these settings.

For LGBTQ+ parents, well infant check-ups delivered in these settings may have fewer advantages, and more disadvantages. Whilst any parent can usually bring their baby to these clinics, most will be brought by their mother, and 99% of Health Visitors themselves are female.[8] Some GBTQ+ trans men will be comfortable in this space, but others may not, and even those who are comfortable in the space may find their presence questioned if they are not accompanied by a partner who is perceived as a woman, forcing them to rapidly assess whether the other parents present are likely to be homophobic or transphobic, and therefore whether to reveal their sexual orientation and/or trans status. Similarly, lesbian, and bisexual women with a same-gender partner may have to decide whether to reveal or conceal the gender of their partner and therefore their sexual orientation, due to the conversation-encouraging set up of the clinic. Non-binary parents are quite likely to be subject to misgendering by other parents, even if the Health Visitors use the correct language, and will have to make similar choices about concealing or revealing their gender to other parents. Health Visitors may not know whether the parent has chosen to conceal or reveal their gender, and so may inadvertently do the opposite within the hearing of other parents during the baby check. The drop-in nature of sessions may also mean that LGBTQ+ parents have less choice in which Health Visitors they interact with, preventing pre-emptive conversations about preferences in terms of language or privacy.

To further promote social connections, Health Visitors may provide postnatal group services for new parents. These might include Breastfeeding Cafes, a series of group sessions for a set number of weeks covering common new parent and infant topics, or one-off weaning or sleep workshops. New LGBTQ+ parents may benefit from both the information delivered in such groups and the social connections, but attending such groups comes with uncertainty about their reception by other parents. Health Visitors cannot make these spaces safe for LGBTQ+ parents, as they cannot prevent homophobic or transphobic comments from other parents from happening, and it is rare that such groups have existing processes for how parents who make and are subject to such comments will be supported after they have occurred. If parents either directly experience a lack of safety in accessing universal services provided by Health Visitors, or if they are concerned about a potential lack of safety based on their own or other LGBTQ+ people's previous experiences, then these universal services are not truly universal.

Specialist services

The Health Visitor's role includes triaging new parents based on their perinatal health needs, and facilitating access to specialist services when necessary. This can include making referrals to lactation support, gynaecological services, and to perinatal mental health services. LGBTQ+ parents may find that their Health Visitor is not able to make appropriate referrals to specialist services for where there is a lack of appropriate provision locally. For example, a Health Visitor may not be able to refer a non-gestational mother for lactation support, a trans gestational father to gynaecological services where a female sex marker is a requirement of referral, or a gay father to a mother and baby specialist perinatal mental health unit.

Where a referral to a specialist service is needed for either the infant or a parent, the Health Visitor cannot guarantee the reception that LGBTQ+ parents will face. Parents may be referred to the appropriately labelled services by the Health Visitor—for example a non-gestational mother to Maternal mental health provision, and a trans gestational father to Paternal mental health services—but may then face cisheterosexist attitudes within those services, which could include rejecting the referral or insisting that the parent accesses inappropriately labelled services, both of which may cause harm to the parent.

Relationships

Building relationships with families with a new baby is the key to a successful Health Visitor relationship. Indeed, WAVE Trust, an international organisation dedicated to reducing child abuse, neglect, and domestic violence, identify

"establishing and maintaining a trustworthy relationship"

between parents and those in a Health Visitor type role as

"absolutely central to effective assessment as well as intervention"[9(pp.37)]

Through the development of a good relationship, the Health Visitor is able to offer a universal service, both advising on normal infant development, and connecting new parents to each other through infant and carer groups. This relationship is also central to the provision of specialist services. Trust that has been developed with the Health Visitor can in part be transferred to other health professionals that the Health Visitor might refer the infant or parents to, such as paediatricians, psychologists, or lactation services, making the transition to these services easier for the parent(s). This relationship is also important in helping the Health Visitor carry out their safeguarding role—if the Health Visitor knows the family well, they are both more likely to confide when there are difficulties, and the Health Visitor is more likely to notice when something is unusual within the family.

Families do not begin their relationship with the Health Visitor with a blank slate. For all families, their experiences of antenatal and intrapartum care will influence their expectations about relationships with the Health Visiting service. Research shows that homophobia, transphobia, and cisheterosexism are quite common experiences for LGBTQ+ people in assisted conception, antenatal, and intrapartum care. The actions of other health care professionals may therefore have predisposed an LGBTQ+ family to be wary of Health Visitors who are trying to build a relationship, and make them wish to maintain some distance. I noticed that during the pandemic, LGBTQ+ families sometimes appeared happier that all contact was online, where a distance was automatically created.

If the Health Visitor is then not able to provide the family with appropriate information and safe access to universal or specialist services, this poses a further challenge to the building of this relationship. Whether information is incorrect (misgendering in information leaflets), not applicable (contraceptive advice for lesbians), or not available (chestfeeding and co-breastfeeding advice, psychological support for non-gestational mothers), the result will be the same. Parents will see the Health Visitor service as not for families like theirs, and—at best—will have less investment in building a relationship. At worst, they may experience psychological harm: through cisheterosexism from the Health Visitor or a specialist service, or homophobic and transphobic encounters when accessing group settings. In such cases LGBTQ+ parents may need to disengage from the Health Visitor service to protect themselves.

WHAT ARE THE ISSUES FOR HEALTH VISITORS?

Many Health Visitors will work with LGBTQ+ parents and be able to provide them with a good service. However, the issues discussed above and in the rest of this book present Health Visitors in some areas with challenges in providing services to some LGBTQ+ parents. These challenges may arise in the context of organisational or professional services, when providing a universal service, or the challenges may relate to the availability of appropriate specialist services to refer parents to. Specific challenges arise from the lack of research into LGBTQ+ parents and Health Visiting, and from the conflation of parental disengagement with Health Visiting as a cause for concern.

Organisational and professional limitations

Health Visitors work within a heavily regulated profession and organisational structure. Different models for the delivery of services exist, which offer some variations in degrees of autonomy, but the safeguarding element of the role means that adherence to policies and procedures about when to make a referral is mandatory. The Health Visitor's remit in supporting parents in a variety of situations with a wide range of issues is broad, and the proscribed training is intensive, and does include consideration of equality and diversity issues. Such training does not however routinely cover any of the structural issues that face LGBTQ+ parents, which are caused by the design of perinatal services, described in this chapter or indeed in this book. This lack of available training is compounded by the dearth of LGBTQ+ specific policies found across perinatal services. Many services will have a policy setting out a general commitment to treat all patients and service users equally. What is required however, are perinatal policies which set out not only a commitment to LGBTQ+ inclusion, but provide an honest appraisal of where exclusion currently exists, specific information about how inclusion will be achieved, and pathways or procedures for professionals to follow on occasions when an issue is recognised. Without these comprehensive policies, Health Visitors and other professionals who raise concerns may find they are unsupported by their line managers, or by senior management. Uncertainty about organisational support may lead Health Visitors to choose not to raise issues in order to protect themselves from being viewed as disruptive or unprofessional. For LGBTQ+ Health Visitors, such choices may involve potential harm both in being complicit in cisheterosexist structures through silence, and through being seen as pushing a personal agenda.

CASE STUDY 1— SURIYA

Suriya regularly brings her baby to the "mum and baby" group run by her Health Visitor, Jan. In the third session, Suriya mentions her wife in a group discussion. Another woman in the group, Helen, is upset that she had breastfed her baby in the group in front of Suriya, not realising that Suriya was a lesbian. She angrily tells Suriya that she should have disclosed her sexual orientation to the group, and a heated argument ensues. Jan ends the session early, and arranges to meet with Helen and Suriya individually later that day.

When Jan meets Helen, Helen is very distressed and also angry. She insists she will not return the group unless either Suriya is banned, or there is a separate place for heterosexual women to breastfeed, without any lesbian parents. Helen wants to make a complaint to Jan's manager because Jan did not tell her that there were lesbian parents in the group.

When Jan meets Suriya, Suriya is very distressed and also angry. She insists she will not return to the group unless Helen is banned and Jan can guarantee that there will not be other homophobic comments made. Suriya wants to make a complaint to Jan's manager because she thinks Jan should have asked Helen to leave as soon as she made the first comment about being uncomfortable breastfeeding in front of a lesbian.

There are no policies about how this situation should be handled.

In deciding what to do, Jan also has to take account of further information that she has:

– Helen is very socially isolated, and Jan has some concerns about her mental health
– There is another lesbian parent in the group
– The existence of the postnatal group is under threat for financial reasons

What should Jan do?

Research

Of all the chapters in this book, this chapter was the most difficult to identify relevant research to draw on. The current literature regarding LGBTQ+ people and Health Visiting is scant, and rarely disaggregated from research into LGBTQ+ people's overall perinatal experiences. This poses a difficulty for making significant improvements, as Health Visiting is theoretically constructed as a research-led, evidence-based practice.[7] Good quality research would be one way for Health Visitors to overcome professional and organisational barriers. In the absence of either a strong evidence base or strong organisational leadership on LGBTQ+ issues, it is difficult for Health Visitors to provide appropriate universal services to LGBTQ+ parents.

Lack of appropriate specialist services to refer to

Earlier in the chapter, the damage to parents of referrals into either inappropriate services, or appropriate services which are governed by cisheterosexist assumptions in referral criteria were discussed. For Health Visitors this poses an ethical conundrum to which there is no easy solution. If an appropriate service does not exist, a referral cannot be made, and the family may suffer harm. If a potentially appropriate service does exist, but the Health Visitor does not know if a referral will be accepted, or whether the service or individual practitioner will be homophobic or transphobic, then either making or not making a referral may result in the family suffering harm. Identifying whether a potentially appropriate service exists, and then establishing whether the service will accept a referral, and whether a parent is likely to experience homophobia or transphobia is likely to take a considerable amount of time. It also has the potential to cause the Health Visitor professional discomfort as this may be seen as acting outside their role, failing to follow standard (cisheterosexist) procedures, or perceptions of accusing fellow professionals of homophobia and/or transphobia. Even a Health Visitor who is well-informed and culturally competent in providing care to LGBTQ+ parents may find that when they need to make a referral to a specialist service, they have no available options that will not cause harm, only a choice of which kind of harm to risk for both parents and themselves.

"Disengagement" as a criterion for concern

Health Visitors' front-line role, involving universal access to young children and families, places them in a key position for the prevention, detection, and monitoring of child maltreatment.[7] This role requires Health Visitors to be skilled in interacting with multiple agencies across the health and social care boundaries. Identifying and reporting appropriate causes for concern, as viewed by a range of different organisations, is challenging. The potential consequences of not reporting a cause for concern are serious—figures from the NSPCC show that over the last 5 years, an average of one child a week was killed by assault, neglect, or undetermined intent in the UK, with children under the age of one being the most likely age group to be killed by another person, most commonly a parent or step-parent.[10]

At the same time, Health Visiting is an optional service, and parents may legitimately choose not to use it. Local policies often set out specific pathways for Health Visitors to follow when parents choose not to engage with the Health Visiting service, or not to attend wellbeing clinics or groups, without formally opting out of the service.[11, 12] Such pathways often include exchanging information with other services, including Children's Services, Housing, and any Early Years' settings, even if there are "no known child/family vulnerabilities."[11]

Parents may not be aware that if they do not want their information shared and discussed in this way, they are required to formally inform the Health Visiting service that they wish to disengage from an optional service. Furthermore, whilst all policies recognise that parents have a right to decline the offered Health Visiting services, the language used, and protocols set out for Health Visitors to follow may make it difficult for parents to formally decline these services. Declining services is variously described in policies aimed at Health Visitors as:

"Refusal of Universal Public Health Services"[13(pp.12)]
"a failure to consent"[13(pp.3)]

Health Visitors are informed that if parents do decline atheir services:

"Total refusal of engagement with universal public health services is rare and usually a compromise can be made… Discussion with the parent/carer is required either by telephone or face to face contact."[13(pp.12)]

The language of "refusal" and "failure" along with the implication that parents are required to engage in discussion about their reasons for declining an optional service are problematic in their own right. For an LGBTQ+ parent, who may choose to disengage with a service for the reasons set out in this chapter, these policies may cause significant harm. Whilst many policies set out various good and bad reasons that parents may disengage from services,[11–14] the authors have been unable to find a single policy that lists lack of appropriate support services due to structural cisheterosexism, homophobia, and/or transphobia as a potential reason for disengagement.

CONSEQUENCES

Taken together, the issues that LGBTQ+ parents face in accessing Health Visiting services, and the issues that Health Visitors face in providing appropriate services to LGBTQ+ parents, have three potential broad categories of negative consequences.

Inappropriate Children's Services referrals

The first potential negative consequence is that if parents choose to disengage with the service, without formally informing the service that they are disengaging, perhaps through lack of awareness that they need to do so, or perhaps through a wish to be polite and avoid confrontation, the Health Visitor may share information with or make a referral to Children's Services in the absence of any concerns about the family outside of withdrawal from services. Inappropriate referrals have negative consequences for all involved—parents are likely to experience anxiety, and to be less receptive to engaging with professionals in future, which may in turn cause the Health Visitor greater problems in building a relationship. Making and receiving an inappropriate referral also takes time for Health Visitors and social workers, both professions where overwork and a lack of sufficient time are pressing concerns.

Unrecognised child developmental problems

If the parent(s) do either successfully disengage from Health Visiting services, or if the Health Visitor is aware of the reasons for disengagement and exercises discretion in not viewing this as a cause for concern then there is the potential for a developmental issue to go unnoticed. Health Visitors have extensive knowledge about child development, and might notice an issue with the child that the parents do not notice. An established relationship with a Health Visitor might also lead parents to have discussions about potential child development concerns at an earlier point than they would seek advice from an unknown professional.

Unsupported parental mental health

Without a good working relationship with their local Health Visitor, some parents' perinatal mental health issues may remain unrecognised, and therefore untreated, for a longer period. Equally, parents might opt into the Health Visiting service, but still be unable to access appropriate support or treatment if the Health Visitor is unable to refer them to an appropriate service.

POTENTIAL IMPROVEMENTS

Most of this chapter has described the challenges facing LGBTQ+ parents and their Health Visitors. Fully overcoming these challenges requires three actions:

1. Further research into the accessibility of Health Visiting Services for LGBTQ+ parents, to establish both quantitatively measurable outcomes for LGBTQ+ parents and their infants, and qualitatively explore experiences for LGBTQ+ parents and their Health Visitors.
2. Introduction of organisational policies and procedures, which acknowledge areas of exclusion, and set out pathways towards inclusion, led by national and international organisations and senior management within services.
3. The redesign of perinatal services, away from a cisheterosexist mono-normative system, so that LGBTQ+ families can be fully included.

These actions are each time and resource intensive, but without them, Health Visitors will continue to face challenges in providing truly universal services to all LGBTQ+ parents.

There are also many actions that can be taken by individual services and practitioners to move towards providing services which exclude fewer LGBTQ+ families, but knowing where to begin can be overwhelming. Over the next three pages, we have created a series of seven mini-workplans, which can each be used alone, or can be used together as a larger workplan. Seven different areas have been identified, and practical actions have been listed within in each area which would improve inclusivity for LGBTQ+ families. The areas do not need to be completed in order—if the actions in one area are not practicable to work on locally, you can pick another area, or even create your own. Working on one area will benefit LGBTQ+ parents, whilst working through all the areas will create more comprehensive change.

GATHER QUANTITATIVE DATA

–   Be aware that you do not know how many LGBTQ+ parents you are working with. The apparent gender of someone's current partner is not an indication of their sexual orientation, in most cases you do not know whether the partner is cis or trans, and they may have more than one partner. Single parents are also not necessarily heterosexual.
–   Find out how many LGBTQ+ parents use your services. Include questions about gender, sexual orientation and partners on your intake forms, alongside other equality data. Use this information locally to monitor outcomes and engagement, as you already use ethnicity or age data.

LGBTQ+ ACCREDITED CONTINUOUS PROFESSIONAL DEVELOPMENT (CPD) FOR HEALTH VISITORS

– Identify any existing training in LGBTQ+ issues for Health Visitors, assess the suitability of the learning outcomes, whether it is accredited, and the cost. If appropriate training is available, consider attending it, or recommending it within the team.
– If no appropriate training is available, consider working with an in-house or external training provider to develop a CPD module.

FORMS AND PARENT-FACING INFORMATION

– Review the forms used locally, ensuring that they differentiate between the information about genetic parents and social parents, and that they have space to collect information about diverse families.
– Collect all the information usually given to new parents. Does it include information suitable for LGBTQ+ parents, such as inclusive sexual health advice and lactation advice for non-gestational parents and chestfeeding parents? If not, identify suitable materials that can be included.

LGBTQ+ PARENT GROUPS

– Gather information about LGBTQ+ voluntary parents' groups at a local or regional level. Ensure this is kept current by annual reviews, and have a timetable for the named person who will do this, how and when they will update all Health Visitors with this information, and who will take over this role if the person is no longer in role.
– If your service provides new parents' groups, consider also providing an LGBTQ+ new parents' group, especially if no voluntary group exists locally. This could be provided on a regional level, across NHS Trusts.

LOCAL POLICY

- For settings and groups which are under the control of a group of Health Visitors, create policies about how issues such as homophobia, transphobia and pronoun/language checking will be carried out. For example, what happens if there is homophobia from a parent within a group? How will Health Visitors ask parents which pronouns they would like to be used for themselves and their partners in group settings, and how will this be communicated to other Health Visitors to avoid misgendering or accidental revealing of someone's gender or sexual orientation against their wishes? These policies need to be agreed by the entire team, and ratified at a senior management level, so that individual Health Visitors are confident that their actions based on these policies will be supported.

  Understand that disengagement might be due to fear of or experiences of homophobia and/or transphobia, or to a lack of appropriate services. Include this information in any local procedures for Health Visitors in reporting disengagement. Request clarification from an appropriate Safeguarding Lead about whether disengagement on these grounds, with no additional concerns about vulnerability, merits data-sharing or referral.

- Consider offering an alternative service configuration to parents who may disengaged from services for these reasons, to promote child development and parental mental health

ANY OTHER AREA YOU IDENTIFY

- How are LGBTQ+ parents currently included or excluded?
- How could inclusion be improved?
- Who could do this work?
- When should it be reviewed, and who by?
- How can you include the views of LGBTQ+ parents in this work?

PRE-EMPTIVE CONTACT WITH SPECIALIST SERVICES

– The point at which a non-gestational mother needs access to lactation support, or a trans man needs a referral to a perinatal mental health team is not the correct point to find out whether those services exist locally and whether they are supportive of LGBTQ+ parents. Obtaining the information at that point will create delays for parents who may need immediate support. If you do not already collect gender and sexual orientation data from parents, it will also mean that you have probably referred LGBTQ+ people who you assumed were cisheterosexuals to services that you do not have inclusivity information about. Within the team, develop a checklist, which can either be physically given to specialist health or voluntary sector services, or discussed over the phone. Contact services and find out who they provide services to, and whether they have expertise in issues affecting LGBTQ+ parents.

– Ensure the information obtained is recorded and shared with all Health Visitors, and that structures are in place to update it.

– If LGBTQ+ parents provide positive or negative feedback about a specialist service, record this information.

– Create a map of the gaps in service provision for LGBTQ+ parents, and consider how these gaps could be filled.

POSTERS WITHIN HEALTH VISITOR SETTINGS

– Are the posters on display exclusive? For example, do they refer to "mums and dads"? If so, change the wording or remove the poster. If the poster is from another organisation, ask them to provide an updated version which is not cisheterosexist.

– Are the posters on display inclusive? Do the photographs used represent a range of families? It is important to consider intersectionality here too, ensuring for example that Black and Asian LGBTQ+ people are represented. If the posters do not represent a range of families, create new ones, or identify another source for such materials.

– Create a new standard for posters on display in each setting, specifying inclusivity criteria. The standard should include a timetable for auditing each location, the names of those who will be responsible for the audit, and a date to review the standard and the audits.

SUMMARY

Health Visitors aim to provide a universal service for families of children aged from 0–5 years old, promoting infant and child wellbeing through familial physical and mental health, creating and strengthening social networks, and offering access to specialist child development, mental health, and safeguarding services when appropriate.

Cisheterosexism and mono-normativity underlie the structure of perinatal services, including Health Visiting. This means that currently the system of Health Visiting is not set up to guarantee either appropriate universal support for LGBTQ+ new parents, or appropriate access to specialist services. Rather, Health Visitors may be faced with choosing which type of harm to risk for parents, and for themselves. Given the evidence-led nature of Health Visiting services, further research should be a priority, however until that evidence base is strengthened, there are improvements that can be made at both an individual practitioner and organisational level.

REFERENCES

1. Institute of Health Visiting. Looking After Your Relationship as New Parents, https://ihv. org.uk/wp-content/uploads/2022/03/PT-Looking-after-your-relationship-as-new-parents-FINAL-VERSION-16.3.22.pdf (2016, accessed 6 December 2023).
2. NHS. Sex and Contraception after Birth, https://www.nhs.uk/conditions/baby/support-and-services/sex-and-contraception-after-birth/ (2023, accessed 6 December 2023).
3. Institute of Health Visiting. Parent Leaflet for Sexual and Reproductive Health, https://ihv. org.uk/parent-leaflet-for-sexual-and-reproductive-health/#/id/600d2f2a2a8c 771bcc98d3c6 (n.d., accessed 6 December 2023).
4. NHS. Chestfeeding if You're Trans or Non-Binary, https://www.nhs.uk/pregnancy/having-a-baby-if-you-are-lgbt-plus/chestfeeding-if-youre-trans-or-non-binary/ (2021, accessed 6 December 2023).
5. NHS. Testosterone and Pregnancy, https://www.nhs.uk/pregnancy/having-a-baby-if-you-are-lgbt-plus/testosterone-and-pregnancy/ (2021, accessed 6 December 2023).
6. Institute of Health Visiting. Supporting Breastfeeding for Everyone, https://ihv.org.uk/wp-content/uploads/2015/10/PT-Supporting-breastfeeding-for-everyone-FINAL-VERSION-31.5.22-1.pdf (2022, accessed 6 December 2023).
7. Peckover S. From 'Public Health' to 'Safeguarding Children': British Health Visiting in Policy, Practice and Research. *Children & Society* 2013; 27: 116–126.
8. Department of Health. *Equality Analysis – Health Visiting Programme*. Department of Health.
9. Wave Trust. *Conception to Age 2: The Age of Opportunity: Addendum to the Government's Vision for the Foundation Years 'Supporting Families in the Foundation Years'*. 2nd ed. Croydon [UK]: Wave Trust, 2013.

10. NSPCC. *Child Deaths Due to Abuse or Neglect: Statistics Briefing*, https://learning.nspcc. org.uk/media/1652/statistics-briefing-child-deaths-abuse-neglect.pdf (December 2021, accessed 6 December 2023).

11. Swindon Borough Council. Health Visiting–Child not Brought / No Access Guidance, https://view.officeapps.live.com/op/view.aspx?src=https%3A%2F%2Fproceduresonline. com%2Ftrixcms1%2Fmedia%2F8186%2Fhealth-visiting-child-not-brought-no-access-guidance.docx&wdOrigin=BROWSELINK (2018, accessed 6 December 2023).

12. Black Country Partnership NHS Trust. Management of did not Attend/Child not Brought, https://www.bcpft.nhs.uk/documents/policies/d/2088-did-not-attend-no-access-visit-cypf-sop-10-management-of-dna-was-not-brought-appointments-health-visiting-and-fnp/ file (n.d., accessed 6 December 2023).

13. Public Health Agency. *Regional Guidance*, https://www.publichealth.hscni.net/sites/ default/files/2021-03/Regional%20Guidance%20on%20Refusal%20to%20Engage%20 Dec%202020%20FINAL.pdf (December 2020, accessed 6 December 2023).

14. Lincolnshire Safeguarding Children Partnership. Recognising Disguised Compliance & Disengagement Among Families: Practice Guidance, https://lincolnshirescb.procedure sonline.com/g_work_uncoop_fams.html (n.d., accessed 6 December 2023).

Chapter 13

The mind-body connection or why an interdisciplinary approach matters

Kate Luxion

INTRODUCTION

As we have seen within the previous chapters, minority stress is prevalent at various stages of reproductive health care, with stressors coming from a variety of sources throughout the process. We have read through example that include a lack of inclusive in-take forms and language options during care to the various forms of stigma and discrimination that take place during reproductive and perinatal care. In LGBTQ+ perinatal research, there is a growing body of qualitative literature that is slowly being supported by inclusive quantitative methods—such as including measures on gender and sexual orientation—while working in tandem to test and refine an understanding of how stigma and discrimination (ie, minority stress) influences reproductive health. These minority stressors, and their negative impacts, can be reduced through the use of more inclusive language and care practices, as have already been evidenced by the other chapters. To better understand why a reduction in minority stressors can improve inclusion and health and well-being outcomes, this chapter explores how the way people are treated cascades through the body; what results is poorer quality of life due to preventable detrimental experiences. The discussions within this chapter will help to highlight both the importance of an intersectional, interdisciplinary approach to reproductive health and why mental and physical health are intrinsically linked. In turn, there will be discussion of the gaps within the literature and recommendations for moving towards reproductive justice for LGBTQ+ parents and their families.

STIGMA, DISCRIMINATION, AND PHYSIOLOGICAL STRESS

When individuals seek health care, they are already under stress from daily life, such as managing a household and/or career and tending to the care and wellbeing of members of their family as well as themselves. For minoritised

DOI: 10.4324/9781003305446-14

individuals, such as LGBTQ+ parents, they must face those daily stresses along with facing an additional layer of stress, because of having to navigate health systems and services that do not always recognise their existence or their relationships. This compounds everyday stressors, alerting the hypothalamic-pituitary-adrenal (HPA) axis to trigger the fight or flight response, also known as our acute stress response. The body is meant to use this response for acute instances of danger (ie, sympathetic nervous system) before returning relatively quickly to baseline once safety is reached (ie, parasympathetic nervous system). However, as gender and sexual minorities, LGBTQ+ people encounter, and have to plan for, the possibility of repeated experiences of stigma and discrimination that make it hard for the body to return to the baseline levels of cortisol production, because of being in a perpetual stressed state. Living in this prolonged state of fight or flight is not ideal and can lead to dysregulation which undermines our health and well-being. If unable to address stress, through reduction or prevention, the body is stuck in a cycle of formerly protective functions that are instead imbalancing the way in which the body's biological systems (ie, biosystems) are functioning. For example, these new "scripts" within each biosystem might result in the production of hormones at non-optimal rates (ie, too high or too low) which the body may not be able to process properly (ie, metabolise and/or produce a feedback response).

The original development of the minority stress theory[1, 2] connected stigma and discrimination as sources of stress, alongside resilience measures (ie, protective factors), to the mental health disparities faced by lesbian, gay, and bisexual (LGB) people when compared to their cisgender heterosexual peers.[1] Connections between mental and physical health have played a role is extending the model,[3, 4] which has since expanded to acknowledge gender minorities along with sexual minorities.[5, 6] These updates aid in understanding the differences and similarities of stigma and discrimination faced when navigating cisheteronormative systems (eg, laws and policies, health systems, educational system, etc.) and societal expectations (eg, levels of acceptance, gender norms, etc.). Additionally, it is important to acknowledge the differences and similarities in life experiences and the fact that individuals can be both gender and sexual minorities simultaneously—experiencing minority stress in multiple, intersecting ways. As laid out in Figure 13.1 below, these sources of stigma and discrimination take place on multiple levels of interaction: intrapersonal, interpersonal, and structural.

Despite removal of homosexuality from the DSM,[7] the assumption has remained that health disparities between LGB people and cisheterosexual people stemmed from strictly individual behaviours (ie, gay sex versus heterosexual sex). As part of this logic, if LGB people had worse health outcomes than cisheterosexual people, it was viewed as their fault in place of recognising that social exclusion

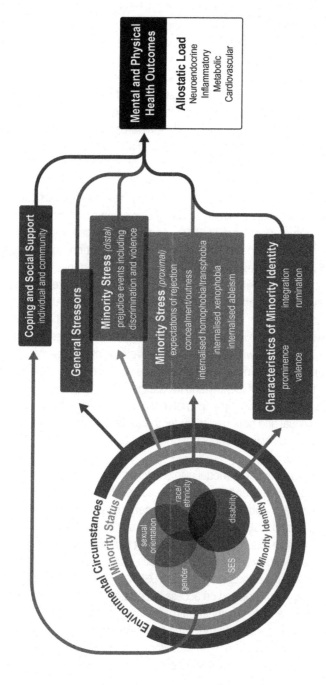

Figure 13.1 Integrated model of minority stress, intersectionality, and allostatic load. Graphic by the author. Adapted from Crenshaw, 1989 and 1991; Meyer 2003; and Sterling et al., 1988.

(ie, the criminalisation and stigmatisation of one's identity) can impact a person's health and well-being. Through the minority stress model as a theoretical framework, research has been able to connect the dots between poorer outcomes and a person's minority status,[1, 8] differentiating between a person's identity and the status held within societal contexts. This key point highlights the sociopolitical responsibility for the poorer health outcomes of LGB people, because of stigma and discrimination; in turn showing that the stressors of stigma and discrimination were built on harmful stereotypes and misinformation. Across all levels of interaction, such as antenatal care designed for heterosexual married individuals (ie, environmental context), social expectations and prejudices result in preventable stressors experienced by marginalised people. However, there is also room within the framework to consider what factors might potentially positively buffer stressors (ie, resilience resources), both in terms of linking individual experiences with health outcomes as well as evaluating health system inclusion and influences. In doing so, it is important to remember that the LGBTQ+ community is itself diverse and any care and research efforts should recognise the impacts of overlapping minority identities. Work by Lisa Bowleg has aptly analogised the importance an intersectional approach as being unable to "unblend" the cake batter; this quote from a Black gay research participant helps to describe how people's own unique, intersecting positions in society cannot be accurately and thoroughly explored if broken down into isolated categories.[9] A selection of these multiple minority identities are seen within Figure 13.1 as overlapping circles, the centre (ie, intersection) of which being where each service user should be seen, meaning that individuals have a mix of identity and lived experiences requiring a unique patient-centred approach. Support and interventions should thus be aimed at the whole of the individual and not operate under the assumption that these characteristics exist solely independent of one another.

An intersectional minority stress model also shows us how the status held in societal contexts can enable and/or amplify stressors while inhibiting resilience resources. At the time of publication, there has been a recent regression of policies and efforts to scale-back LGBTQ+ inclusion in general, though much of it is specifically in relation to reproductive and parenting rights. The latter is indicative of most reproductive health systems experienced still, particularly with recent regression of policies and efforts to scale-back LGBTQ+ inclusion. Within the UK there have been legal limits placed on access to certain roles on birth certificates, as well as changes in access to gender-affirming care for transgender youth—despite retaining access to the same treatments for cisgender youths. This trend can also be observed in Italy with the removal of previous granted rights for non-gestational mothers and within the recent increases in attempts to limit access to gender-affirming care in the United States. These are all examples of how a change to the status held in, socio-legal contexts—as an example of environmental influences—are interacting with and causing individual level stress and diminished autonomy which adds to the minority stress already experienced by LGBTQ+ people. These limitations to rights and access to health care contribute to preventable negative outcomes through discrimination and the stigmatisation of labelling LGBTQ+ reproductive health as non-normative, despite the only niche component being awareness of how, when, and why people are needing certain health services. Environmental factors are part of a cycle in which people might internalise experiences of stigma and discrimination, taking responsibility for external forces outsides of their control—a compounding of minority stressors across multiple unpredictable sources. As such, there is also a complex interplay between intrapersonal (proximal), interpersonal (distal), and structural stressors that are constantly shifting and changing, contributing to the uncertainty of experience.

Social and medical stigma which can be part of LGBTQ+ people's experiences of discrimination can lead to the internalisation of these preventable events. This movement of prejudice and stigma "under the skin" means LGBTQ+ people are processing higher rates of stress, which can dysregulate the body over time, contributing to poorer outcomes.[3] This can be further complicated and compounded through the complex intersections of identity, contributing to the layers of social[10] and/or medical expectations of service users. Measuring these impacts of stressors, both acutely and chronically, helps to operationalise this framework, which in turn can help us to better grasp the importance of LGBTQ+ inclusive reproductive health care.

Allostatic load

Making the connection between mental and physical health outcomes and experiences requires an approach to health and wellbeing that takes into account the role that the social world plays on the body. Homeostasis is used as a measure of understanding balance within the body, assessing for proper regulation of the body's biosystems. For example, this would view the body as waiting for an issue (eg, increase in blood sugar) before providing a solution (eg, the pancreas creates insulin). Allostasis instead considers both where the body is situated (ie, environmental context and historical experiences)[11, 12] and what it might need to be prepared for based on what it has already gone through (ie, the ability to adapt to changes). Thus, Allostasis is the approach of looking at the body as a series of dynamic systems that exists within and reacts to the world around it, both environmentally and socially. Allostasis was first mentioned by Sterling and

Eyer in 1988,[13] who recommended biomedical research look beyond isolated organs and instead assess the arousal of biosystems allowing for complexities in the feedback process that acknowledged negative health outcomes when overloaded (ie, allostatic overload) by chronic stress or strains. Sterling clarifies it is the reliance on the body's maintenance of uncorrupted information to continue processing without being over taxed which can require adaptation over time.[14] Allostasis also helps to address biological processes as part of the open system of the social world.[15, 16] Serving as a biopsychosocial model of ageing, morbidity, and mortality, allostatic load helps to assess for strain in biosystems (ie, cardiovascular, neuroendocrine, metabolic, and inflammatory) to adjust in accordance with events to avoid dysregulation and overloaded biosystems, the presence of which would increase risk of illness and disease. Research on allostatic load has also helped to highlight the importance of moving beyond "sex-based differences," supporting the importance of non-binary methodologies as they strengthen results. For example, evidence has shown associations of higher levels of allostatic load based on gender roles and presentation that depart from cisheterosexual expectations which expands what is possible to understand through a sex-specific analysis alone, particularly within the space of health research and practice.[10] To give an instance, facing additional stressors for being a man who is considered more feminine or navigating health spaces that are gendered while being non-binary and/or androgynous. There are also findings for LGB adults that counter the expected higher levels when compared with their heterosexual peers, despite individual biomarkers falling in-line with higher prevalence of health inequalities for LGB adults.[17] Results highlight that there can be unique health disparities for lesbian women when compared to bisexual women with varying associations to allostatic load and/or its components, which points to the need of unique solutions to rectify those disparities. These findings are part of a larger body of research that signal for more inclusive and comprehensive research methods in order to better understand the roles of stressors and protective factors.

Impacts of biosystem dysregulation within the stages of reproduction

As clarified within the previous chapters, we know that the impacts of pregnancy and birth experiences go beyond one individual in influencing the health and wellbeing of the entire family for both LGBTQ+ families and cisheteronormative families. While sexual health and conception should be the choice of the individual, there are still interpersonal and societal dynamics that need to be navigated and thus every facet of reproductive health can be a source of internal and external stress. Because of limitations in past research, primarily what is known presently about the impacts of stigma and discrimination during pregnancy is based upon experiences with racial discrimination. For example, Black women who experience higher rates of discrimination and prejudice have a higher rate of preterm births, which in turn also influences the preterm birth rates of the next generation while highlighting a preventable cause (ie, prejudice and discrimination).[18] In hopes of addressing the health disparities highlighted above, inclusive of gender and sexual minorities at the intersection of multiple minoritised groups, current research practices must go beyond cisheterosexual-centred approaches taking into consideration a person's reproductive life course throughout all stages of reproductive health care services. For health systems, this means ensuring that LGBTQ+ families are visible within data monitoring and administrative practices.

Throughout the course of a person's reproductive health journey, there are instances in which we are aware of how stressors impact outcomes, such as the links between prejudice and discrimination and poorer pregnancy outcomes.[18] Thus, there is much that needs to be considered within research and clinical care spaces when taking preventative measures to improve the health and wellbeing of LGBTQ+ parents and their families. The academic literature helps to present what is known about complications, caused by biosystem dysregulation (eg, augmented stress response), for marginalised groups within reproductive health care throughout the life course in an effort to improve the overall quality of care received. In instances where there are gaps in the literature for LGBTQ+ individuals, research centred on other minoritised groups is discussed because of similarities in sources of stress and the biological pathways that can be affected. Additionally, knowledge at the intersection of minoritised groups must remain a key consideration in the improvement of inclusion in reproductive health care.

For LGBTQ+ people who want to avoid pregnancy, or need to access contraceptives for medical purposes, it is important to consider how increased levels of stress impact overall health, in part due to said stress leading to a strained baseline that can impact health and healing. The use of contraceptives can be life-changing and lifesaving, which can account for their widespread use. This value is balanced with recent studies that highlight the increased oxidative stress levels[19, 20] and how they can change how the body processes stress.[21] The ability to reduce external sources of stress could help to ameliorate some of these elevated stress levels by reducing minority stressors, which would have both short- and long-term health benefits. The role of this higher stress can cascade in other aspects of life through the dysregulation of various biosystems within the body. For example, in part due to changes within the inflammatory biosystem as well as the neuroendocrine system, higher levels of stress are shown to slow the process of healing and recovery post-wound and/or surgery.[22] So for patients who need to access surgical care, the higher levels of preventable stress can impede their recovery and extend the time necessary to heal. While more research is necessary, it is important to then consider what this might mean for the higher levels of stress faced by gender and sexual minorities and their recovery from health interventions such as abortion care.

Similar considerations continue for LGBTQ+ individuals waiting until later in life to become pregnant. While there is a complex understanding of the role that preconception allostatic load plays on fertility and pregnancy outcomes,[23–25] evidence suggests that stress plays a role in reducing the probability of becoming pregnant.[26] In the instance of biosystems during pregnancy, there are heightened processes (eg, elevated cortisol) that are necessary for foetal development.[27] What the literature suggests is that the levels of stress experienced while pregnant, including stigma and discrimination, can have a tangible impact on infants being born pre-term and/or with non-ideal birth weights. These are examples of how disruption or dysregulation would result in negative pregnancy and birth outcomes,[27–29] which Sterling clarifies is counter to the biosystems evolving for reproductive success.[14] Research has shown an association between higher allostatic load and adverse pregnancy outcomes.[30–33] This can manifest as shortened gestational length.[23, 24, 34, 35] Gestational parents with racial/ethnic minority status show higher levels of allostatic load,[23, 25, 27] with higher levels linked to gestational parents' likelihood in experiencing cardiovascular disease later in life due to adverse pregnancy outcomes (ie, preeclampsia).[32, 33] For differences based on social characteristics, two studies show unanticipated allostatic load scores, where Black women had similar or lower allostatic load than their white peers.[24, 34] The complex interplay between minoritised status and allostatic load provides an understanding of how stress impacts outcomes while also bringing forward the importance of taking a longitudinal approach to enable translational research and improved clinical outcomes.

Even more evidence is available when looking at the various biosystems considered beyond the concept of allostatic load within the literature (ie, looking at only cardiovascular health or the role of inflammation, etc.). For example, negative outcomes are prevalent for both the gestational parent's health, as Black mothers have higher rates of maternal mortality than white mothers, and for the outcome of the pregnancy as well. Black mothers have higher rates of low weight and preterm births being linked with higher rates of discrimination.[18, 36, 37] Part of these disparities can be accounted for the role that dysregulation can play in key hormonal processes related to stress (ie, stigma, prejudice, and discrimination), such as the role of cortisol discussed above. For women of colour in Ireland and the UK, having a minoritised status based on ethnicity translates to a 3.7 times increase in maternal death for Black women and 1.8 times for Asian mothers when compared to their white peers.[37] In the United States, there are similar patterns of outcomes, with a 2.6 times increase in maternal mortality for Black mothers when compared to their White peers.[38] Additionally, for pregnancies later in life, there is a higher level of poorer outcomes when comparing the outcomes for Black and white women, associating longer lived experiences facing discrimination with the higher risk as an ever-widening health disparity.[i] While there is currently no published research on pregnancy outcomes and allostatic load using LGBTQ+ inclusive samples, available literature does show similar disparities in outcomes for gender and sexual minorities,[39-42] with considerations for multiple minority statuses (eg, racial and sexual minorities) highlighting poorer outcomes when belonging to more than one minoritised group.[39] As part of making improvements to care for marginalised groups, it is key that inclusive data monitoring be put in place to help understand as/when there are preventative losses at the local level, both within the clinical provision of care and within ensuring that gender and sexual orientation are considered alongside race/ethnicity, among other factors (ie, an inclusive intersectional approach), during the perinatal period.

During the postpartum period, there are various facets of parenthood that are negatively influenced by higher levels of allostatic load as well. While there are higher levels of allostatic load for people with higher postpartum poor health symptoms, this higher level of allostatic load can show a trend of decreasing with time through the monitoring and mitigation of symptoms.[43] Scroggins et al.[43] highlight the importance of the reduction of allostatic load both for long-term health, but also because the average time between each pregnancy can place the subsequent pregnancy during the recovery period, resulting in an additional layer of risk. In other words, another pregnancy at 18-months postpartum can mean the subsequent pregnancy comes with antenatal health beginning with a higher baseline of allostatic load resulting in a higher likelihood of more interpregnancy risks[43] and higher health risks later in life.[eg, 44] These higher levels of stress can also compound when there are physiological barriers to lactation[45, 46] and healing[22] which can in turn become a source of stress in and of itself. However, it is possible to mitigate this additional risk through making sure that the proper support is in place (eg, doula support to help with sleep duration, therapeutic support for psychological symptoms, contraception for autonomy in spacing pregnancies, etc.). It is key then to be aware of when and where stressors can be prevented or avoided during the postpartum period to improve health and well-being outcomes, both at the time and as a means of reducing longer term risks through evidence-based, trauma informed postnatal care.

PROTECTIVE POSSIBILITIES

An awareness of the negative impacts, as well as the better understanding of allostatic load, enables an understanding of the ways in which LGBTQ+ people are able to adapt (ie, be resilient) to help diminish negative outcomes. As emphasised within the other chapters, it is the preventative and inclusive measures that can be taken at the institutional level that enables the most protective factors known: counting LGBTQ+ parents as a regular part of the diversity present within reproductive health care. While more often than not the negation of minority stressors is not due to the actions of the individual, there are protective ways in which LGBTQ+ families are less likely to replicate harmful cisheterosexist norms.

There are ways in which gender and sexual minorities navigate reproductive health spaces with the hopes that the outcome will mean lower levels of stress and less uncertainty overall because of their approach. This might include preplanning for appointments and/or seeking out health care providers who are known to have the knowledge necessary to support them. Additionally, certain minority identity characteristics can lead to in the moment "protective behaviours" to diminish the stress faced while accessing reproductive health care. Like hypervigilance and experiences with stigma and discrimination resulting in being more discerning about health care options, in some cases changing where antenatal care is being accessed mid-pregnancy to ensure they feel safe during childbirth.[47] For some individuals, this can also translate into self-advocacy through researching and preparing for appointments to ensure clinical discussions remain on topic and are not dismissed due to presumptions that the issue is relevant only to heterosexual individuals. Lactation is one such space that is complex in how it is viewed socially, having both short- and long-term protective factors (eg, reduction in allostatic load) for parents who chose to breast/chestfeed.[48] So in some instances it is the use of resilience resources with the aim of accessing desired experiences (ie, breast/chestfeeding) in order to access spaces of care and support that cisheterosexual people are ushered into because of the overwhelming importance for the parent-infant dyad. Facilitating these relationships can be supported through stress-reduction and reduction in allostatic load for marginalised parents,[45, 49] which can at least in part be achieved through creating more inclusive reproductive health spaces.

Another example is the distribution of parenting responsibilities and parental stress levels. Within lesbian couples, this is seen to be protective against some of the stress that is faced postpartum due to the balance of shared responsibilities in place of gender norms in parenting and household maintenance.[50] A similar pattern of equitable sharing of responsibilities is also noted for gender minorities,[51] with additional research suggesting that there are overall protective elements for LGBTQ+ parents when compared to cisheterosexual parents and LGBTQ+ people without children.[52]

While these and other means of adapting to less than ideal circumstances are protective, they are not completely preventative of the negative influences of minority stress. The ideal solution would be to identify and remove the sources of stigma and discrimination present, such as expanding options on intake forms and ensuring that there are resources available for all different parents and families. When it is not possible to come to a universal solution, there should then be programs and resources in place that provide access to protective factors (eg, LGBTQ+ inclusive antenatal education) to help reduce the impacts of the stressors that are more difficult to adjust or remove. Taking an intersectional lens meaning that these benefits are also acknowledging that other marginalised groups would benefit, with some overlapping resources and a wider, deeper pool of options to support all of the service user groups present (eg, support for LGBTQ+ people of colour, educational resources based on various religious and cultural background, etc.). Without these changes, and without monitoring and evaluation, what can result is the on-going presence of preventable stressors that diminish the quality of care being accessed. Additionally, more needs to be done in research to champion ways in which LGBTQ+ people are resilient and able to adapt, so that more immediate policies can support those means for the health and wellbeing of LGBTQ+ people. As such, these examples should serve to highlight that there are beneficial elements that come along with parenthood despite the additional stigma faced as LGBTQ+ people, meaning that those who envision a future as a parent should be supported in enabling these outcomes and in better understanding additional protective and preventative factors.

IMPLICATIONS FOR HEALTH POLICY AND PRACTICE

Awareness of the impacts of clinical policies and procedures, specifically those catering to a cisheteronormative health care system, should hopefully result in an improvement for LGBTQ+ individuals. The chapters within this book provide a starting point for considerations throughout potential reproductive health journeys. Within sexual and reproductive health care, it is key that policies and medical education curricula acknowledge that LGBTQ+ individuals need access to contraception and screenings that are offered and provided with a minimising of gendered interactions (see Chapter 1). For example, being able to provision cervical screenings for patients with M/male as their gender marker whenever relevant and without the burden on the patient to have to correct the system regularly because they would otherwise be denied necessary screenings. As a starting point, an audit of these processes—inclusive of participatory and community-based methods—can also assist in reviewing if additional barriers are in place for people accessing assisted reproductive care, including differences within and between groups (ie, LGBTQ+ versus cisheterosexual, married/partnered versus unpartnered). Possible solutions can include both provisions of care as well as understanding when and where care might not necessitate additional barriers (ie, irrelevant counselling requirements applied only to LGBTQ+ individuals) which ultimately limit or slow access, among others (see Chapter 2). These are examples of direct interactions of policies at the individual level which increases minority stressors while not always being medically or administratively necessary.

For individuals needing access to abortion care (see Chapter 4), it is essential that health services are aware of the complexities between access, rights, and identity. Similarly, it is key to acknowledge and provide culturally-humble and -competent bereavement care in the case of pregnancy losses for all parents (see Chapter 3). Along with access to care, it is paramount that there be equal access to supportive and knowledgeable antenatal education (see Chapter 5), particularly as this plays an integral role in decision-making and preparedness during pregnancy and childbirth. For the process of making choices during the ante- and perinatal periods, it should be ensured that the process of discussing risk and informed consent recognises how/if risk and side effects differ for LGBTQ+ individuals (see Chapter 6). Without these elements of care available, it is possible to compound increased levels of fear of childbirth for gender and sexual minorities (see Chapter 7), additional stressors that the literature suggests will impact overall outcomes as well. For partners' and non-gestational parents, these parents must be counted within the health systems and services for the roles that they play in reproductive health care as well as in understanding the intricacies of LGBTQ+ relationships that are often flattened within through limited literature (see Chapter 8).

Within the postpartum period, the need for nuanced support and health care continues, requiring perspectives and knowledge on how best to provide those services for LGBTQ+ families. The variety of parents that may seek to breast/chestfeed their children (see Chapter 9) are at times being socially and medically excluded due to a lack of knowledge and awareness alone. While families will ideally have positive experiences, the complexities of childbirth and becoming a parent need to be treated as ongoing, liminal spaces where recovering and processing (see Chapter 10) and postnatal mental health support (see Chapter 11) may be required. Last, but certainly not least, it must be ensured that the idealised home life is not reinforcing heterosexual, monogamous norms (see Chapter 12)—meaning that community midwives, general practitioners, and health visitors must be critical of social expectations which may be outdated and/or irrelevant for LGBTQ+ families.

It is our hope that this text will raise awareness of known exclusionary practices and gaps in knowledge to provide points at which reproductive health care services and research can be improved (ie, result in fewer minority stressors). As clinicians and members of health systems administration, it is possible to inadvertently perpetuate some of the key sources of stress, stigma, and discrimination that are inherent in cisheteronormative policy structures (eg, assumptions about who needs what health care and why). These preventable stressors, as discussed throughout this chapter and the others, might be done by enacting policies and practice driven assumptions that are yet to reflect the diversity of families accessing reproductive health services across the life course. Just as patient centred care needs to be tailored to the wants and needs of the individual, from a policy perspective, local health systems need to conduct needs assessments to ensure that there is a recognition of both the diverse populations accessing health services. In turn, a supportive and inclusive health system is more likely to encourage a culture of patient-centred care. Thus, one potential starting point for those seeking to improve their quality of care is an audit of the current administrative and clinical pathways. Through this process of evaluation, it will enable awareness and ensure measurable efforts towards the reduction of stressors for minoritised groups either through removal and/or alternate pathways among other forms of improve support and accessibility during reproductive health care.

Key Points

- The experiences of LGBTQ+ people can be directly linked to their health and wellbeing, including mental and physical health as intrinsically linked components of those outcomes.
- The minority stress model, bolstered by intersectionality, can be used with allostatic load to measure health outcomes, as well as evaluate the provision of interventions. This can be both for helping with translational research and also for implementing and measuring changes within various health systems.
- Local health services audits should be conducted regularly using participatory methods alongside sexual orientation and gender inclusive data monitoring to help to understand where improvements can be made and to ensure that the right programs are available to local service users.
- Preventative approaches include inclusive language and clinical practice as a means of lowering the presence of general and minority stressors, with patient-led care helping to support and guide these efforts.
- Provider awareness and training, using an intersectional approach, can help to facilitate improvements in care for marginalised services users by understanding how current practices are moving or keeping certain groups at the margins.

- Protective factors are present within LGBTQ+ families and should be supported through clinical practice and policies.
- Existing health system policies should be audited and needs assessments should be conducted to enable local health services that support the diverse populations accessing reproductive health services.

NOTE

i   This is known as the Weathering hypothesis. In some instances, this is reserved for the discussion of allostatic load later in the life course, but the initial research is focused on maternal health differences and should be recognised as a consideration for taking intersectional approaches to research if lasting change is to be achieved.

REFERENCES

1.   Meyer IH. Prejudice, Social Stress, and Mental Health in Lesbian, Gay, and Bisexual Populations: Conceptual Issues and Research Evidence. *Psychol Bull*. 2003;129(5):674–697. doi:10.1037/0033-2909.129.5.674
2.   Brooks VR. *Minority Stress and Lesbian Women*. Lexington Books; 1981.
3.   Hatzenbuehler ML, Nolen-Hoeksema S, Dovidio J. How Does Stigma "Get Under the Skin"?: The Mediating Role of Emotion Regulation. *Psychol Sci*. 2009;20(10):1282–1289. doi:10.1111/j.1467-9280.2009.02441.x
4.   Flentje A, Heck NC, Brennan JM, Meyer IH. The Relationship between Minority Stress and Biological Outcomes: A Systematic Review. *J Behav Med*. 2020;43(5):673–694. doi:10.1007/s10865-019-00120-6
5.   Hendricks ML, Testa RJ. A Conceptual Framework for Clinical Work with Transgender and Gender Nonconforming Clients: An Adaptation of the Minority Stress Model. *Prof Psychol Res Pract*. 2012;43(5):460–467. doi:10.1037/a0029597
6.   Testa RJ, Habarth J, Peta J, Balsam K, Bockting W. Development of the Gender Minority Stress and Resilience Measure. *Psychol Sex Orientat Gend Divers*. 2015;2(1):65–77. doi:10.1037/sgd0000081
7.   Bayer R. *Homosexuality and American Psychiatry: The Politics of Diagnosis*. Princeton University Press; 1987.
8.   Meyer IH, Frost DM. Minority Stress and the Health of Sexual Minorities. In: Patterson CJ, D'Augelli AR, eds. *Handbook of Psychology and Sexual Orientation*. Oxford University Press; 2012:252–266. doi:10.1093/acprof:oso/9780199765218.003.0018
9.   Bowleg L. "Once You've Blended the Cake, You Can't Take the Parts Back to the Main Ingredients": Black Gay and Bisexual Men's Descriptions and Experiences of Intersectionality. *Sex Roles*. 2013;68(11):754–767. doi:10.1007/s11199-012-0152-4
10.   Juster RP, de Torre MB, Kerr P, Kheloui S, Rossi M, Bourdon O. Sex Differences and Gender Diversity in Stress Responses and Allostatic Load Among Workers and LGBT People. *Curr Psychiatry Rep*. 2019;21(11):110. doi:10.1007/s11920-019-1104-2
11.   Bernard C. *An Introduction to the Study of Experimental Medicine*. (Henderson LJ, ed.). Dover Publications Inc.; 1927.

12. Walter CB. *Wisdom Of The Body*. Rev. and Enl. Ed Edition. W. W. Norton and Company, Inc.; 1963.

13. Sterling P, Eyer J. Allostasis: A New Paradigm to Explain Arousal Pathology. In: Fisher S, Reason J, eds. *Handbook of Life Stress, Cognition and Health*. John Wiley & Sons; 1988:629–649.

14. Sterling P. Allostasis: A Model of Predictive Regulation. *Physiol Behav*. 2012;106(1):5–15. doi:10.1016/j.physbeh.2011.06.004

15. McEwen BS, Stellar E. Stress and the Individual: Mechanisms Leading to Disease. *Arch Intern Med*. 1993;153(18):2093–2101. doi:10.1001/archinte.1993.00410180039004

16. McEwen BS, Wingfield JC. The Concept of Allostasis in Biology and Biomedicine. *Horm Behav*. 2003;43(1):2–15. doi:10.1016/S0018-506X(02)00024-7

17. Mays VM, Juster RP, Williamson TJ, Seeman TE, Cochran SD. Chronic Physiologic Effects of Stress among Lesbian, Gay, and Bisexual Adults: Results from the National Health and Nutrition Examination Survey. *Psychosom Med*. 2018;80(6):551–563. doi:10.1097/PSY.000 0000000000600

18. Collins JW, David RJ, Handler A, Wall S, Andes S. Very Low Birthweight in African American Infants: The Role of Maternal Exposure to Interpersonal Racial Discrimination. *Am J Public Health*. 2004;94(12):2132–2138. doi:10.2105/AJPH.94.12.2132

19. Cauci S, Xodo S, Buligan C, et al. Oxidative Stress Is Increased in Combined Oral Contraceptives Users and Is Positively Associated with High-Sensitivity C-Reactive Protein. *Molecules*. 2021;26(4):1070. doi:10.3390/molecules26041070

20. Masama C, Jarkas DA, Thaw E, et al. Hormone Contraceptive Use in Young Women: Altered Mood States, Neuroendocrine and Inflammatory Biomarkers. *Horm Behav*. 2022;144:105229. doi:10.1016/j.yhbeh.2022.105229

21. Pedersen MV, Hansen LMB, Garforth B, Zak PJ, Winterdahl M. Adrenocorticotropic Hormone Secretion in Response to Anticipatory Stress and Venepuncture: The Role of Menstrual Phase and Oral Contraceptive Use. *Behav Brain Res*. 2023;452:114550. doi:10.1016/j.bbr.2023.114550

22. Robinson H, Norton S, Jarrett P, Broadbent E. The Effects of Psychological Interventions on Wound Healing: A Systematic Review of Randomized Trials. *Br J Health Psychol*. 2017;22(4):805–835. doi:10.1111/bjhp.12257

23. Wallace M, Harville E, Theall K, Webber L, Chen W, Berenson G. Preconception Biomarkers of Allostatic Load and Racial Disparities in Adverse Birth Outcomes: The Bogalusa Heart Study. *Paediatr Perinat Epidemiol*. 2013;27(6):587–597. doi:10.1111/ppe.12091

24. Wallace ME, Harville EW. Allostatic Load and Birth Outcomes Among White and Black Women in New Orleans. *Matern Child Health J*. 2013;17(6):1025–1029. doi:10.1007/s10995-012-1083-y

25. McKee KS, Seplaki C, Fisher S, Groth S, Fernandez ID. Cumulative Physiologic Dysfunction and Pregnancy: Characterization and Association with Birth Outcomes. *Matern Child Health J*. 2017;21(1):147–155. doi:10.1007/s10995-016-2103-0

26. Buck Louis GM, Lum KJ, Sundaram R, et al. Stress Reduces Conception Probabilities across the Fertile Window: Evidence in Support of Relaxation. *Fertil Steril*. 2011;95(7):2184–2189. doi:10.1016/j.fertnstert.2010.06.078

27. Li Y, Dalton VK, Lee SJ, Rosemberg MAS, Seng JS. Exploring the Validity of Allostatic Load in Pregnant Women. *Midwifery*. 2020;82:102621. doi:10.1016/j.midw.2019.102621

28. Olson D, Severson E, Verstraeten B, Ng J, McCreary J, Metz G. Allostatic Load and Preterm Birth. *Int J Mol Sci*. 2015;16(12):29856–29874. doi:10.3390/ijms161226209

29. Rubin LP. Maternal and Pediatric Health and Disease: Integrating Biopsychosocial Models and Epigenetics. *Pediatr Res*. 2016;79(1):127–135. doi:10.1038/pr.2015.203

30. Accortt EE, Mirocha J, Dunkel Schetter C, Hobel CJ. Adverse Perinatal Outcomes and Postpartum Multi-Systemic Dysregulation: Adding Vitamin D Deficiency to the Allostatic Load Index. *Matern Child Health J*. 2017;21(3):398–406. doi:10.1007/s10995-016-2226-3

31. Barrett ES, Vitek W, Mbowe O, et al. Allostatic Load, a Measure of Chronic Physiological Stress, is Associated with Pregnancy Outcomes, but not Fertility, among Women with Unexplained Infertility. *Hum Reprod*. 2018;33(9):1757–1766. doi:10.1093/humrep/dey261

32. Hux VJ, Catov JM, Roberts JM. Allostatic Load in Women with a History of Low Birth Weight Infants: The National Health and Nutrition Examination Survey. *J Womens Health*. 2014;23(12):1039–1045. doi:10.1089/jwh.2013.4572

33. Hux VJ, Roberts JM. A Potential Role for Allostatic Load in Preeclampsia. *Matern Child Health J*. 2015;19(3):591–597. doi:10.1007/s10995-014-1543-7

34. Morrison S, Shenassa ED, Mendola P, Wu T, Schoendorf K. Allostatic Load may not be Associated with Chronic Stress in Pregnant Women, NHANES 1999–2006. *Ann Epidemiol*. 2013;23(5):294–297. doi:10.1016/j.annepidem.2013.03.006

35. Sayre MM. *Maternal Allostatic Load during Pregnancy: Predicting Length of Gestation*. Ph.D. University of Kentucky; 2016. Accessed October 16, 2020. http://search.proquest.com/docview/1798477678/abstract/72CB164C84A447B9PQ/1

36. Datta-Nemdharry P, Dattani N, Macfarlane AJ. Birth Outcomes for African and Caribbean Babies in England and Wales: Retrospective Analysis of Routinely Collected Data. *BMJ Open*. 2012;2(3):e001088. doi:10.1136/bmjopen-2012-001088

37. on behalf of MBRRACE-UK. *Saving Lives, Improving Mothers' Care Core Report –Lessons Learned to Inform Maternity Care from the UK and Ireland Confidential Enquiries into Maternal Deaths and Morbidity 2018–20*. (Marian Knight, Kathryn Bunch, Roshni Patel, et al., eds.). National Perinatal Epidemiology Unit, University of Oxford; 2022. Accessed April 16, 2023. https://www.npeu.ox.ac.uk/assets/downloads/mbrrace-uk/reports/maternal-report-2022/MBRRACE-UK_Maternal_MAIN_Report_2022_v10.pdf

38. Hoyert DL. *Maternal Mortality Rates in the United States, 2021*. Published online 2023.

39. Everett BG, Limburg A, Charlton BM, Downing JM, Matthews PA. Sexual Identity and Birth Outcomes: A Focus on the Moderating Role of Race-Ethnicity. *J Health Soc Behav*. 2021;62(2):183–201. doi:10.1177/0022146521997811

40. Everett BG, Kominiarek MA, Mollborn S, Adkins DE, Hughes TL. Sexual Orientation Disparities in Pregnancy and Infant Outcomes. *Matern Child Health J*. 2019;23(1):72–81. doi:10.1007/s10995-018-2595-x

41. Downing J, Everett B, Snowden JM. Differences in Perinatal Outcomes of Birthing People in Same-Sex and Different-Sex Marriages. *Am J Epidemiol*. 2021;190(11):2350–2359. doi:10.1093/aje/kwab148

42. Barcelona V, Jenkins V, Britton LE, Everett BG. Adverse Pregnancy and Birth Outcomes in Sexual Minority Women from the National Survey of Family Growth. *BMC Pregnancy Childbirth*. 2022;22(1):923. doi:10.1186/s12884-022-05271-0

43. Scroggins JK, Yang Q, Dotters-Katz SK, Brandon D, Reuter-Rice K. Examination of Maternal Allostatic Load Among Postpartum Women with Distinct Postpartum Symptom Typologies. *Biol Res Nurs*. 2024;26(2):279–292. doi:10.1177/10998004231217680

44. Lueth AJ, Allshouse AA, Blue NM, et al. Can Allostatic Load in Pregnancy Explain the Association between Race and Subsequent Cardiovascular Disease Risk: A Cohort Study. *BJOG Int J Obstet Gynaecol*. 2023;130(10):1197–1206. doi:10.1111/1471-0528.17486

45. Isiguzo C, Mendez DD, Demirci JR, et al. Stress, Social Support, and Racial Differences: Dominant Drivers of Exclusive Breastfeeding. *Matern Child Nutr*. 2023;19(2):e13459. doi:10.1111/mcn.13459

46. Nagel EM, Howland MA, Pando C, et al. Maternal Psychological Distress and Lactation and Breastfeeding Outcomes: A Narrative Review. *Clin Ther*. 2022;44(2):215–227. doi:10.1016/j.clinthera.2021.11.007

47. Luxion K. Serving LGBT+ Parents: How Patient Experiences Influence Birth Outcomes. In: Southeastern Women's Studies Association; 2018.

48. Hsiao B sek J, Sibeko L. Breastfeeding Is Inversely Associated with Allostatic Load in Postpartum Women: Cross-Sectional Data from Nationally Representative US Women. *J Nutr*. 2021;151(12):3801–3810. doi:10.1093/jn/nxab302

49. Riggan KA, Gilbert A, Allyse MA. Acknowledging and Addressing Allostatic Load in Pregnancy Care. *J Racial Ethn Health Disparities*. 2021;8(1):69–79. doi:10.1007/s40615-020-00757-z

50. Ross LE. Perinatal Mental Health in Lesbian Mothers: A Review of Potential Risk and Protective Factors. *Women Health*. 2005;41(3). doi:10.1300/J013v41n03_07

51. Tornello SL. Division of Labor Among Transgender and Gender Non-binary Parents: Association with Individual, Couple, and Children's Behavioral Outcomes. *Front Psychol*. 2020;11. doi:10.3389/fpsyg.2020.00015

52. Luxion K. Reframing Discourse: Using BRFSS Data to Deconstruct Influences of Parenthood on Depression and LGBTQ+ Mental Health. Poster presented at: GW Research Days; 2018; Washington, DC. https://hsrc.himmelfarb.gwu.edu/gw_research_days/2018/GWSPH/64/

Index

Printed in the United States
by Baker & Taylor Publisher Services